Sharing Clinic

MAXIMIZING BE

M000287495

Committee on Strategies for Responsible Sharing of Clinical Trial Data

Board on Health Sciences Policy

INSTITUTE OF MEDICINE
OF THE NATIONAL ACADEMIES

THE NATIONAL ACADEMIES PRESS
Washington, D.C.
www.nap.edu

THE NATIONAL ACADEMIES PRESS   500 Fifth Street, NW   Washington, DC 20001

NOTICE: The project that is the subject of this report was approved by the Governing Board of the National Research Council, whose members are drawn from the councils of the National Academy of Sciences, the National Academy of Engineering, and the Institute of Medicine. The members of the committee responsible for the report were chosen for their special competences and with regard for appropriate balance.

This study was supported by contracts between the National Academy of Sciences and the U.S. National Institutes of Health (HHSN263201200074I), U.S. Food and Drug Administration, AbbVie Inc., Amgen Inc., AstraZeneca Pharmaceuticals, Bayer, Biogen Idec, Bristol-Myers Squibb, Burroughs Wellcome Fund, Doris Duke Charitable Foundation, Eli Lilly and Company, EMD Serono, Genentech, GlaxoSmithKline, Johnson & Johnson, Medical Research Council (UK), Merck & Co., Inc., Novartis Pharmaceuticals Corporation, Novo Nordisk, Pfizer Inc., Sanofi-Aventis, Takeda, and The Wellcome Trust. Any opinions, findings, conclusions, or recommendations expressed in this publication are those of the author(s) and do not necessarily reflect the views of the organizations or agencies that provided support for the project.

International Standard Book Number-13:   978-0-309-31629-3
International Standard Book Number-10:   0-309-31629-4
Library of Congress Control Number: 2015934702

Additional copies of this report are available for sale from the National Academies Press, 500 Fifth Street, NW, Keck 360, Washington, DC 20001; (800) 624-6242 or (202) 334-3313; http://www.nap.edu.

For more information about the Institute of Medicine, visit the IOM home page at: **www.iom.edu.**

Printed in the United States of America

The serpent has been a symbol of long life, healing, and knowledge among almost all cultures and religions since the beginning of recorded history. The serpent adopted as a logotype by the Institute of Medicine is a relief carving from ancient Greece, now held by the Staatliche Museum in Berlin.

Front cover designed by Ovaitt Health Media LLC.

Suggested citation: Institute of Medicine (IOM). 2015. *Sharing clinical trial data: Maximizing benefits, minimizing risk.* Washington, DC: The National Academies Press.

"Knowing is not enough; we must apply.
Willing is not enough; we must do."
—Goethe

INSTITUTE OF MEDICINE
OF THE NATIONAL ACADEMIES

Advising the Nation. Improving Health.

THE NATIONAL ACADEMIES
Advisers to the Nation on Science, Engineering, and Medicine

The **National Academy of Sciences** is a private, nonprofit, self-perpetuating society of distinguished scholars engaged in scientific and engineering research, dedicated to the furtherance of science and technology and to their use for the general welfare. Upon the authority of the charter granted to it by the Congress in 1863, the Academy has a mandate that requires it to advise the federal government on scientific and technical matters. Dr. Ralph J. Cicerone is president of the National Academy of Sciences.

The **National Academy of Engineering** was established in 1964, under the charter of the National Academy of Sciences, as a parallel organization of outstanding engineers. It is autonomous in its administration and in the selection of its members, sharing with the National Academy of Sciences the responsibility for advising the federal government. The National Academy of Engineering also sponsors engineering programs aimed at meeting national needs, encourages education and research, and recognizes the superior achievements of engineers. Dr. C. D. Mote, Jr., is president of the National Academy of Engineering.

The **Institute of Medicine** was established in 1970 by the National Academy of Sciences to secure the services of eminent members of appropriate professions in the examination of policy matters pertaining to the health of the public. The Institute acts under the responsibility given to the National Academy of Sciences by its congressional charter to be an adviser to the federal government and, upon its own initiative, to identify issues of medical care, research, and education. Dr. Victor J. Dzau is president of the Institute of Medicine.

The **National Research Council** was organized by the National Academy of Sciences in 1916 to associate the broad community of science and technology with the Academy's purposes of furthering knowledge and advising the federal government. Functioning in accordance with general policies determined by the Academy, the Council has become the principal operating agency of both the National Academy of Sciences and the National Academy of Engineering in providing services to the government, the public, and the scientific and engineering communities. The Council is administered jointly by both Academies and the Institute of Medicine. Dr. Ralph J. Cicerone and Dr. C. D. Mote, Jr., are chair and vice chair, respectively, of the National Research Council.

www.national-academies.org

COMMITTEE ON STRATEGIES FOR RESPONSIBLE SHARING OF CLINICAL TRIAL DATA

BERNARD LO (*Chair*), President, The Greenwall Foundation
TIMOTHY COETZEE, Chief Research Officer, National Multiple Sclerosis Society
DAVID L. DeMETS, Professor and Chair, Department of Biostatistics and Medical Informatics, University of Wisconsin–Madison
JEFFREY DRAZEN, Editor-in-Chief, *New England Journal of Medicine*
STEVEN N. GOODMAN, Professor, Medicine & Health Research & Policy, Stanford University School of Medicine
PATRICIA A. KING, Carmack Waterhouse Professor of Law, Medicine, Ethics and Public Policy, Georgetown University Law Center
TRUDIE LANG, Principal Investigator, Global Health Network, Nuffield Department of Medicine, University of Oxford
DEVEN McGRAW, Partner, Healthcare Practice, Manatt, Phelps & Phillips, LLP
ELIZABETH NABEL, President, Brigham and Women's Hospital
ARTI RAI, Elvin R. Latty Professor of Law, Duke University School of Law
IDA SIM, Professor of Medicine and Co-Director of Biomedical Informatics of the Clinical and Translational Science Institute, University of California, San Francisco
SHARON TERRY, President and CEO, Genetic Alliance
JOANNE WALDSTREICHER, Chief Medical Officer, Johnson & Johnson

IOM Staff

ANNE B. CLAIBORNE, Senior Program Officer
INDIA HOOK-BARNARD, Study Director (July 2014 to February 2015)
LEIGHANNE OLSEN, Study Director (until November 2013)
REBECCA N. LENZI, Study Director (November 2013 to April 2014)
MICHELLE MANCHER, Associate Program Officer
ELIZABETH CORNETT, Research Assistant (from October 2014)
RACHEL KIRKLAND, Senior Program Assistant (until October 2013)
BARRET ZIMMERMANN, Senior Program Assistant (from October 2013)
MICHAEL BERRIOS, Senior Program Assistant (from September 2014)
SCOTT D. HALPERN, IOM Anniversary Fellow
ANDREW M. POPE, Director, Board on Health Sciences Policy

Reviewers

This report has been reviewed in draft form by individuals chosen for their diverse perspectives and technical expertise, in accordance with procedures approved by the National Research Council's Report Review Committee. The purpose of this independent review is to provide candid and critical comments that will assist the institution in making its published report as sound as possible and to ensure that the report meets institutional standards for objectivity, evidence, and responsiveness to the study charge. The review comments and draft manuscript remain confidential to protect the integrity of the deliberative process. We wish to thank the following individuals for their review of this report:

Lawrence J. Appel, Johns Hopkins Medical Institutions
Virginia Barbour, *PLoS Medicine*
Mark Barnes, Multi-Regional Clinical Trials Center at Harvard
Cynthia Dwork, Microsoft Research
Ezekiel J. Emanuel, University of Pennsylvania
David Harrington, Harvard School of Public Health
David Korn, Harvard University
Ronald L. Krall, University of Pittsburgh
Harlan M. Krumholz, Yale University School of Medicine
Christine Laine, *Annals of Internal Medicine*
Erika Lietzan, University of Missouri School of Law
Alexa T. McCray, Center for Biomedical Informatics

John J. Orloff, Baxter BioScience
Gary Puckrein, National Minority Quality Forum
Sir Michael Rawlins, Royal Society of Medicine

Although the reviewers listed above provided many constructive comments and suggestions, they were not asked to endorse the report's conclusions or recommendations, nor did they see the final draft of the report before its release. The review of this report was overseen by **Enriqueta Bond,** Burroughs Wellcome Fund, and **Sara Rosenbaum,** George Washington University. Appointed by the National Research Council and the Institute of Medicine, they were responsible for making certain that an independent examination of this report was carried out in accordance with institutional procedures and that all review comments were carefully considered. Responsibility for the final content of this report rests entirely with the authoring committee and the institution.

Preface

Patients and their physicians depend on clinical trials for reliable evidence on what therapies are effective and safe. Responsible sharing of the data gleaned from clinical trials will increase the validity and extent of this evidence. Several large pharmaceutical companies and some academic investigators already are sharing clinical trial data, and the European Medicines Agency will soon do so as well. The issue is no longer whether to share clinical trial data, but what specific data to share, at what time, and under what conditions.

Responsible sharing of clinical trial data raises complex challenges. Key stakeholders—clinical trial participants, sponsors and funders, clinical trialists, and regulatory authorities—have concerns and interests that need to be addressed and balanced. Because clinical trials are conducted worldwide, laws and regulations of different jurisdictions will need to be followed. Moreover, the very nature of clinical trials may change dramatically as data from personal sensors and devices and electronic medical records are increasingly used and new trial designs are introduced. In the face of these changes, sponsors, investigators, clinical trial participants, and regulators may feel that familiar, established practices and expectations are being overturned and that the future is uncomfortably uncertain. If sharing of clinical trial data is to be responsible and sustainable, there will need to be new business models for data sharing, changes in the culture of academic medicine, and incentives for sponsors and investigators to continue to develop new therapies and carry out clinical trials.

In this rapidly changing landscape of clinical trials, how can this report play a constructive and enduring role? The committee that conducted this study could not anticipate, much less try to resolve, the many practical issues that will arise as the sharing of clinical trial data unfolds. Nor could we provide a detailed roadmap for terrain that is unknown and under development. We could, however, provide guiding principles, outline operational considerations, and offer specific recommendations regarding what data should be shared at key milestones in the life cycle of a clinical trial, and we could also recommend conditions that will increase the benefits and minimize the risks of data sharing. Our recommendations represent an attempt to balance the interests of different stakeholders with the public interest of having the best information possible regarding the effectiveness and safety of therapies.

Our committee comprised people with different professional backgrounds and experiences. Their varied interdisciplinary perspectives deepened our discussions and our appreciation for the complexity of clinical trial data sharing. This report is better because of this richness of viewpoints. As chair I wish to thank the committee members for their hard work, their willingness to reconsider their views in light of evidence and persuasion, and their good humor. I believe our deliberations can serve as a model for how stakeholders can learn from each other and find common ground.

This report would not have been possible without the dedicated and expert work of the Institute of Medicine (IOM) staff, including India Hook-Barnard, Michelle Mancher, Anne Claiborne, Andrew Pope, Elizabeth Cornett, and Michael Berrios, whom the committee gratefully acknowledges and thanks. Scott Halpern, IOM Anniversary Fellow, sponsored by the American Board of Internal Medicine Foundation in honor of Dr. John Benson, made many important contributions to the committee's work as well. I would also like to thank Chelsea Ott for her skilled research assistance.

Bernard Lo, M.D., *Chair*
Committee on Strategies for Responsible Sharing of Clinical Trial Data

Contents

Abstract   xiii

Summary   1

1 Introduction   17
  Study Context, 19
  Charge to the Committee and Study Scope, 22
  Study Approach, 24
  Organization of the Report, 27
  References, 28

2 Guiding Principles for Sharing Clinical Trial Data   31
  Overview of Key Potential Benefits and Risks, 31
  Guiding Principles, 34
  The Committee's Approach to Applying the Principles, 41
  References, 43

**3 The Roles and Responsibilities of Stakeholders in the
    Sharing of Clinical Trial Data**   47
  Participants, 47
  Funders and Sponsors, 58
  Regulatory Agencies, 67
  Investigators, 72
  Research Institutions and Universities, 75

xi

Journals, 77
Professional Societies, 79
Recommendation, 80
References, 82

4 **The Clinical Trial Life Cycle and When to Share Data**   91
The Clinical Trial Life Cycle, 92
What Data Should Be Shared, 96
When Data Packages Should Be Shared, 113
Recommendation, 132
References, 134

5 **Access to Clinical Trial Data: Governance**   139
Open Access, 141
Approaches to Mitigating the Risks of Data Sharing, 142
Creating a Learning System, 156
Recommendation, 157
References, 158

6 **The Future of Data Sharing in a Changing Landscape**   163
Looking Forward, 163
Infrastructure Challenges, 164
Technical Challenges, 167
Workforce Challenges, 168
Sustainability Challenges, 170
Structure for Collaborative Next Steps, 173
Recommendation, 176
References, 177

Appendixes

A Study Approach   179
B Concepts and Methods for De-identifying Clinical Trial Data   203
C Legal Discussion of Risks to Industry Sponsors   257
D Clinical Trial Data Sharing Policies: Top 1-12 Pharmaceutical
    Companies Ranked by 2013 Market Capitalization   267
E Biosketches of Committee Members   281

Abstract

In response to 23 public- and private-sector sponsors, the Institute of Medicine assembled an ad hoc committee to develop guiding principles and a framework (activities and strategies) for the responsible sharing of clinical trial data. Responsible sharing of clinical trial data will allow other investigators to carry out additional analyses and reproduce published findings, strengthen the evidence base for regulatory and clinical decisions, and increase the scientific knowledge gained from investments by the funders of clinical trials. Data sharing can accelerate new discoveries by avoiding duplicative trials, stimulating new ideas for research, and enabling the maximal scientific knowledge and benefits to be gained from the efforts of clinical trial participants and investigators.

At the same time, sharing clinical trial data presents risks, burdens, and challenges. These include the need to (1) protect the privacy and honor the consent of clinical trial participants; (2) safeguard the legitimate economic interests of sponsors (e.g., intellectual property and commercially confidential information); (3) guard against invalid secondary analyses, which could undermine trust in clinical trials or otherwise harm public health; (4) give researchers who put effort and time into planning, organizing, and running clinical trials adequate time to analyze the data they have collected and appropriate recognition for their intellectual contributions; and (5) assuage the fear of research institutions that requirements for sharing clinical trial data will be unfunded mandates.

With the goal of ensuring responsible sharing of clinical trial data to increase scientific knowledge and ultimately lead to better therapies for patients, the committee that conducted this study identified the following guiding principles for data sharing: (1) maximize the benefits of clinical trials while minimizing the risks of sharing clinical trial data, (2) respect individual participants whose data are shared, (3) increase public trust in clinical trials and the sharing of trial data, and (4) conduct the sharing of clinical trial data in a fair manner. The committee drew on these guiding principles in developing its recommendations and believes they will be useful in the future as circumstances change and unforeseen issues emerge.

In this report, the committee analyzes how key stakeholders (including participants, sponsors, regulators, investigators, research institutions, journals, and professional societies) assess the benefits, risks, and challenges of data sharing and concludes that all stakeholders have roles and responsibilities in responsible sharing of clinical trial data. The report presents four recommendations designed to maximize the benefits and minimize the risks associated with data sharing:

> **Recommendation 1: Stakeholders in clinical trials should foster a culture in which data sharing is the expected norm, and should commit to responsible strategies aimed at maximizing the benefits, minimizing the risks, and overcoming the challenges of sharing clinical trial data for all parties.**

> **Recommendation 2: Sponsors and investigators should share the various types of clinical trial data no later than the times specified in this report (e.g., the full analyzable data set with metadata no later than 18 months after study completion—with specified exceptions for trials intended to support a regulatory application—and the analytic data set supporting publication results no later than 6 months after publication).**

> **Recommendation 3: Holders of clinical trial data should mitigate the risks and enhance the benefits of sharing sensitive clinical trial data by implementing operational strategies that include employing data use agreements, designating an independent review panel, including members of the lay public in governance, and making access to clinical trial data transparent.**

> **Recommendation 4: The sponsors of this study should take the lead, together with or via a trusted impartial organization(s), to convene a multistakeholder body with global reach and broad representation to address, in an ongoing process, the key infrastructure, technological, sustainability, and workforce challenges associated with the sharing of clinical trial data.**

Summary

Responsible sharing of clinical trial data is in the public interest. It maximizes the contributions made by clinical trial participants to scientific knowledge that benefits future patients and society as a whole. Results from many clinical trials are not published in peer-reviewed journals in a timely manner. Even when findings are published, large amounts of data remain unanalyzed. Data sharing makes data from clinical trials available to other investigators for secondary uses, which include carrying out additional analyses, analyzing unpublished data, reproducing published findings, and conducting exploratory analyses to generate new research hypotheses. In several highly publicized cases, independent investigators who have reanalyzed the data underlying published results of clinical trials have challenged the published results as invalid or incomplete. These allegations have sparked debates, additional analyses, and new clinical trials. Further, they have caused regulators to limit marketing of the products or led sponsors to withdraw them. This back-and-forth discussion, while complex and perhaps confusing to the public, is how scientific knowledge progresses, and it has resulted in a broader evidence base for regulatory and clinical decisions.

Taken together, these are compelling justifications for sharing clinical trial data to benefit society and future patients. The challenge is to set clear expectations that clinical trial data should be shared and to agree on how to do so in a responsible manner that mitigates the risks involved. Stakeholders have concerns about data sharing. Clinical trial participants want assurance that data will be shared in a way that protects privacy and is consistent with informed consent. Sponsors want a quiet period for regulators to evaluate the entire body of evidence submitted to them, appropriate safeguards for intellectual property and commercially confidential information, and protections from invalid secondary analyses. Academic clinical trialists want time to analyze and publish the data they have collected and thereby gain appropriate professional recognition for planning, organizing, and running clinical trials whose data are subsequently used by other investigators. Research institutions fear that requirements for sharing clinical trial data will be unfunded mandates. Participant and patient advocates want clinical trial data to be widely available in order to advance the development of new treatments. If data sharing is to be broadly accepted and fulfill its promise, these concerns of key stakeholders will need to be acknowledged and addressed. Moreover, the sharing of clinical trial data needs to be carried out in a way that maintains incentives for sponsors and researchers to develop new therapies and carry out future clinical trials and that sustains participants' willingness to participate in trials.

In addressing its statement of task (see Box S-1), the committee that conducted this study worked to craft a report that would be useful well into the future, as well as addressing specific issues that need attention in the short term. The committee acknowledges that no body or authority currently is capable of enforcing the recommendations offered in this report for all stakeholders; rather, the committee interpreted its charge as helping to establish professional standards and set expectations for responsible sharing of clinical trial data.

GUIDING PRINCIPLES FOR SHARING CLINICAL TRIAL DATA

The goal of responsible sharing of clinical trial data should be to increase scientific knowledge that leads to better therapies for patients. The committee formulated the following guiding principles for responsible sharing of clinical trial data:

- Maximize the benefits of clinical trials while minimizing the risks of sharing clinical trial data.
- Respect individual participants whose data are shared.
- Increase public trust in clinical trials and the sharing of trial data.
- Conduct the sharing of clinical trial data in a fair manner.

These guiding principles need to be specified and balanced in the context of specific issues associated with the sharing of clinical trial data. The committee determined that the public should benefit from the sharing of clinical trial data in the form of valid scientific knowledge and

BOX S-1
Statement of Task for This Study

An ad hoc committee of the Institute of Medicine will conduct a study to develop guiding principles and a framework (activities and strategies) for the responsible sharing of clinical trial data. For the purposes of the study, the scope will be limited to interventional clinical trials, and "data sharing" will include the responsible entity (data generator) making the data available via open or restricted access, or exchanged among parties. For the purposes of this study, data generator will include industry sponsors, data repositories, and researchers conducting clinical trials. Specifically, the committee will:

- Articulate guiding principles that underpin the responsible sharing of clinical trial data.
- Describe a selected set of data and data sharing activities, including but not limited to:
  - Types of data (e.g., summary, participant).
  - Provider(s) and recipient(s) of shared data.
  - Whether and when data are disclosed publicly, with or without restrictions, or exchanged privately among parties.
- For each data sharing activity, the committee will:
  - Identify key benefits of sharing and risks of not sharing for research sponsors and investigators, study participants, regulatory agencies, patient groups, and the public.
  - Address key challenges and risks of sharing (e.g., resource constraints, implementation, disincentives in the academic research model, changing norms, protection of human subjects and patient privacy, intellectual property/legal issues, preservation of scientific standards and data quality).
  - Outline strategies and suggest practical approaches to facilitate responsible data sharing.
- Make recommendations to enhance responsible sharing of clinical trial data. The committee will identify guiding principles and characteristics for the optimal infrastructure and governance for sharing clinical trial data, taking into consideration a variety of approaches (e.g., a distributed/federated data system).

In developing the principles and framework and in defining the rights, responsibilities, and limitations underpinning the responsible sharing of clinical trial data, the committee will take into account the benefits of data sharing, the potential adverse consequences of both sharing and not sharing data, and the landscape of regulations and policies under which data sharing occurs. Focused consideration will also be given to the ethical standards and to integrating core principles and values, including privacy. The committee is not expected to develop or define specific technical data standards.

A discussion framework will be released for public comment, which will include tentative findings regarding (a) guiding principles and (b) a selected set of data sharing activities. Based on the public comments received and further deliberations, the committee will prepare a final report with its findings and recommendations.

improved clinical practice and public health; at the same time, however, the legitimate interests of stakeholders—particularly their concerns about the potential harms and costs of data sharing—need to be recognized and addressed in a fair manner.

KEY STAKEHOLDERS INVOLVED IN DATA SHARING

In Chapter 3, the committee analyzes the perspectives of key stakeholders regarding the sharing of clinical trial data and their assessment of the associated benefits, risks, and challenges.

No stakeholder can single-handedly create a clinical trial ecosystem in which sharing data is expected and the risks of sharing are minimized. But all stakeholders have crucial roles and responsibilities in creating a culture of responsible sharing of clinical trial data and in providing effective incentives for such sharing. The committee envisaged that different approaches to sharing clinical trial data will be developed and urges learning from experience with these approaches.

Recommendation 1: Stakeholders in clinical trials should foster a culture in which data sharing is the expected norm, and should commit to responsible strategies aimed at maximizing the benefits, minimizing the risks, and overcoming the challenges of sharing clinical trial data for all parties.

Funders and sponsors should
- promote the development of a sustainable infrastructure and mechanism by which data can be shared, in accordance with the terms and conditions of grants and contracts;
- provide funding to investigators for sharing of clinical trial data as a line item in grants and contracts;
- include prior data sharing as a measure of impact when deciding about future funding;
- include and enforce requirements in the terms and conditions of grants and contracts that investigators will make clinical trial data available for sharing under the conditions recommended in this report; and
- fund and promote the development and adoption of common data elements.

Disease advocacy organizations should
- require data sharing plans as part of protocol reviews and criteria for funding grants;

- provide guidance and educational programs on data sharing for clinical trial participants;
- require data sharing plans as a condition for promoting clinical trials to their constituents; and
- contribute funding to enable data sharing.

Regulatory and research oversight bodies should
- work with industry and other stakeholders to develop and harmonize new clinical study report (CSR) templates that do not include commercially confidential information or personally identifiable data;
- work with regulatory authorities around the world to harmonize requirements and practices to support the responsible sharing of clinical trial data; and
- issue clear guidance that the sharing of clinical trial data is expected and that the role of Research Ethics Committees or Institutional Review Boards (IRBs) is to encourage and facilitate the responsible and ethical conduct of data sharing through the adoption of protections such as those recommended by this committee and the emerging best practices of clinical trial data sharing initiatives.

Research Ethics Committees or IRBs should
- provide guidance for clinical trialists and templates for informed consent for participants that enable responsible data sharing;
- consider data sharing plans when assessing the benefits and risks of clinical trials; and
- adopt protections for participants as recommended by this committee and the emerging best practices of clinical trial data sharing initiatives.

Investigators and sponsors should
- design clinical trials and manage trial data with the expectation that data will be shared;
- adopt common data elements in new clinical trial protocols unless there is a compelling scientific reason not to do so;
- explain to participants during the informed consent process
  - what data will (and will not) be shared with the individual participants during and after the trial,
  - the potential risks to privacy associated with the collection and sharing of data during and after the trial and a summary of the types of protections employed to mitigate this risk, and
  - under what conditions the trial data may be shared (with regulators, investigators, etc.) beyond the trial team; and

- make clinical trial data available at the times and under the conditions recommended in this report.

Research institutions and universities should
- ensure that investigators from their institutions share data from clinical trials in accordance with the recommendations in this report and the terms and conditions of grants and contracts;
- promote the development of a sustainable infrastructure and mechanisms for data sharing;
- make sharing of clinical trial data a consideration in promotion of faculty members and assessment of programs; and
- provide training for data science and quantitative scientists to facilitate sharing and analysis of clinical trial data.

Journals should
- require authors of both primary and secondary analyses of clinical trial data to
  - document that they have submitted a data sharing plan at a site that shares data with and meets the data requirements of the World Health Organization's International Clinical Trials Registry Platform before enrolling participants, and
  - commit to releasing the analytic data set underlying published analyses, tables, figures, and results no later than the times specified in this report;
- require that submitted manuscripts using existing data sets from clinical trials, in whole or in part, cite these data appropriately; and
- require that any published secondary analyses provide the data and metadata at the same level as in the original publication.

Membership and professional societies should
- establish as policy that members should participate in sharing clinical trial data as part of their professional responsibilities;
- require as a condition of submitting abstracts to a meeting of the society and manuscripts to the journal of the society that clinical trial data will be shared in accordance with the recommendations in this report; and
- collaborate on and promote the development and use of common data elements relevant to their members.

WHAT DATA SHOULD BE SHARED AND WHEN
IN THE LIFE CYCLE OF A CLINICAL TRIAL

In Chapter 4, the committee analyzes the benefits, risks, and challenges of sharing the various types of clinical trial data that are generated at different times during the clinical trial life cycle.

Data sharing can refer to various types of data, including individual participant data (i.e., raw data and the analyzable data set); metadata, or "data about the data" (e.g., protocol, statistical analysis plan, and analytic code); and summary-level data (e.g., summary-level results posted on registries, lay summaries, publications, and CSRs). Therefore, a clinical trial data sharing policy needs to specify what data will be shared, when, and under what conditions.

The committee recognizes that sharing the various types of data presents different benefits and risks.

- Sharing summary results helps protect against publication bias but does not enable new analysis.
- Sharing the analyzable data set allows for reanalysis, meta-analysis, and scientific discovery through hypothesis generation, but this data set needs to be accompanied by metadata in order for secondary analyses to be rigorous and efficient, and sharing it could also lead to privacy risks and inappropriate analyses.
- Sharing the CSR allows for better understanding of regulatory decisions and facilitates use of the analyzable data set, but the CSR may contain commercially confidential information or be used for unfair commercial purposes.
- Sharing raw data is useful in certain circumstances but is overly burdensome in most cases and also presents risks to privacy.
- Summary results may be posted on public websites with few risks, but the risks of sharing individual participant data and CSRs are significant and may need to be mitigated in most cases through appropriate controls.
- Explaining to trial participants what data will be shared during the informed consent process and making their own data available to them following study completion and data analysis help uphold public trust in clinical trials.

The committee applied these considerations to clinical trial data for trials initiated after this report only, recognizing that sharing data from legacy trials may present greater risks and burdens and thus needs to be deliberated on a case-by-case basis. Sponsors and investigators are strongly urged to give priority to sharing of data from legacy trials whose findings influence decisions about clinical care.

Next, the committee considered the timing of data sharing. The committee sought to balance several goals: (1) providing to trial investigators a fair opportunity to publish their analyses; (2) allowing other investigators to analyze and use data that are otherwise not being published in a timely manner and to reproduce the findings of a published paper; and (3) reducing the risks of data sharing, including risks to participants and sponsors and the risk of invalid analyses of shared data. The committee appreciated that many clinical trialists feel strongly that, after years of effort carrying out a clinical trial, they should have the opportunity to write a series of papers analyzing the collected data before other investigators have access to the data. The committee concluded that after completion of a clinical trial, a moratorium of 18 months is generally appropriate before data are shared to allow trialists to carry out their analyses.

The committee paid particular attention to sharing of the analytic data set that supports a published paper reporting results of a clinical trial. Once the results of a study have been published, the scientific process is best served by allowing other investigators immediate access to the analytic data set supporting the publication so they can reproduce the published findings and carry out additional analyses to test the robustness of the conclusions.

In an ideal clinical trials ecosystem, the committee would favor sharing the analytic data set supporting a publication immediately upon publication. However, the committee recognized that there currently are many associated practical constraints and challenges that need to be addressed. The committee therefore has recommended a pragmatic compromise time frame of 6 months after publication at this time, with the expectation that the standard ultimately will become sharing the analytic data set simultaneously with publication. The committee hopes that the evolution of responsible sharing of clinical trial data will be guided by empirical evidence.

At the same time, the committee recognized that there will be justifiable exceptions to its recommendations in light of the wide variation in clinical trials. The recommended time periods at which specific data are to be shared are not intended to be hard-and-fast, inflexible rules. For trials that are likely to have a major clinical, public health, or policy impact, the committee favors sharing the analytic data set supporting a publication sooner than the 6-month guideline.

The committee next considered clinical trials submitted to a regulatory agency. Regulatory agencies review data from many trials and may carry out further analyses or require additional data. There are advantages to allowing regulatory agencies a "quiet period" to review the totality of evidence without being influenced by multiple analyses of just a portion of the data under review. However, if the sponsor publishes results from a trial prior to regulatory approval, the analytic data set supporting the publication should be shared as recommended, even if that occurs before the end of the regulators' quiet period.

Turning to clinical trials of products that are abandoned, the committee distinguished situations in which the sponsor transfers rights to develop the product to another company from situations in which it does not. The committee also considered sharing of data with trial participants and the public, distinguishing summary results of a trial from results of measurements on individual participants made during the trial.

Drawing together these considerations, the committee formulated the following recommendation for what data should be shared after key points in a clinical trial. The committee believes that this recommendation will set professional standards and establish expectations that clinical trial data should be shared (see also Figure S-1):

Recommendation 2: Sponsors and investigators should share the various types of clinical trial data no later than the times specified below. Sponsors and investigators who decide to make data available for sharing before these times are encouraged to do so.

Trial registration:
- The data sharing plan for a clinical trial (i.e., what data will be shared when and under what conditions) should be publicly available at a third-party site that shares data with and meets the data requirements of the World Health Organization's International Clinical Trials Registry Platform; this should occur before the first participant is enrolled.

Study completion:
- Summary-level results of clinical trials (including adverse event summaries) should be made publicly available no later than 12 months after study completion.
- Lay summaries of results should be made available to trial participants concurrently with the sharing of summary-level results, no later than 12 months after study completion.
- The "full data package"[1] should be shared no later than 18 months after study completion (unless the trial is in support of a regulatory application).

---

[1] See the notes to Figure S-1 for definitions of "full data package," "post-publication data package," and "post-regulatory data package."

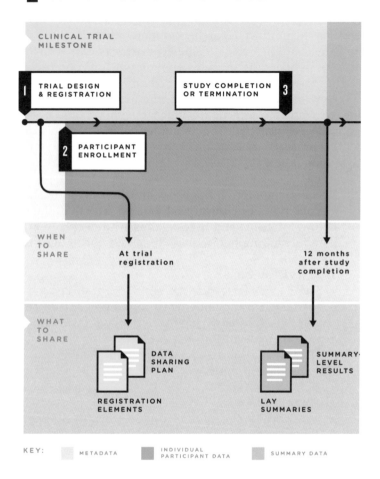

FIGURE S-1 The clinical trial life cycle: When to share data.
NOTES: Full data package = the full analyzable data set, full protocol (including initial version, final version, and all amendments), full statistical analysis plan (including all amendments and all documentation for additional work processes), and analytic code. Post-publication data package = a subset of the full data package supporting the findings, tables, and figures in the publication. Post-regulatory

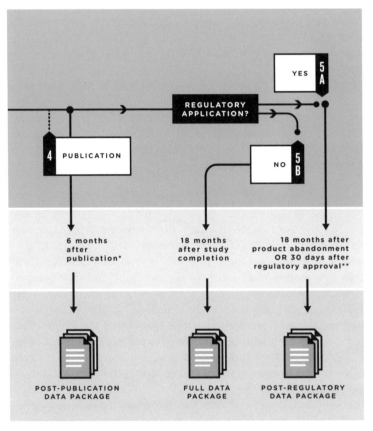

YES 5A

REGULATORY APPLICATION?

4 PUBLICATION

NO 5B

6 months after publication*

18 months after study completion

18 months after product abandonment OR 30 days after regulatory approval**

POST-PUBLICATION DATA PACKAGE

FULL DATA PACKAGE

POST-REGULATORY DATA PACKAGE

* No later than 6 months after publication applies to all studies, whether intended or not intended to support regulatory applications and regardless of publication timing relative to study completion, though publication is most likely to occur after study completion.
** Sharing the post-regulatory data package should occur 30 days after approval or 18 months after study completion, whichever is later; 18 months after abandonment of the product or indication. This applies to all studies intended and to support regulatory applications, even if abandonment occurs prior to actual regulatory application.

data package = the full data package plus the clinical study report (redacted for commercially or personal confidential information). Legacy trials: For trials initiated prior to the publication of these recommendations, sponsors and principal investigators should decide on a case-by-case basis whether to share data from the completed trials. They are strongly urged to do so for major and significant clinical trials whose findings will influence decisions about clinical care.

Publication:
- The "post-publication data package" should be shared no later than 6 months after publication.

Regulatory application:
- For studies of products or new indications that are approved, the "post-regulatory data package" should be shared 30 days after regulatory approval or 18 months after study completion, whichever occurs later.
- For studies of new products or new indications for a marketed product that are abandoned, the "post-regulatory data package" should be shared no later than 18 months after abandonment. However, if the product is licensed to another party for further development, these data need be shared only after publication, approval, or final abandonment.

ACCESS TO CLINICAL TRIAL DATA

In Chapter 5, the committee analyzes how several risks associated with sharing clinical trial data (in particular individual participant data and CSRs) might be addressed through controls on data access (i.e., with whom the data are shared and under what conditions) without compromising the usefulness of data sharing for the generation of additional scientific knowledge. Arrangements for determining access to clinical trial data need to balance several goals: protecting the privacy of research participants, reducing the likelihood of invalid analyses or misuse of the shared data, avoiding undue burdens on secondary users seeking access, avoiding undue harms to investigators and sponsors that share data, and enhancing public trust in the sharing of clinical trial data.

The committee noted support for open and free access to scientific publications immediately upon publication, as well as the requirement of the U.S. Food and Drug Administration (FDA) to make a summary of clinical trial results available to the public. The committee believes that open access (to the public with no controls) is appropriate and desirable for clinical trial results, and, in some cases, no or few controls on sharing other types of clinical trial data may be the preferred approach when all stakeholders involved in a trial (i.e., sponsors, investigators, and participants) are comfortable with this approach and believe the benefits outweigh the risks. In many cases, however, sponsors, investigators, and/or participants may have concerns about an open access model for certain clinical trial data and may wish to place some conditions on access to or uses of the data.

In reviewing protections for privacy, the committee noted that while de-identification is commonly used to protect privacy, it has limitations. Different jurisdictions have different de-identification standards. Moreover, the risk of re-identification depends on the context in which data are released, the type of data, and the additional information that might be combined with the shared data. In the case of genome-wide sequencing data and "big data" analyses, for example, de-identification and data security alone may not provide adequate protection; additional privacy and security techniques are being developed for these cases.

The committee determined that data use agreements are a promising vehicle for reducing these risks and related disincentives for sharing clinical trial data. The committee reviewed a variety of provisions in existing data use agreements aimed at reducing risks to various parties, enhancing the scientific value of secondary analyses, and protecting the public health. The committee does not endorse all the specific provisions that were reviewed but believes they should be considered as potential options. Although it is unclear whether and how data use agreements will be enforced, the committee believes these agreements have significant normative, symbolic, and deterrent value, setting professional expectations and standards for responsible behavior.

The committee considered the review of requests for data access and reached several conclusions. Access restrictions based on the composition of the secondary analysis team—for example, requiring a biostatistician with particular qualifications or excluding lawyers—would not further the goals of responsible sharing of clinical trial data. Review of research proposals could mitigate risks, but overly restrictive controls would inhibit valid secondary analyses and innovative scientific proposals. If the trial sponsor or investigator, rather than an independent review panel, reviewed data requests and made decisions regarding access, concerns about conflicts of interest could lead to mistrust. Representatives of communities and patient and disease advocacy groups could serve as useful members of such review panels. Furthermore, making the policies and procedures regarding access to clinical trial data transparent would enhance the trustworthiness of data sharing programs.

Finally, the committee concluded that the experience of early adopters of the sharing of clinical trial data will undoubtedly offer lessons and best practices from which others can learn. As sponsors try different approaches to data sharing, collecting empirical data that allow comparison of different approaches will provide crucial information on what does and does not work in various contexts.

In light of the above considerations, the committee formulated the following recommendation regarding data access:

Recommendation 3: Holders of clinical trial data should mitigate the risks and enhance the benefits of sharing sensitive clinical trial data by implementing operational strategies that include employing data use agreements, designating an independent review panel, including members of the lay public in governance, and making access to clinical trial data transparent. Specifically, they should take the following actions:

- Employ data use agreements that include provisions aimed at protecting clinical trial participants, advancing the goal of producing scientifically valid secondary analyses, giving credit to the investigators who collected the clinical trial data, protecting the intellectual property interests of sponsors, and ultimately improving patient care.
- Employ other appropriate techniques for protecting privacy, in addition to de-identification and data security.
- Designate an independent review panel—in lieu of the sponsor or investigator of a clinical trial—if requests for access to clinical trial data will be reviewed for approval.
- Include lay representatives (e.g., patients, members of the public, and/or representatives of disease advocacy groups) on the independent review panel that reviews and approves data access requests.
- Make access to clinical trial data transparent by publicly reporting
  - the organizational structure, policies, procedures (e.g., criteria for determining access and conditions of use), and membership of the independent review panel that makes decisions about access to clinical trial data; and
  - a summary of the decisions regarding requests for data access, including the number of requests and approvals and the reasons for disapprovals.
- Learn from experience by collecting data on the outcomes of data sharing policies, procedures, and technical approaches (including the benefits, risks, and costs), and share information and lessons learned with clinical trial sponsors, the public, and other organizations sharing clinical trial data.

THE FUTURE OF CLINICAL TRIAL DATA SHARING IN A CHANGING LANDSCAPE

Chapter 6 presents the committee's vision for responsible sharing of clinical trial data in the future. In this vision, all stakeholders are committed to sharing data responsibly, have modified their work processes to facilitate data sharing, and possess the resources and tools necessary to do so.

- A culture of sharing clinical trial data with effective incentives for sharing emerges.
- There are more platforms for sharing clinical trial data, with different data access models and with sufficient total capacity to meet demand. The different platforms are interoperable: data obtained from various platforms can easily be searched and combined to allow further analyses.
- There is adequate financial support for sharing clinical trial data, and costs are fairly allocated among stakeholders.
- Protections are in place to minimize the risks of data sharing and to reduce disincentives for sharing.
- Best practices for sharing clinical trial data are identified and modified in response to ongoing experience and feedback. The sharing of clinical trial data forms a "learning" ecosystem in which data on data sharing outcomes are routinely collected and continually used to improve how data sharing is conducted.

Next the committee identified remaining key challenges to responsible sharing of clinical trial data, which include the following:

- Infrastructure challenges—Currently there are insufficient platforms to store and manage clinical trial data under a variety of access models.
- Technological challenges—Current data sharing platforms are not consistently discoverable, searchable, and interoperable. Special attention is needed to the development and adoption of common protocol data models and common data elements to ensure meaningful computation across disparate trials and databases. A federated query system of "bringing the data to the question" may offer effective ways of achieving the benefits of sharing clinical trial data while mitigating its risks.
- Workforce challenges—A sufficient workforce with the skills and knowledge to manage the operational and technical aspects of data sharing needs to be developed.
- Sustainability challenges—Currently the costs of data sharing are borne by a small subset of sponsors, funders, and clinical trialists; for data sharing to be sustainable, costs will need to be distributed equitably across both data generators and users.

The committee gave particular attention to the need for a sustainable and equitable business model for responsible sharing of clinical trial data and developed the following conceptual framework:

- Responsible sharing of clinical trial data benefits the public and multiple stakeholders, including payers of health care as well as patients, their physicians, and researchers.
- As a matter of fairness, those who benefit from responsible sharing of clinical trial data, including the users of shared data, should also bear some of the costs of sharing. Additional sources of funding for responsible sharing of clinical trial data, such as private philanthropies, need to be identified.
- Policies on equitable distribution of the costs of responsible sharing of clinical trial data among stakeholders should be based on accurate information on the costs of data sharing for various kinds of clinical trials.
- The costs of responsible sharing of clinical trial data will decrease in the future if data collection and management are designed to facilitate sharing.

The committee concluded that a market analysis of the costs of sharing clinical trial data and an economic analysis of options for funding data sharing would provide an evidence base for developing sustainable and equitable models for responsible sharing of clinical trial data.

Finally, the committee considered the ecosystem of responsible sharing of clinical trial data. Individual sponsors and trusted intermediaries can do a great deal to make sharing clinical trial data more responsible, effective, and efficient. For responsible sharing of clinical trial data to become pervasive, sustained, and rooted as a professional norm, however, many challenges need to be addressed in collaboration with other institutions and stakeholders. The committee recommends a next step to promote discussion and exchange of ideas among a wide range of stakeholders in order to forge agreement on best practices, standards, and incentives:

Recommendation 4: The sponsors of this study should take the lead, together with or via a trusted impartial organization(s), to convene a multistakeholder body with global reach and broad representation to address, in an ongoing process, the key infrastructure, technological, sustainability, and workforce challenges associated with the sharing of clinical trial data.

1

Introduction

The clinical trials enterprise,[1] tasked with testing the safety and efficacy of health interventions and informing medical decisions, is poised to undergo important changes in response to significant and sustained challenges, including the lengthy time frame, high cost, and often limited relevance of the research it produces (NRC and IOM, 2011). A key driver of the changes on the horizon for clinical trials is the increasingly consumer- and patient-driven nature of research and health care (NRC and IOM, 2011). The traditional system of investigators, sponsors, and journal editors as gatekeepers of clinical trials and their results is being tested as calls for "open science" and the democratization of clinical research intensify. Although a large-scale transition is still under way and significant challenges remain, many observers note that early adopters of the principles and practices of open science will be rewarded (Boulton et al., 2011; Walport and Brest, 2011).

The movement toward greater transparency is being further accelerated by trial participants who have emerged from behind the veil of being termed and treated only as "research subjects" to assume the roles of full partners, leaders, and funders of research. Organized and motivated groups of patients and healthy individuals can and are moving beyond the traditional research and health systems to publicly generate

---

[1] The clinical trials enterprise encompasses the full spectrum of clinical trials and their applications. It includes the processes, institutions, and individuals that participate in research, as well as those who eventually apply clinical trial findings in a care setting.

data about themselves and/or the treatments they choose, compare and analyze these data, and share the results (Kaye et al., 2012; Terry and Terry, 2011; Wicks et al., 2014). These efforts suggest a larger cultural shift already under way, one in which the results of research are deemed a public good that can benefit society only when shared in a timely and responsible manner (Loder, 2013; Mello et al., 2013; Ross et al., 2012). Exploring the implementation of this broad societal desire to extract maximal benefit from the data generated by volunteers in a clinical trial reveals a number of benefits and risks to the sharing of clinical trial data. There is significant potential to share these data successfully in a responsible manner that does not entail complete, unfettered access to individual participant data (ClinicalStudyDataRequest.com, 2014; YODA Project, 2014), but determining the appropriate sharing strategy for various types of clinical trial data will require identifying, evaluating, and addressing the benefits and risks involved.

Clinical trials are crucial to determining the safety and efficacy of health interventions. Vast amounts of data are generated over the course of a clinical trial; however, a large portion of these data is never published in peer-reviewed journals (Doshi et al., 2013b; Zarin, 2013). Today, moreover, researchers other than the trialists have limited access to clinical trial data that could be used to reproduce published results, carry out secondary analyses, or combine data from different trials in systematic reviews (Rathi et al., 2012). Public well-being would be enhanced by the additional knowledge that could be gained from these analyses. Furthermore, sharing clinical trial data might accelerate the drug discovery and development process, reducing redundancies and facilitating the identification and validation of new drug targets or surrogate endpoints. In short, there are today many missed opportunities to gain scientific knowledge from clinical trial data that could strengthen the evidence base for the treatment decisions of physicians and patients. In economic terms, these missed opportunities result in a suboptimal return on the altruism and contributions of clinical trial participants, the efforts of clinical trialists and research staff, and the financial resources invested by study funders and sponsors (Doshi et al., 2013a). At the same time, however, the sharing of clinical trial data presents risks to various important stakeholders and raises complex challenges regarding the consent and privacy of participants, protection of the legitimate interests of stakeholders, and the development of a sustainable and equitable business model for sharing (IOM, 2013b).

STUDY CONTEXT

Historical Highlights

Before 2012, the evolution of enhanced transparency in clinical research involved a number of research stakeholders, including international regulatory and funding organizations such as the European Medicines Agency (EMA), the U.S. Food and Drug Administration (FDA), the U.S. National Institutes of Health (NIH), and The Wellcome Trust; biomedical journals; and participant groups.

The Food and Drug Administration Modernization Act of 1997 mandated registration on ClinicalTrials.gov of federally or privately funded clinical trials conducted under Investigational New Drug applications (INDs) to test the effectiveness of experimental drugs for patients with serious or life-threatening diseases or conditions (Zarin, 2007). The International Committee of Medical Journal Editors further supported trial registration by requiring it as a condition of consideration for publication in 2004 (De Angelis et al., 2004). In 2003, NIH issued its *Final Statement on Sharing Research Data*, which states that "all investigator-initiated applications with direct costs greater than $500,000 in any single year will be expected to address data sharing in their application" (NIH, 2003). In 2007, the Food and Drug Administration Amendments Act (FDAAA) required reporting of summary results from certain trials (e.g., non-phase 1) of FDA-approved drugs, biologics, and devices to ClinicalTrials.gov, whether the results have been published or not (Zarin, 2011).[2] Also in 2007, the *Annals of Internal Medicine* launched a Reproducible Research initiative, requiring that all original articles include a statement indicating the authors' willingness to share with the public the study protocol (original and amendments), the statistical code used to generate results, and the data set from which the results were derived (Laine et al., 2007). And in 2009 the *British Medical Journal* required that authors include data sharing statements at the end of each published article, indicating what data are available, to whom, and how (FDA, 2010; Groves, 2009; Roehr, 2009).

In November 2010, the EMA created an "access to documents" policy and agreed to release clinical study reports (CSRs) to external persons who submit a freedom of information request (EMA, 2014). In 2011, an international group of funders (Inserm, The Wellcome Trust, the UK Medical Research Council, NIH, The World Bank, and others) issued a statement endorsing "making research data sets available to investigators beyond the original research team in a timely and responsible manner, subject to appropriate safeguards" (The Wellcome Trust, 2011). Also in

---

[2] 42 U.S.C. § 282(j)(3)(C).

2011, the health data sharing platform PatientsLikeMe released the results of a patient-initiated observational study of amyotrophic lateral sclerosis (ALS) patients experimenting with lithium carbonate treatment—the first time a social network of patients convened to evaluate a treatment in real time (PatientsLikeMe, 2011; Wicks et al., 2011).

2012 Institute of Medicine (IOM) Workshop on Sharing Clinical Research Data

In October 2012, the IOM convened a broad range of experts and stakeholders to discuss the sharing of clinical research data. As highlighted by participants at the workshop, data sharing can have important benefits for industry, nonprofit funders of research, academic investigators, patient advocacy groups, and ultimately patients and the public. These benefits include, for example, accelerating medical innovation by reducing redundancies, facilitating the identification and validation of new drug targets, identifying new indications for use, and improving understanding of the safety and efficacy of therapies (IOM, 2013b). Workshop participants suggested that the conversation around sharing clinical research data has evolved from whether the data should be shared to how best to facilitate sharing, and cited examples of data sharing activities that had been established or proposed at the time (EMA, 2014; Krumholz and Ross, 2011; Nisen and Rockhold, 2013; Zarin, 2013). Concerns were raised, however, that the potential benefits of data sharing may not be realized if the sharing is fragmented or conducted largely through uncoordinated initiatives. Further, data sharing involves costs, burdens, risks, lack of incentives, and even disincentives that need to be addressed from the perspectives of multiple stakeholders.

Progress Since the 2012 IOM Workshop

Since the 2012 workshop was held, momentum has continued to build for sharing clinical trial data. Major developments include the following:

- Medtronic and Johnson & Johnson partnered with Yale University Open Data Access (YODA). Medtronic agreed to release all clinical trial data on one product widely used in spine surgery, rBMP2, to academic investigators for reanalysis (YODA Project, 2013). Johnson & Johnson transferred authority to YODA for making decisions on data requests for all Janssen pharmaceutical trials (Johnson & Johnson, 2014).
- The EMA issued a draft policy, modified it in response to consultation and feedback, and has now issued requirements for sharing

clinical trial data submitted to the agency[3] once a marketing decision on the study products has been made (EMA, 2014).

- The AllTrials campaign was launched, calling for "all past and present clinical trials to be registered and their full methods and summary results reported" (AllTrials, 2013). As of December 2014, more than 81,000 people had signed the AllTrials petition, and 532 organizations had joined AllTrials (AllTrials, 2014).
- Astellas, Bayer, Boehringer Ingelheim, GlaxoSmithKline, Lilly, Novartis, Roche, Sanofi, Takeda, UCB, and ViiV Healthcare committed to sharing clinical trial data through ClinicalStudyDataRequest.com and allowing an independent review panel to make decisions on data requests (ClinicalStudyDataRequest.com, 2014).
- The *British Medical Journal* issued a policy requiring data sharing for clinical trials it publishes (BMJ, 2013).
- The Pharmaceutical Research and Manufacturers of America (PhRMA), the European Federation of Pharmaceutical Industries and Associations (EFPIA), and the Biotechnology Industry Organization (BIO) released principles documents signaling their support for sharing clinical trial data (BIO, 2014; PhRMA, 2013).
- The National Institute of Allergy and Infectious Diseases (NIAID) made de-identified data from 11 clinical trials available through the Immunology Database and Analysis Portal (ImmPort) (ImmPort, 2013).
- NIH issued a new policy on sharing of genomic data. The new policy outlines and emphasizes the expectation that investigators will obtain informed consent from study participants for potential future use of the participants' de-identified data for both research and broad sharing, and commit to sharing data no later than the date of first publication of the study results (NIH, 2014).

Numerous approaches and models for sharing clinical trial data are being implemented with varying levels of access control. At one end of the spectrum, ImmPort in the United States and the FreeBIRD website (FreeBIRD, 2014) in the United Kingdom make available some de-identified data sets from publicly funded clinical trials (NIAID and CRASH trials, respectively) with minimal restrictions; the data sets can be downloaded from the Web upon registration and acceptance of their terms

---

[3] Clinical trial sponsors seeking regulatory approval from authorities such as the EMA and the FDA must submit detailed CSRs and individual participant data as required, which form the basis of the marketing application for a product. In trials not conducted for regulatory approval of a product, detailed CSRs may or may not be prepared (Doshi et al., 2012; Teden, 2013).

of use. At the other end of the spectrum, many programs for sharing of clinical trial data from private sponsors (e.g., GlaxoSmithKline, Johnson & Johnson) place various restrictions on data access—for example, requiring review of requests by an independent scientific review board and access through a format that cannot be downloaded. As an increasing number of organizations take the initiative to share their data more actively, the time is right to develop broadly accepted guidance for responsible sharing of clinical trial data that will increase the availability and usefulness of the data while mitigating the risks of data sharing.

CHARGE TO THE COMMITTEE AND STUDY SCOPE

As a follow-up to the 2012 IOM workshop, a group of federal, industry, and U.S. and international foundation sponsors[4] asked the IOM to conduct a consensus study that would generate guiding principles and a framework for the responsible sharing of clinical trial data.

As described in the committee's statement of task (see Box 1-1), over a 17-month study period, the committee was charged with releasing two reports:

- a discussion framework document ("the Framework") that was released in January 2014 for public comment, summarizing the committee's tentative findings regarding guiding principles and describing a selected set of data sharing activities; and
- a final report containing conclusions and recommendations related to the committee's full charge.

To respond to this charge, the IOM convened a 13-member committee comprising experts in key scientific and research-related domains, including academia, industry, funding bodies, regulatory activities, scientific publications, clinicians, and patients. Individual committee members' expertise spans academic clinical trial design, performance, and dissemination; pharmaceutical product development; statistics, informatics, and data security; ethics of human subjects research; and law and regulatory requirements (including privacy, security, and intellectual property). Committee members also have insight into the global context of data sharing; the concerns of research participants, patients, and their families; and

---

[4] AbbVie Inc., Amgen Inc., AstraZeneca Pharmaceuticals, Bayer, Biogen Idec, Bristol-Myers Squibb, Burroughs Wellcome Fund, Doris Duke Charitable Foundation, Eli Lilly and Company, EMD Serono, Genentech, GlaxoSmithKline, Johnson & Johnson, Medical Research Council (UK), Merck & Co., Inc., Novartis Pharmaceuticals Corporation, Novo Nordisk, Pfizer Inc., Sanofi-Aventis, Takeda, U.S. Food and Drug Administration, U.S. National Institutes of Health, and The Wellcome Trust.

BOX 1-1
Statement of Task for This Study

An ad hoc committee of the Institute of Medicine will conduct a study to develop guiding principles and a framework (activities and strategies) for the responsible sharing of clinical trial data. For the purposes of the study, the scope will be limited to interventional clinical trials, and "data sharing" will include the responsible entity (data generator) making the data available via open or restricted access, or exchanged among parties. For the purposes of this study, data generator will include industry sponsors, data repositories, and researchers conducting clinical trials. Specifically, the committee will:

- Articulate guiding principles that underpin the responsible sharing of clinical trial data.
- Describe a selected set of data and data sharing activities, including but not limited to:
  - Types of data (e.g., summary, participant).
  - Provider(s) and recipient(s) of shared data.
  - Whether and when data are disclosed publicly, with or without restrictions, or exchanged privately among parties.
- For each data sharing activity, the committee will:
  - Identify key benefits of sharing and risks of not sharing for research sponsors and investigators, study participants, regulatory agencies, patient groups, and the public.
  - Address key challenges and risks of sharing (e.g., resource constraints, implementation, disincentives in the academic research model, changing norms, protection of human subjects and patient privacy, intellectual property/legal issues, preservation of scientific standards and data quality).
  - Outline strategies and suggest practical approaches to facilitate responsible data sharing.
- Make recommendations to enhance responsible sharing of clinical trial data. The committee will identify guiding principles and characteristics for the optimal infrastructure and governance for sharing clinical trial data, taking into consideration a variety of approaches (e.g., a distributed/federated data system).

In developing the principles and framework and in defining the rights, responsibilities, and limitations underpinning the responsible sharing of clinical trial data, the committee will take into account the benefits of data sharing, the potential adverse consequences of both sharing and not sharing data, and the landscape of regulations and policies under which data sharing occurs. Focused consideration will also be given to the ethical standards and to integrating core principles and values, including privacy. The committee is not expected to develop or define specific technical data standards.

A discussion framework will be released for public comment, which will include tentative findings regarding (a) guiding principles and (b) a selected set of data sharing activities. Based on the public comments received and further deliberations, the committee will prepare a final report with its findings and recommendations.

BOX 1-2
Key Definitions

For the purposes of this study, **interventional clinical trials** are defined as "research in which participants are assigned to receive one or more interventions (or no intervention) so that the effects of the interventions on biomedical or health-related outcomes can be evaluated. Assignments to treatment groups are determined by the study protocol" (ClinicalTrials.gov, 2012). An **intervention** is a "process or action that is the focus of a clinical trial. This can include giving participants drugs, medical devices, procedures, vaccines, and other products that are either investigational or already available" (ClinicalTrials.gov, 2012). For the purposes of this study, **intervention types** are limited to drugs, devices, biologics, surgical procedures, behavioral interventions, and changes in the administration or delivery of clinical care. The committee further found it useful to consider interventional clinical trials in two broad categories—those studies intended and those not intended to support a **regulatory application**.

Data sharing is the practice of making data* from scientific research available for secondary uses. This report distinguishes between **primary and secondary uses of data**. The former include analyses addressing research questions the trial was originally designed to address; these questions would be delineated in the analysis plan that is registered prior to enrollment of the first participant. The latter include (1) reanalyses of questions addressed in the primary uses to check for replicability/validity, (2) meta-analyses, and (3) de novo analyses designed to address questions the trial was not explicitly designed to address. Data may be shared either proactively (e.g., by posting to a website or providing to a repository) or upon request.

---

* Many different types of data may be shared, including individual participant data (i.e., raw data and the analyzable data set); metadata, or "data about the data" (e.g., protocol, statistical analysis plan, and analytic code); and summary-level data (e.g., summary-level results posted on registries, lay summaries, publications, and clinical study reports). See Chapter 4 for the committee's analysis of the benefits and risks of sharing different types of data.

other relevant issues. As specified in the statement of task (see Box 1-1), the scope of the study was limited to interventional clinical trials (see the definitions in Box 1-2).

STUDY APPROACH

Study Process

During the course of its deliberations, the committee gathered information through a variety of mechanisms: (1) three 1.5-day face-to-face workshops held in Washington, DC, in October 2013, February 2014, and May 2014 and one virtual workshop held in April 2014, all of which were open to the public (see Appendix A for the workshop agendas and speaker information); (2) release in January 2014 of the Framework document, which invited public feedback on a set of issues relevant to this report and is described in greater detail in the section below; (3) reviews of the scientific literature and commissioning of two papers on special topics—the de-identification of clinical trial data (see Appendix B) and drug regulation in selected developing countries[5]; and (4) personal communication between committee members and staff and individuals who have been directly involved in or have special knowledge of the issues under consideration.

Framework for Discussion and Public Feedback

In accordance with the study charge, the Framework was publicly released in January 2014. The Framework articulated the committee's preliminary observations on guiding principles for the responsible sharing of clinical trial data, a nomenclature for data sharing, and a description of a selected set of data sharing activities. The Framework did not contain conclusions or recommendations but rather served to elicit feedback from a variety of stakeholders to inform the second phase of this study and the conclusions and recommendations contained in this final report. The committee invited comments on a set of difficult issues that were likely to be complex and on which stakeholders were likely to have differing perspectives (see Appendix A).

In addition to the public release of the Framework, several medical journals—including the *New England Journal of Medicine*, the *British Medical Journal*, and the *Journal of the American Medical Association*—wrote editorials or otherwise published on the committee's work and encouraged their readership to send comments (Drazen, 2014; Kuehn, 2014; McCarthy, 2014). In response to these efforts, the committee received 85 written comments from a variety of individuals and organizations, including academic researchers from across the globe, industry representatives (pharmaceutical, device, and biologic from both individual companies and trade associations), clinicians and health care organizations, patient/ disease advocacy representatives, and others (a complete list of these individuals and organizations is provided in Appendix A). IOM staff collected and compiled all comments for the committee's review, calling particular attention to cross-cutting themes and unique perspectives.

---

[5] The commissioned paper "The Interaction Between Open Trial Data and Drug Regulation in Selected Developing Countries" was used by the committee in support of its analysis in this report. This paper is available on this report's website (www.iom.edu/datasharing).

Formulation and Applicability of the Committee's Recommendations

Sharing of clinical trial data is a relatively new and evolving field, with a limited evidence base in the scientific literature. Consequently, although the committee drew on the literature when possible, its conclusions and recommendations were formulated largely on the basis of knowledge gained through its extensive information gathering process, as described above, as well as its members' own expertise.

It is the committee's hope that the rationale for data sharing, the guiding principles, and the recommendations articulated in this report will apply to a broad range of current and future trials. Although much current discussion has focused on trials conducted by large pharmaceutical companies and publicly funded trials conducted in academic medical centers, the committee also considered, consistent with its charge,

- clinical trials involving educational interventions, quality improvement, behavioral interventions, and health care delivery modifications as well as drug trials;
- trials carried out in resource-poor settings, where unfunded mandates or expectations for data would be particularly burdensome; and
- clinical trials sponsored by small nonprofits and small companies without a revenue stream and investigator-initiated trials with no external funding, cases in which resources for data sharing will be very limited.

Additionally, as a result of advances in methods and technology, the way clinical trials are conducted is undergoing a major transformation (Munos, 2014), and clinical trials are likely to continue to change dramatically:

- Trials will increasingly collect patient-centered data directly from participants and from personal sensors, social media, and other digital information technologies (IOM, 2013a; Munos, 2014).
- Trials will progressively use electronic health records as data sources, for example, to assess simple clinical endpoints in large pragmatic trials (IOM, 2013a; Munos, 2014).
- Many trials will be embedded into clinical care. Examples include quality improvement and prevention trials, prompted optional randomized trials (PORTs) (e.g., trials using point-of-care randomization), and n-of-1 studies (Flory and Karlawish, 2012; Pletcher et al., 2014).
- Innovative clinical trial designs are increasingly being used, including adaptive designs (e.g., stepped wedge, PORTs).

- Also likely are more hybrid methodology trials (i.e., those that collect both quantitative and qualitative data).
- Citizen-scientists and patient advocacy groups will become active collaborators with traditional sponsors in designing and implementing clinical trials.

Policies regarding responsible sharing of clinical trial data will need to take these new developments into account. For example, data collected from clinical care and from personal devices and sensors will present additional opportunities for secondary research but also new challenges regarding consent and sharing of private and identifiable data. In its analyses and recommendations, the committee focused on present-day challenges and constraints while also attempting to account for such potential changes in the landscape in which clinical trials are conducted and in the attitudes of clinical trial investigators, sponsors, and the public toward data sharing, which cannot be fully anticipated.

ORGANIZATION OF THE REPORT

Following this introduction, Chapter 2 presents the major potential benefits and risks of sharing clinical trial data and the guiding principles set forth in the Framework document. Informed by these principles and the committee's consideration of the various sources of information detailed above, Chapters 3 through 5 address the "who, what, when, and how" of data sharing. Chapter 3 addresses the question of "who." It identifies the stakeholders in clinical trials, their roles and responsibilities with respect to the clinical trials enterprise, and the benefits and risks of data sharing from their perspectives. In this chapter, the committee recommends actions each stakeholder could take to help foster a culture in which data sharing is the expected norm. Chapter 4 articulates professional and community standards for "what" data should be shared and "when" in the clinical trials process. Chapter 5 addresses the question of "how" these data should be shared. It presents various approaches for controlling access to data, ranging from less to more restrictive, and explores their associated implications. Throughout Chapters 4 and 5, the committee delineates the salient benefits and risks associated with sharing different types of data at different timepoints and under various conditions; this discussion serves as the foundation for the committee's conclusions and recommendations in these two chapters. Finally, Chapter 6 presents a vision for data sharing based on the discussion in the preceding chapters and outlines remaining challenges that need to be addressed before this vision can be realized. This chapter offers the committee's recommendation for beginning to address these challenges and moving forward.

REFERENCES

AllTrials. 2013. *What does all trials registered and reported mean?* http://www.alltrials.net/find-out-more/all-trials (accessed October 14, 2014).

AllTrials. 2014. *Supporters.* http://www.alltrials.net/supporters (accessed October 14, 2014).

BIO (Biotechnology Industry Organization). 2014. *BIO principles on clinical trial data sharing.* http://www.bio.org/articles/bio-principles-clinical-trial-data-sharing (accessed October 14, 2014).

BMJ (*British Medical Journal*). 2013. *Open data.* http://www.bmj.com/open-data (accessed October 14, 2014).

Boulton, G., M. Rawlins, P. Vallance, and M. Walport. 2011. Science as a public enterprise: The case for open data. *Lancet* 377(9778):1633-1635.

ClinicalStudyDataRequest.com. 2014. *Home.* https://clinicalstudydatarequest.com/Default.aspx (accessed October 15, 2014).

ClinicalTrials.gov. 2012. *Glossary of common site terms.* http://clinicaltrials.gov/ct2/about-studies/glossary (accessed October 15, 2014).

De Angelis, C., J. M. Drazen, F. A. Frizelle, C. Haug, J. Hoey, R. Horton, S. Kotzin, C. Laine, A. Marusic, A. J. P. M. Overbeke, T. V. Schroeder, H. C. Sox, and M. B. Van Der Weyden. 2004. Clinical trial registration: A statement from the International Committee of Medical Journal Editors. *New England Journal of Medicine* 351(12):1250-1251.

Doshi, P., T. Jefferson, and C. Del Mar. 2012. The imperative to share clinical study reports: Recommendations from the Tamiflu experience. *PLoS Medicine* 9(4):e1001201.

Doshi, P., K. Dickersin, D. Healy, S. S. Vedula, and T. Jefferson. 2013a. Restoring invisible and abandoned trials: A call for people to publish the findings. *British Medical Journal* 346:f2865.

Doshi, P., S. N. Goodman, and J. P. A. Ioannidis. 2013b. Raw data from clinical trials: Within reach? *Trends in Pharmacological Sciences* 34(12):645-647.

Drazen, J. M. 2014. Open data. *New England Journal of Medicine* 370(7):662.

EMA (European Medicines Agency). 2014. *Release of data from clinical trials.* http://www.ema.europa.eu/ema/index.jsp?curl=pages/special_topics/general/general_content_000555.jsp&mid=WC0b01ac0580607bfa (accessed October 14, 2014).

FDA (U.S. Food and Drug Administration). 2010. *Transparency task force.* http://www.fda.gov/AboutFDA/Transparency/PublicDisclosure/TransparencyTaskForce/default.htm (accessed October 23, 2014).

Flory, J., and J. Karlawish. 2012. The prompted optional randomization trial: A new design for comparative effectiveness research. *American Journal of Public Health* 102(12):e8-e10.

FreeBIRD. 2014. *Welcome to FreeBIRD.* https://ctu-web.lshtm.ac.uk/freebird (accessed October 30, 2014).

Groves, T. 2009. Managing UK research data for future use. *British Medical Journal* 338(7697):729-730.

ImmPort (Immunology Database and Analysis Portal). 2013. *News and events.* https://immport.niaid.nih.gov/immportWeb/display.do?content=News (accessed October 14, 2014).

IOM (Institute of Medicine). 2013a. *Digital data improvement priorities for continuous learning in health and health care: Workshop summary.* Washington, DC: The National Academies Press.

IOM. 2013b. *Sharing clinical research data: Workshop summary.* Washington, DC: The National Academies Press.

Johnson & Johnson. 2014. *Johnson & Johnson announces clinical trial data sharing agreement with Yale School of Medicine.* http://www.jnj.com/news/all/johnson-and-johnson-announces-clinical-trial-data-sharing-agreement-with-yale-school-of-medicine (accessed October 15, 2014).

Kaye, J., L. Curren, N. Anderson, K. Edwards, S. M. Fullerton, N. Kanellopoulou, D. Lund, D. G. MacArthur, D. Mascalzoni, and J. Shepherd. 2012. From patients to partners: Participant-centric initiatives in biomedical research. *Nature Reviews Genetics* 13(5):371-376.

Krumholz, H. M., and J. S. Ross. 2011. A model for dissemination and independent analysis of industry data. *Journal of the American Medical Association* 306(14):1593-1594.

Kuehn, B. M. 2014. IOM outlines framework for clinical data sharing, solicits input. *Journal of the American Medical Association* 311(7):665.

Laine, C., S. N. Goodman, M. E. Griswold, and H. C. Sox. 2007. Reproducible research: Moving toward research the public can really trust. *Annals of Internal Medicine* 146(6):450-453.

Loder, E. 2013. Sharing data from clinical trials: Where we are and what lies ahead. *British Medical Journal* 347:f4794.

McCarthy, M. 2014. US committee calls for comments on how to share clinical trial data. *British Medical Journal* 348:g1135.

Mello, M. M., J. K. Francer, M. Wilenzick, P. Teden, B. E. Bierer, and M. Barnes. 2013. Preparing for responsible sharing of clinical trial data. *New England Journal of Medicine* 369(17):1651-1658.

Munos, B. 2014. *The future of clinical trials: Impacts for data-sharing.* Paper presented at IOM Committee on Strategies for Responsible Sharing of Clinical Trial Data: Meeting Four, May 5-7, Washington, DC.

NIH (U.S. National Institutes of Health). 2003. *Final NIH statement on sharing research data.* http://grants1.nih.gov/grants/guide/notice-files/NOT-OD-03-032.html (accessed October 14, 2014).

NIH. 2014. *NIH issues finalized policy on genomic data sharing.* http://www.nih.gov/news/health/aug2014/od-27.htm (accessed October 14, 2014).

Nisen, P., and F. Rockhold. 2013. Access to patient-level data from glaxosmithkline clinical trials. *New England Journal of Medicine* 369(5):475-478.

NRC (National Research Council) and IOM. 2011. *Toward precision medicine: Building a knowledge network for biomedical research and a new taxonomy of disease.* Washington, DC: The National Academies Press.

PatientsLikeMe. 2011. *Nature biotechnology paper details breakthrough in real world outcomes measurement.* https://www.patientslikeme.com/press/20110425/27-patientslikeme-social-network-refutes-published-clinical-trial-br-bri-nature-biotechnology-paper-details-breakthrough-in-real-world-outcomes-measurement-i- (accessed October 14, 2014).

PhRMA (Pharmaceutical Research and Manufacturers of America). 2013. *EFPIA and PhRMA release joint principles for responsible clinical trial data sharing to benefit patients.* http://www.phrma.org/press-release/EFPIA-and-phrma-release-joint-principles-for-responsible-clinical-trial-data-sharing-to-benefit-patients (accessed October 14, 2014).

Pletcher, M. J., B. Lo, and D. Grady. 2014. Informed consent in randomized quality improvement trials: A critical barrier for learning health systems. *JAMA Internal Medicine* 174(5):668-670.

Rathi, V., K. Dzara, C. P. Gross, I. Hrynaszkiewicz, S. Joffe, H. M. Krumholz, K. M. Strait, and J. S. Ross. 2012. Sharing of clinical trial data among trialists: A cross sectional survey. *British Medical Journal* 345:e7570.

Roehr, B. 2009. FDA creates task force to make its work more transparent. *British Medical Journal* 338:b2618.

Ross, J. S., R. Lehman, and C. P. Gross. 2012. The importance of clinical trial data sharing: Toward more open science. *Circulation: Cardiovascular Quality and Outcomes* 5(2):238-240.

Teden, P. 2013. *Types of clinical trial data to be shared*. Paper presented at IOM Committee on Strategies for Responsible Sharing of Clinical Trial Data: Meeting One, October 22-23, Washington, DC.

Terry, S. F., and P. F. Terry. 2011. Power to the people: Participant ownership of clinical trial data. *Science Translational Medicine* 3(69):69cm63.

Walport, M., and P. Brest. 2011. Sharing research data to improve public health. *Lancet* 377(9765):537-539.

The Wellcome Trust. 2011. *Sharing research data to improve public health: Full joint statement by funders of health research*. http://www.wellcome.ac.uk/About-us/Policy/Spotlight-issues/Data-sharing/Public-health-and-epidemiology/WTDV030690.htm (accessed October 14, 2014).

Wicks, P., T. E. Vaughan, M. P. Massagli, and J. Heywood. 2011. Accelerated clinical discovery using self-reported patient data collected online and a patient-matching algorithm. *Nature Biotechnology* 29(5):411-414.

Wicks, P., T. Vaughan, and J. Heywood. 2014. Subjects no more: What happens when trial participants realize they hold the power? *British Medical Journal* 348:g3383.

YODA (Yale University Open Data Access) Project. 2013. *Medtronic/rhBMP-2*. http://medicine.yale.edu/core/projects/yodap/datasharing/medtronic/index.aspx (accessed October 14, 2014).

YODA Project. 2014. *Welcome to the YODA Project*. http://yoda.yale.edu/welcome-yoda-project (accessed October 15, 2014).

Zarin, D. A. 2007. Issues in the registration of clinical trials. *Journal of the American Medical Association* 297(19):2112-2120.

Zarin, D. A. 2011. *Overview of ClinicalTrials.gov reporting requirements*. Paper presented at Secretary's Advisory Committee on Human Research Protections (SACHRP) Meeting, March 8-9, Rockville, MD.

Zarin, D. A. 2013. Participant-level data and the new frontier in trial transparency. *New England Journal of Medicine* 369(5):468-469.

2

Guiding Principles for Sharing Clinical Trial Data

This chapter provides an overview of the key potential benefits and risks of data sharing and sets forth the guiding principles (as evolved from the Framework document; see Box 2-1) that informed the committee's thinking as it considered the issues presented throughout the remainder of this report. These principles served as a lens through which the committee weighed the benefits and risks of data sharing and considered the roles and responsibilities of individuals and organizations that participate in and benefit from the clinical trials enterprise. Additionally, this chapter describes the committee's approach for applying these principles to develop the conclusions and recommendations offered in the following chapters.

OVERVIEW OF KEY POTENTIAL BENEFITS AND RISKS

Potential Benefits of Data Sharing

Sharing of clinical trial data has great potential to accelerate scientific progress and ultimately improve public health by generating better evidence on the safety and effectiveness of therapies for patients. There have been some notable examples of how secondary analyses of shared data have benefited the public, for example, by showing that widely used interventions are ineffective or unsafe (Chan et al., 2014; Doshi et al., 2012; Kaiser et al., 2003; Nissen and Wolski, 2007) or by improving clinical care (Farrar et al., 2014; Gabler et al., 2012a,b; Ventetuolo et al., 2014a,b).

BOX 2-1
Evolution of Guiding Principles from the Framework Document

In the Framework document, released in January 2014, the committee set forth guiding principles that underpin responsible sharing of clinical trial data and posed a question to help direct its thinking for this final report: To whom do the benefits of clinical trial data belong? As detailed in Chapter 1, the Framework document encouraged the public and interested stakeholders to submit written comments, and the committee gathered further commentary through its public workshops. This chapter incorporates the insights and knowledge the committee gained over the course of the study and updates the guiding principles and approach to their application accordingly. The committee did not delete or add any principles after the Framework was released but did revise the supporting text to better align with this new understanding.

From the perspective of clinical trial participants, data sharing increases their contributions to generalizable knowledge about human health by potentially facilitating additional findings beyond the original, prespecified clinical trial outcomes. Conversely, if data are not shared, opportunities to generate additional knowledge from participants' contributions are missed (Califf, 2013; Collyar, 2013; Hamblett, 2013; IOM, 2013; Mello et al., 2013; Terry and Terry, 2011).

From the perspective of society as a whole, sharing of data from clinical trials could provide a more comprehensive picture of the benefits and risks of an intervention and allow health care professionals and patients to make more informed decisions about clinical care. Moreover, sharing clinical trial data could potentially lead to enhanced efficiency and safety of the clinical research process by, for example, reducing unnecessary duplication of effort and the costs of future studies, reducing exposure of participants in future trials to avoidable harms identified through the data sharing, and providing a deeper knowledge base for regulatory decisions (Califf, 2013; Doshi et al., 2013; Eichler et al., 2012; Goldacre, 2013; IOM, 2013; Krumholz et al., 2014; Mello et al., 2013; Ross et al., 2012).

In the long run, sharing clinical trial data could potentially improve public health and patient outcomes, reduce the incidence of adverse effects from therapies, and decrease expenditures for medical interventions that are ineffective or less effective than alternatives. In addition, data sharing could open up opportunities for exploratory research that might lead to new hypotheses about the mechanisms of disease, more effective therapies, or alternative uses of existing or abandoned therapies that could then be tested in additional research (Califf, 2013; IOM, 2013;

Mello et al., 2013; Zarin, 2013). The risks of not sharing are inverse to these benefits and include unnecessary duplication of trials, which unduly exposes additional participants to experimentation; increased unwillingness of individuals to participate in clinical trials if the data resulting from those trials are withheld; bias in the body of evidence; and the inability of investigators to build on previous work, thereby slowing progress in understanding of human health.

Risks of Data Sharing

The potential benefits of sharing clinical trial data and the risks of not sharing need to be weighed against any potential harms from sharing.

First, data sharing could put clinical trial participants at increased risk of invasions of privacy or breaches of confidentiality. As a result, participants could suffer social or economic harms (IOM, 2013; Malin, 2014; Mello et al., 2013).[1]

Data sharing also could result in potential harms to society. For example, shared clinical trial data might be analyzed in a manner that would lead to distorted effect estimates or incorrect conclusions (although this could also occur with the original analyses) (Krumholz and Ross, 2011). For example, if multiple secondary analyses are carried out in an attempt to establish serious adverse effects but statistical analyses do not take these multiple analyses into account, some apparent adverse effects may be identified on the basis of chance alone. A potential consequence is that invalid analyses will lead to claims of risk that are not scientifically valid, which may in turn lead to lawsuits for negligence that, while without merit, are expensive to respond to and defend against.[2] If spurious claims of risk are publicized in the lay media, they may be difficult to refute even if they are disproved in peer-reviewed articles. Such claims may harm the public by deterring appropriate use of beneficial therapies. Furthermore, investigators may find it highly burdensome in terms of time and effort to respond to invalid secondary analyses, as the investigators in the PLATO (Platelet Inhibition and Patient Outcomes) trial have documented (Wallentin et al., 2014). To further complicate matters, such invalid analyses may result not only from inadvertent errors in data analysis but also from conflicts of interest, including, in the United States, the prospect of monetary gain through *qui tam* lawsuits. Incorrect conclu-

---

[1] This section draws on a paper commissioned by the Committee on Strategies for Responsible Sharing of Clinical Trial Data on "Concepts and Methods for De-identifying Clinical Trials Data," by Khaled El Emam and Bradley Malin (see Appendix B).

[2] Personal communication, Virtual WebEx Open Session, G. Fleming, to Committee on Strategies for Responsible Sharing of Clinical Trial Data, Institute of Medicine, regarding clinical trial data sharing: product liability, April 9, 2014.

sions or treatment recommendations for either whole patient populations or subgroups could produce suboptimal care, avoidable adverse effects, and unnecessary anxiety and result in possible discrimination (IOM, 2013; Spertus, 2012). Concerns about such future uses of their clinical trial data might also deter some individuals and/or communities from participating in future clinical trials (IOM, 2013).

The manner in which data are shared might undermine the incentives of clinical trial sponsors, clinical investigators, researchers, and other essential stakeholders to invest their time and resources in the development and clinical testing of potential new treatment practices (Dickersin, 2013; Rathi et al., 2012). For example, data sharing might allow confidential commercial information to be discerned from the data (EMA, 2014; Teden, 2013).[3] Competitors might use shared data to seek regulatory approval for competing products in countries that do not recognize data exclusivity periods or do not grant patents for certain types of research (Kapczynski, 2014). The manner in which clinical trial data are shared also might harm the intellectual capital and professional recognition of academic clinical investigators who devote considerable effort and time to designing a clinical trial, recruiting and retaining participants, and collecting the primary data. If subsequent independent analyses failed to give appropriate recognition to the original investigators, those investigators would not have incentives to conduct clinical trials in the future.

GUIDING PRINCIPLES

The committee offers the following guiding principles as an essential foundation for any approach to sharing clinical trial data.

Maximize the Benefits of Clinical Trials While Minimizing the Risks of Sharing Clinical Trial Data

Understanding and balancing the benefits and risks of health interventions is an essential component of health care, clinical research, and the development of therapies. Similarly, sharing clinical trial data entails potential benefits and harms, as outlined above. Strategies for data sharing should maximize the benefits of sharing to those who give of themselves to participate and to society as a whole while minimizing the potential harms for all stakeholders. This guiding principle for responsible sharing of clinical trial data is derived from the ethical concept of beneficence.

---

[3] E-mail communication, Advanced Medical Technology Association (AdvaMed), to A. Claiborne, Institute of Medicine, regarding strategies for responsible sharing of clinical trial data, March 21, 2014.

The International Conference on Harmonisation's (ICH's) Guideline for Good Clinical Practice (GCP) declares: "Before a trial is initiated, foreseeable risks and inconveniences should be weighed against the anticipated benefit for the individual trial subject and society. A trial should be initiated and continued only if the anticipated benefits justify the risks," and "the rights, safety, and well-being of the trial subjects are the most important considerations and should prevail over interests of science and society" (ICH, 1996). Likewise, the U.S. Belmont Report articulates beneficence as a basic ethical principle and obligation of research involving human subjects. With respect to persons involved in clinical trials, beneficent actions "(1) do not harm and (2) maximize possible benefits and minimize possible harms" (National Commission for the Protection of Human Subjects of Biomedical and Behavioral Research, 1979, p. 6). Benefits include both the immediate knowledge gained from testing the hypothesis of a particular clinical trial and the broader utility of the study data in informing the development of effective and safe clinical care. As discussed in the Belmont Report, practitioners are faced with deciding "when it is justifiable to seek certain benefits despite the risks involved" (National Commission for the Protection of Human Subjects of Biomedical and Behavioral Research, 1979, p. 7). The potential utility of data should be factored into the balance of potential benefits and risks in making the decision whether to expose individual clinical trial participants to risk in order to seek benefits to society as a whole.

Internationally, the right "to share in scientific advancement and its benefits" and "to the protection of the moral and material interests resulting from any scientific . . . production of which [a person] is the author" are both recognized in the 1948 United Nations Universal Declaration of Human Rights.[4] Of particular importance is that rights can be framed as positive access to the fruits of scientific research (Knoppers et al., 2014) as well as negative rights to privacy and antidiscrimination. The right of patients and the public to the benefits of scientific research is an alternative way of framing the idea that responsible sharing of clinical trial data should be guided by the goal of increasing scientific knowledge that leads to better therapies for patients (Knoppers et al., 2014).

Respect Individual Participants Whose Data Are Shared

The committee's second guiding principle stems from the broadly articulated concept that respect for research participants is a fundamental principle of research ethics (ICH, 1996; National Commission for the Protection of Human Subjects of Biomedical and Behavioral Research, 1979).

---

[4] *Universal Declaration of Human Rights*, G.A. res. 217A (III), U.N. Doc A/810 (1948).

"Respect for research participants" is a term used to describe a bundle of obligations that researchers owe to clinical trial participants. This bundle is commonly understood to include informed consent to participate in a trial and protection of privacy and confidentiality; the committee adds to these components participant engagement throughout a research project.

Clinical trials are designed and carried out to answer research questions about the safety and efficacy of specific health interventions. The interventions that participants receive are determined by the study protocol, not by what their personal physicians consider best for them as individuals. In consenting to participate, clinical trial participants also accept that complying with the study protocol potentially entails inconvenience and risks (Lidz et al., 2004). Although participation in clinical trials, on the whole, may not be significantly more risky than ordinary clinical care or receiving the study intervention outside of the trial (Gross et al., 2006), the benefits and risks of the study arms in a specific trial are not known at the outset. In some instances, the intervention arm of a trial will be shown to have significantly worse outcomes than the control arm, a finding that cannot be predicted at the time of enrollment.

Respect Through Protections for Research Participants

Respect for research participants requires protecting their dignity, integrity, and right to self-determination; this includes, at a minimum, compliance with applicable regulations and ethical standards for the conduct of clinical trials and handling of the resulting data. Respect for research participants has historically been understood to require specific informed consent from participants (including consent for how their data will be used) before they enroll in a clinical trial in which the intervention will be carried out at the individual participant level (Childress et al., 2005; CIOMS, 2002; WMA, 2013).[5] In addition, it could be argued that respect for clinical trial participants requires a broader concept of sharing information with participants and obtaining their ongoing consent or concurrence throughout the trial. For example, clinical trial staff might educate participants about the condition being studied, provide more information about study interventions over the course of the trial, and offer additional opportunities for participants to learn more. In addition, respect for participants might require that clinical trialists offer to inform participants of the overall results of the trial, in language that they can understand (Brealey et al., 2010; Fernandez et al., 2003, 2009); studies

---

[5] Specific informed consent is not necessarily required for trials at the group level, such as certain cluster randomized trials (Weijer and Emanuel, 2000), or for certain comparative effectiveness trials (Faden et al., 2013).

indicate that this information is desired by most clinical trial participants. Respect for participants also requires that professional staff in a clinical trial prevent serious and imminent harms that they are uniquely situated to identify and prevent (NRC, 2005).

For existing trials, data sharing (particularly sharing beyond other investigators in the trial) may not have been discussed explicitly with participants during the consent process. Sharing of data without specific participant consent may be ethically acceptable and legally permitted in certain instances. If the shared data are anonymized, for example, current U.S. federal regulations on human research protections and U.S. health information privacy regulations (e.g., the Health Insurance Portability and Accountability Act [HIPAA])[6] allow other researchers to use the data for research under certain conditions without consent from the original participants.[7]

Respect also suggests a need to protect the confidentiality and privacy of trial participants when data are shared. For example, additional protections may be needed when participant identifiers cannot be removed from data or must be included in shared data in order to address an important research question.

Respect Through Engagement

Respect also can be demonstrated and advanced through efforts to engage participants and their representatives in the development of the processes for sharing of clinical trial data, so as to build public trust in the value and importance of data sharing (CTSA, 2011). It is important to remember that individuals participating in clinical trials come from cultures and communities around the world in which power may be unequally and perhaps unfairly distributed (NRC, 2005). Representatives of communities and groups from which clinical trial participants are recruited can provide insight into the cultural and societal values and concerns pertinent to sharing of clinical trial data. Proactive input and feedback on plans for sharing clinical trial data can be obtained from representatives of research participants, disease advocacy groups, community advisory boards, and the public (Jiang et al., 2013). Such engagement also can help sponsors and investigators explain the rationale for data sharing to participants and the public in an accessible and understand-

---

[6] Health Insurance Portability and Accountability Act of 1996, Public Law 104-191, 104th Cong. (August 21, 1996).

[7] The U.S. example has been described here for illustrative purposes. The European Union also has strong data privacy protections that must be observed when clinical trial data are shared by its member states (European Commission, 2013).

able manner. The act of seeking and obtaining such input does not in itself constitute surrogate consent or authorization for data sharing. Rather, it demonstrates respect for participants by actively soliciting their concerns about data sharing, identifying its unappreciated benefits and risks that were not previously taken into account, and allowing participants or their advocates to suggest how the data sharing process might be improved (Stiles and Petrila, 2011).

Increase Public Trust in Clinical Trials and the Sharing of Trial Data

Public trust is an intrinsic value undergirding the biomedical science and health research enterprise, which is fundamentally aimed at improving human health. At a more instrumental level, trust also is essential for ensuring continued public support for clinical research and for fostering participation in clinical trials. The concept of public trust in clinical trials encompasses trust both in the scientific process of generating the data (i.e., that there is accountability for how the trials are carried out) and in the validity of the trials (i.e., that the reported findings are an accurate representation of the underlying data) (IOM, 2013). Sharing of clinical trial data could either enhance or reduce public trust in clinical research. The process used for data sharing should therefore be undertaken in a manner that enhances public trust in both the clinical trial process and the data sharing process.

Trust in Clinical Trial Data

By increasing the transparency of how a trial was designed and carried out and of the pathway to the conclusions derived from the trial, sharing of clinical trial data could increase public trust in the outcomes of that particular trial and of trials generally (Loder, 2013). Data sharing also could increase the usefulness and trustworthiness of clinical trial data and analyses of the data because clinical researchers who know that others will be using their data may be more thorough and more careful in their methodology and its documentation. Such additional attention to detail could also help reduce bias in the data and findings (Mello et al., 2013).

Sharing clinical trial data could enhance public trust by facilitating secondary analyses that could determine whether the final conclusions and summaries of clinical trials are robust, valid inferences from the original evidence, although this must be done in a credible and fair manner (Laine et al., 2007). Whether the inferences drawn from a particular trial are strong or called into question, efforts to demonstrate the widespread applicability of the study findings could enhance overall trust in the scientific process and result in more evidence-based recommendations for clinical care.

Trust in clinical research could further be enhanced if sharing of clinical trial data were accompanied by public outreach and engagement to help the public understand that numerous judgments are needed to transform source data into analyzable data (CTSA, 2011), and that highly trained researchers may take different approaches to answering a research question or to analyzing a given data set. Discrepancies in researchers' analytical approaches and interpretations are an expected part of scientific processes and discussions. Such outreach also could help the public better understand that findings from early clinical trials (i.e., phase I and early phase II trials) often are not definitive and that attempts to reproduce original analyses or to conduct meta-analyses using pooled data from multiple clinical trials can strengthen, modify, refute, or extend the original reports from a trial.

Trust in the Data Sharing Process

Sharing clinical trial data could carry the risk of undermining public trust in clinical trials under certain circumstances, for example, if multiple analyses were to yield conflicting conclusions (Califf, 2013). Public trust in clinical trials whose data are shared could be undermined unless the processes for sharing the data are clear, transparent, and accountable. To this end, established criteria for sharing clinical trial data, procedures for fairly adjudicating requests for data against those criteria, and accountability for both data holders and requesters in adhering to those standards are necessary. Clear, transparent, and accountable processes for data sharing also must include protection of participant privacy and respectful handling of individual participant data.

Sharing of clinical trial data should be carried out in such a manner that it does not repeat, in the data sharing context, well-documented historical examples of imposing disproportionate risks of clinical research on vulnerable groups and thereby undermining the trust of those groups in the overall clinical trial process (Bioethics Commission, 2011; Emanuel et al., 2008; Jones, 2008; Wertheimer, 2008). For example, data sharing ought to include protections for participant subgroups that are particularly vulnerable to breaches of confidentiality or other adverse consequences of data sharing. Clinical trial participants may be particularly vulnerable to harm if they have conditions, or are members of groups, that are commonly stigmatized (Bioethics Commission, 2011; Emanuel et al., 2008; Jones, 2008). In this regard, there may be justifiable and ethical reasons for handling some types of clinical trial data differently with respect to sharing so as to reduce the potential for unfair treatment of participants. For example, whole genome sequencing data could be identifiable (Gymrek et al., 2013) and might be viewed as putting participants at heightened risk and warranting additional safeguards or protections for participants whose genomic data could be shared. As another example, persons with mental illness, communicable diseases such as HIV infection, injection drug use, and other conditions suffer severe stigma and discrimination in some communities and societies (Bierer et al., 2013; Emanuel et al., 2008).

Further, public trust could be increased if the public saw evidence that their perspectives had been incorporated into the data sharing process (whether by employing the mechanisms described above or by addressing specific community concerns). If analyses of shared data used methods and statistics that were not scientifically valid and led to biased conclusions, they could inappropriately undermine patient trust in valid conclusions about the trial intervention. Such mistrust could ultimately lead to seriously flawed clinical care decisions, unwarranted patient concerns about the quality of care, or avoidable patient anxiety.

Conduct the Sharing of Clinical Trial Data in a Fair Manner

Fairness, broadly articulated, is a core ethical principle that is applicable to the sharing of clinical trial data. In general terms, fairness entails persons receiving what is due to them or what they deserve (Beauchamp and Childress, 2009). Fairness requires similar treatment of people (whether as individuals or as part of groups, entities, processes, etc.) unless there are justifiable reasons to treat them differently. Where disagreements arise is in specifying what an individual or group is due or deserves, identifying sufficient reasons for differential treatment under what might be perceived by some as similar circumstances, and determining whether inequity (i.e., unfairness, unethical conduct) has occurred. Participants, sponsors, and investigators, in particular, have a stake in the fairness of data sharing.

Clinical trial participants could perceive fairness as including equitable distribution of the benefits of clinical research across different groups of participants and different communities. Pooling of shared data from several clinical trials could, for example, benefit groups that have been enrolled in clinical trials in such small numbers that the statistical power to draw valid inferences about risks and benefits for them in any single trial is limited. Among the underserved groups for whom data sharing might accelerate research are individuals with rare conditions or rare subtypes of common conditions and members of certain ethnic groups that historically have had low enrollment in clinical trials. Underrepresentation of these groups in clinical trials can lead to a weaker evidence base for clinical care decisions, as well as health disparities and discrimination (IOM, 2002).

Clinical trial sponsors and investigators who design and carry out clinical trials might believe that fairness includes appropriate recognition and reward for their work and protection of their legitimate interests. Investigators who make substantial investments of intellectual capital, time, and resources in a trial have an interest in carrying out additional analyses of the data they have collected and in receiving due credit when other researchers take advantage of those data. Sponsors that bring a new therapy to market have an interest in competitors not using shared data to gain an unfair competitive advantage or as the sole means of obtaining licensing in other countries without carrying out any original clinical studies. Appropriate protection of these interests could help provide incentives (or reduce disincentives) to share data and to conduct future clinical trials.

THE COMMITTEE'S APPROACH TO APPLYING THE PRINCIPLES

The committee next considered its approach for practical application of the above principles to the issues entailed in sharing clinical trial data. If each principle were to be given equal weight, many issues would be unresolvable, as the principles would be in conflict. For example, the principle of maximizing benefits to society could conflict with the principle of respecting participants in addressing the issue of whether participants should be given the opportunity to opt out of data sharing in the consent process. Therefore, the committee needed to develop a practical approach for weighing the principles, particularly in cases in which two or more are in tension.

To develop this approach, the committee returned to the original question posed in the Framework document: "To whom do the benefits of clinical trial data belong?" Note that this is a separate question from who has ownership of the data (described in Box 2-2). The benefits of clinical trial data could be regarded as belonging primarily to the public: the data benefit patients and the public through the advancement of science and clinical knowledge that leads to improved patient care. From this perspective, some might argue that sharing clinical trial data ought to be a prima facie obligation. That is, the default policy—the presumption—should be sharing, with justification needed to restrict or recognize an exception to sharing.

On the other hand, the benefits of clinical trial data could be regarded as belonging primarily to the organizations and individuals who invested resources and time to plan and carry out the clinical trial and analyze the data. The rationale here could be providing fair rewards for investment and work, or it could be instrumental: new tests and therapies would not be developed if organizations and individuals lacked appropriate incen-

---

BOX 2-2
Ownership of Clinical Trial Data

With respect to ownership of clinical trial data, academic institutions that receive research grants might claim ownership over the data collected during the research in order to comply with regulatory requirements (Drazen, 2002). Private funders of clinical trials might claim they own the resulting data, particularly if the data will form part of a submission to the U.S. Food and Drug Administration (FDA) for regulatory approval. The language of research grants and contracts and the wording of informed consent forms signed by participants in clinical trials also could delineate ownership or disposition of the data. For example, the U.S. National Institutes of Health (NIH) includes data sharing requirements in the terms and conditions of research grants (NIH, 2003).

It is also important to note that the owner of property does not always have absolute dominion over it; others may have legal access to it under certain conditions for certain purposes. Moreover, property may be taken for public use without consent of the owner, subject to constitutional requirements for due process and fair compensation (Evans, 2011). Ultimately, the question of who owns the data is less important than the question of the rights and responsibilities of data holders.

---

tives to do so. From this perspective, the policy presumption could be that sharing of clinical trial data should be undertaken only if those who carried out the trial are appropriately incentivized and their interests and rights are protected. Some might argue that sharing of clinical trial data should be optional and voluntary, at the discretion of the organization and individuals who invested resources and time in conducting the trial.

The committee's position is that the benefits of data sharing belong primarily to the public in the form of valid scientific knowledge and improvement of clinical practice and public health. However, these benefits are not necessarily best attained by full open transparency. Rather, transparency is a means to these goals of scientific knowledge and improvements in clinical care and public health, not a goal in and of itself (Schauer, 2011). The legitimate interests of stakeholders—particularly their concerns about the potential risks and costs of data sharing—need to be recognized and addressed in a fair manner. If full open transparency of clinical trial data carries on balance more risks than benefits, it does not serve the public good.

Rather, the public good is served by policies that seek to attain the benefits of data sharing to advance science and improve clinical care while mitigating its risks to stakeholders.

Finally, the committee was mindful that its estimation of the balance of benefits and risks will likely change over time. As discussed in

Chapter 1, the clinical trial ecosystem—the methods and technologies for conducting and reporting trials; the expectations of participants and the public for increased involvement and transparency; and the attitudes of clinical trial investigators, sponsors, and funders toward sharing clinical trial data—is rapidly evolving. Consideration of the benefits and risks of data sharing needs to be forward looking and take into account not only the risks of sharing but also the potential harms of not sharing in this changing environment.

REFERENCES

Beauchamp, T. L., and J. F. Childress. 2009. *Principles of biomedical ethics*. 6th ed. New York: Oxford University Press.

Bierer, B. E., R. Li, M. Barnes, and J. S. Scott. 2013. Submission of comments on "Policy 0070 on publication and access to clinical-trial data" to IOM Committee on Strategies for Responsible Sharing of Clinical Trial Data, October 23, Washington, DC.

Bioethics Commission. 2011. *"Ethically impossible" STD research in Guatemala from 1946 to 1948*. http://bioethics.gov/node/654 (accessed October 15, 2014).

Brealey, S., L. Andronis, L. Dennis, C. Atwell, S. Bryan, S. Coulton, H. Cox, B. Cross, F. Fylan, A. Garratt, F. Gilbert, M. Gillan, M. Hendry, K. Hood, H. Houston, D. King, V. Morton, M. Robling, I. Russell, and C. Wilkinson. 2010. Participants' preference for type of leaflet used to feed back the results of a randomised trial: A survey. *Trials* 11:116.

Califf, R. M. 2013. *Clinical trial data sharing and challenges to data sharing: Current and future*. Paper presented at IOM Committee on Strategies for Responsible Sharing of Clinical Trial Data: Meeting One, October 22-23, Washington, DC.

Chan, A. W., F. Song, A. Vickers, T. Jefferson, K. Dickersin, P. C. Gøtzsche, H. M. Krumholz, D. Ghersi, and H. B. van der Worp. 2014. Increasing value and reducing waste: Addressing inaccessible research. *Lancet* 383(9913):257-266.

Childress, J. F., E. M. Meslin, and H. T. Shapiro. 2005. *Belmont revisited: Ethical principles for research with human subjects*. Washington, DC: Georgetown University Press.

CIOMS (Council for International Organizations of Medical Sciences). 2002. *International ethical guidelines for biomedical research involving human subjects*. Geneva: CIOMS.

Collyar, D. 2013. *What patients want from clinical trials—results from data!* Paper presented at IOM Committee on Strategies for Responsible Sharing of Clinical Trial Data: Meeting One, October 22-23, Washington, DC.

CTSA (Clinical & Translational® Science Awards). 2011. *Principles of community engagement*. 2nd ed. Washington, DC: NIH.

Dickersin, K. 2013. *Principles of responsible data sharing*. Paper presented at IOM Committee on Strategies for Responsible Sharing of Clinical Trial Data: Meeting One, October 22-23, Washington, DC.

Doshi, P., T. Jefferson, and C. Del Mar. 2012. The imperative to share clinical study reports: Recommendations from the Tamiflu experience. *PLoS Medicine* 9(4):e1001201.

Doshi, P., K. Dickersin, D. Healy, S. S. Vedula, and T. Jefferson. 2013. Restoring invisible and abandoned trials: A call for people to publish the findings. *British Medical Journal* 346:f2865.

Drazen, J. M. 2002. Who owns the data in clinical trial? *Science and Engineering Ethics* 8(3):407-411.

Eichler, H. G., E. Abadie, A. Breckenridge, H. Leufkens, and G. Rasi. 2012. Open clinical trial data for all? A view from regulators. *PLoS Medicine* 9(4):e1001202.

EMA (European Medicines Agency). 2014. *Redaction principles.* http://www.google.com/ url?sa=t&rct=j&q=&esrc=s&frm=1&source=web&cd=2&ved=0CCgQFjAB&url=h ttp%3A%2F%2Fwww.ombudsman.europa.eu%2FshowResource%3FresourceId% 3D1402406006491_INC2014-003908_2_Redaction%2520principles%2520DRAFT.pdf% 26type%3Dpdf%26download%3Dtrue%26lang%3Den&ei=Qj9OVKPOO8uxyATzl4K YBw&usg=AFQjCNHYKYQJ1X47URHVduc2cr7gutNEEQ&bvm=bv.77880786,d.aWw (accessed October 27, 2014).

Emanuel, E. J., D. Wendler, and C. Grady. 2008. An ethical framework for biomedical research. In *The Oxford textbook of research ethics*, edited by E. J. Emanuel, C. Grady, R. A. Crouch, R. K. Lie, F. G. Miller and D. Wendler. New York: Oxford University Press. Pp. 123-135.

European Commission. 2013. *Protection of personal data.* http://ec.europa.eu/justice/data-protection (accessed October 15, 2014).

Evans, B. J. 2011. Much ado about data ownership. *Harvard Journal of Law and Technology* 25. http://jolt.law.harvard.edu/articles/pdf/v25/25HarvJLTech69.pdf (accessed October 15, 2014).

Faden, R., N. Kass, D. Whicher, W. Stewart, and S. Tunis. 2013. Ethics and informed consent for comparative effectiveness research with prospective electronic clinical data. *Medical Care* 51(8, Suppl. 3):S53-S57.

Farrar, J. T., A. B. Troxel, K. Haynes, I. Gilron, R. D. Kerns, N. P. Katz, B. A. Rappaport, M. C. Rowbotham, A. M. Tierney, D. C. Turk, and R. H. Dworkin. 2014. Effect of variability in the 7-day baseline pain diary on the assay sensitivity of neuropathic pain randomized clinical trials: An action study. *Pain* 155(8):1622-1631.

Fernandez, C. V., E. Kodish, and C. Weijer. 2003. Informing study participants of research results: An ethical imperative. *IRB: Ethics and Human Research* 25(3):12-19.

Fernandez, C. V., J. Gao, C. Strahlendorf, A. Moghrabi, R. D. Pentz, R. C. Barfield, J. N. Baker, D. Santor, C. Weijer, and E. Kodish. 2009. Providing research results to participants: Attitudes and needs of adolescents and parents of children with cancer. *Journal of Clinical Oncology* 27(6):878-883.

Gabler, N. B., B. French, B. L. Strom, Z. Liu, H. I. Palevsky, D. B. Taichman, S. M. Kawut, and S. D. Halpern. 2012a. Race and sex differences in response to endothelin receptor antagonists for pulmonary arterial hypertension. *Chest* 141(1):20-26.

Gabler, N. B., B. French, B. L. Strom, H. I. Palevsky, D. B. Taichman, S. M. Kawut, and S. D. Halpern. 2012b. Validation of 6-minute walk distance as a surrogate end point in pulmonary arterial hypertension trials. *Circulation* 126(3):349-356.

Goldacre, B. 2013. My comments to IOM on IPD sharing. In *bengoldacre: passing thoughts.* http://bengoldacre.tumblr.com/post/64880190003/my-comments-to-iom-on-ipd-sharing (accessed December 16, 2014).

Gross, C. P., H. M. Krumholz, G. Van Wye, E. J. Emanuel, and D. Wendler. 2006. Does random treatment assignment cause harm to research participants? *PLoS Medicine* 3(6):e188.

Gymrek, M., A. L. McGuire, D. Golan, E. Halperin, and Y. Erlich. 2013. Identifying personal genomes by surname inference. *Science* 339(6117):321-324.

Hamblett, N. 2013. *Study sponsor perspectives: Cystic Fibrosis Therapeutics Development Network—Seattle Children's Hospital.* Paper presented at IOM Committee on Strategies for Responsible Sharing of Clinical Trial Data: Meeting One, October 22-23, Washington, DC.

ICH (International Conference on Harmonisation of Technical Requirements for Registration of Pharmaceuticals for Human Use). 1996. *Guideline for good clinical practice E6(R1).* http://www.ich.org/fileadmin/Public_Web_Site/ICH_Products/Guidelines/ Efficacy/E6/E6_R1_Guideline.pdf (accessed December 16, 2014).

IOM (Institute of Medicine). 2002. *Unequal treatment: Confronting racial and ethnic disparities in health care.* Washington, DC: National Academy Press.

IOM. 2013. *Sharing clinical research data: Workshop summary*. Washington, DC: The National Academies Press.

Jiang, X., A. D. Sarwate, and L. Ohno-Machado. 2013. Privacy technology to support data sharing for comparative effectiveness research: A systematic review. *Medical Care* 51(8):S58-S65.

Jones, J. H. 2008. Tuskegee syphilis experiment. In *The Oxford textbook of clinical research ethics*, edited by E. J. Emanuel, C. Grady, R. A. Crouch, R. K. Lie, F. G. Miller, and D. Wendler. New York: Oxford University Press. Pp. 86-96.

Kaiser, L., C. Wat, T. Mills, P. Mahoney, P. Ward, and F. Hayden. 2003. Impact of oseltamivir treatment on influenza-related lower respiratory tract complications and hospitalizations. *Archives of Internal Medicine* 163(14):1667-1672.

Kapczynski, A. 2014. *The interaction between open trial data and drug regulation in selected developing countries*. Paper commissioned by the Committee on Strategies for Responsible Sharing of Clinical Trial Data. www.iom.edu/datasharing (accessed December 19, 2014).

Knoppers, B. M., J. R. Harris, I. Budin-Ljosne, and E. S. Dove. 2014. A human rights approach to an international code of conduct for genomic and clinical data sharing. *Human Genetics* 133(7):895-903.

Krumholz, H. M., and J. S. Ross. 2011. A model for dissemination and independent analysis of industry data. *Journal of the American Medical Association* 306(14):1593-1594.

Krumholz, H. M., C. P. Gross, K. L. Blount, J. D. Ritchie, B. Hodshon, R. Lehman, and J. S. Ross. 2014. Sea change in open science and data sharing: Leadership by industry. *Circulation: Cardiovascular Quality and Outcomes* 7(4):499-504.

Laine, C., S. N. Goodman, M. E. Griswold, and H. C. Sox. 2007. Reproducible research: Moving toward research the public can really trust. *Annals of Internal Medicine* 146(6):450-453.

Lidz, C. W., P. S. Appelbaum, T. Grisso, and M. Renaud. 2004. Therapeutic misconception and the appreciation of risks in clinical trials. *Social Science & Medicine* 58(9):1689-1697.

Loder, E. 2013. Sharing data from clinical trials: Where we are and what lies ahead. *British Medical Journal* 347:f4794.

Malin, B. 2014. *De-identification and clinical trials data: Oh the possibilities!* Paper presented at IOM Committee on Strategies for Responsible Sharing of Clinical Trial Data: Meeting Two, February 3-4, Washington, DC.

Mello, M. M., J. K. Francer, M. Wilenzick, P. Teden, B. E. Bierer, and M. Barnes. 2013. Preparing for responsible sharing of clinical trial data. *New England Journal of Medicine* 369(17):1651-1658.

National Commission for the Protection of Human Subjects of Biomedical and Behavioral Research. 1979. *The Belmont Report: Ethical principles and guidelines for the protection of human subjects of research*. Washington, DC: HHS.

NIH (U.S. National Institutes of Health). 2003. *Final NIH statement on sharing research data*. http://grants1.nih.gov/grants/guide/notice-files/NOT-OD-03-032.html (accessed October 14, 2014).

Nissen, S. E., and K. Wolski. 2007. Effect of rosiglitazone on the risk of myocardial infarction and death from cardiovascular causes. *New England Journal of Medicine* 356(24):2457-2471.

NRC (National Research Council). 2005. *Ethical considerations for research on housing-related health hazards involving children*. Washington, DC: The National Academies Press.

Rathi, V., K. Dzara, C. P. Gross, I. Hrynaszkiewicz, S. Joffe, H. M. Krumholz, K. M. Strait, and J. S. Ross. 2012. Sharing of clinical trial data among trialists: A cross sectional survey. *British Medical Journal* 345:e7570.

Ross, J. S., R. Lehman, and C. P. Gross. 2012. The importance of clinical trial data sharing: Toward more open science. *Circulation: Cardiovascular Quality and Outcomes* 5(2):238-240.

Schauer, F. 2011. Transparency in three dimensions. *University of Illinois Law Review* 1339:1342-1343.

Spertus, J. A. 2012. The double-edged sword of open access to research data. *Circulation: Cardiovascular Quality and Outcomes* 5(2):143-144.

Stiles, P. G., and J. Petrila. 2011. Research and confidentiality: Legal issues and risk management strategies. *Psychology, Public Policy, and Law* 17(3):333-356.

Teden, P. 2013. *Types of clinical trial data to be shared.* Paper presented at IOM Committee on Strategies for Responsible Sharing of Clinical Trial Data: Meeting One, October 22-23, Washington, DC.

Terry, S. F., and P. F. Terry. 2011. Power to the people: Participant ownership of clinical trial data. *Science Translational Medicine* 3(69):69cm63.

Ventetuolo, C. E., N. B. Gabler, J. S. Fritz, K. A. Smith, H. I. Palevsky, J. R. Klinger, S. D. Halpern, and S. M. Kawut. 2014a. Are hemodynamics surrogate endpoints in pulmonary arterial hypertension? *Circulation* 130(9):768-775.

Ventetuolo, C. E., A. Praestgaard, H. I. Palevsky, J. R. Klinger, S. D. Halpern, and S. M. Kawut. 2014b. Sex and haemodynamics in pulmonary arterial hypertension. *European Respiratory Journal* 43(2):523-530.

Wallentin, L., R. C. Becker, C. P. Cannon, C. Held, A. Himmelmann, S. Husted, S. K. James, H. S. Katus, K. W. Mahaffey, K. S. Pieper, R. F. Storey, P. G. Steg, and R. A. Harrington. 2014. Review of the accumulated PLATO documentation supports reliable and consistent superiority of ticagrelor over clopidogrel in patients with acute coronary syndrome. Commentary on: DiNicolantonio JJ, Tomek A, Inactivations, deletions, nonadjudications, and downgrades of clinical endpoints on ticagrelor: Serious concerns over the reliability of the PLATO trial, International Journal of Cardiology, 2013. *International Journal of Cardiology* 170(3):E59-E62.

Weijer, C., and E. J. Emanuel. 2000. Ethics. Protecting communities in biomedical research. *Science* 289(5482):1142-1144.

Wertheimer, A. 2008. Exploitation in clinical research. In *The Oxford textbook of clinical research ethics*, edited by E. J. Emanuel, C. Grady, R. A. Crouch, R. K. Lie, F. G. Miller, and D. Wendler. New York: Oxford University Press. Pp. 201-210.

WMA (World Medical Association). 2013. *Declaration of Helsinki: Ethical principles for medical research involving human subjects.* Helsinki: WMA.

Zarin, D. A. 2013. Participant-level data and the new frontier in trial transparency. *New England Journal of Medicine* 369(5):468-469.

3

The Roles and Responsibilities of Stakeholders in the Sharing of Clinical Trial Data

This chapter describes the roles and responsibilities of the key stakeholders involved in the sharing of clinical trial data: (1) participants in clinical trials, (2) funders and sponsors of trials, (3) regulatory agencies, (4) investigators, (5) research institutions and universities, (6) journals, and (7) professional societies (see Box 3-1). These parties have differing perspectives on the benefits, risks, and challenges associated with sharing clinical trial data. Further, all stakeholders have a role and responsibility in helping to maximize the benefits and minimize the risks of data sharing for others, as well as themselves.

PARTICIPANTS

As outlined in Box 3-1, participants in clinical trials include individual patients and healthy volunteers. Research Ethics Committees (called Institutional Review Boards [IRBs] in the United States), Data Monitoring Committees (DMCs)/Data and Safety Monitoring Boards, and disease advocacy organizations—which oversee the informed consent process, help recruit participants for trials, and monitor the quality and safety of trials during the course of participant recruitment and follow-up—are integral to the participant experience and hence are discussed in this section as well.

BOX 3-1
Key Stakeholders Involved in Sharing Clinical Trial Data

- **Participants in clinical trials**
  - Individual patients and healthy volunteers*
  - Research Ethics Committees (termed Institutional Review Boards [IRBs] in the United States)
  - Data Monitoring Committees (DMCs), also called Data and Safety Monitoring Boards (DSMBs)
  - Disease advocacy organizations
- **Funders and sponsors of trials**
  - Public and nonprofit funders/sponsors (including disease advocacy organizations in this role)
  - Industry sponsors (including large and small private sponsors of pharmaceutical, device, and biologic clinical trials)
- **Regulatory agencies**
  - European Medicines Agency (EMA)
  - U.S. Food and Drug Administration (FDA)
- **Investigators**
  - Clinical trialists
  - Secondary users (e.g., reanalysts, meta-analysts)
- **Research institutions and universities**
- **Journals**
- **Professional societies**

---

* Individual participants in a clinical trial (who are the initial "providers" of data to researchers) may hold data to the extent that they self-generate the data and transmit them (from self-quantifying devices), retain copies of their data, or receive information from investigators. Participants may, in turn, share their data with organizations that aggregate data from many participants (e.g., disease advocacy groups, research platforms such as PatientsLikeMe, Reg4ALL, or Sage Bionetwork's Bridge).

Individual Patients and Healthy Volunteers

Clinical trial participants are the initial "providers" of data to investigators in clinical trials; they may be either patients or healthy volunteers, depending on the condition being studied. Without willing participants, sponsors and investigators would be unable to carry out clinical trials to advance science and improve clinical care. Thus, it is vital to the clinical trials enterprise that participants be respected, that trust be maintained, and that data sharing not become a barrier (and ideally that it become an incentive) to broad participation in clinical trials (Terry and Terry, 2011).

Participants' attitudes toward data sharing are mixed for a variety of reasons. First, participants are not monolithic, and certain individuals and groups are more or less supportive of data sharing than others. Second, individual participants may have positive attitudes toward some types of data sharing and negative attitudes toward others. Third, individuals' attitudes may change over time with changes in real or perceived benefits and risks.

In its October 2013 public workshop, the committee heard testimony from Sharon Hesterlee, Vice President of Research for Parent Project Muscular Dystrophy, which focuses on this rare fatal disease that affects boys. Ms. Hesterlee stated that this group of participants and their families have expressed the belief that it would be "morally repugnant to not share that data given the burden of participating in trials" and the urgency to find treatments (Hesterlee, 2013). On the other hand, healthy participants may not feel the same urgency and may therefore place greater weight on the protection of their data (Hesterlee, 2013).

According to Deborah Collyar, founder of the Patients Advocates in Research (PAIR) International Communication Network (primarily a cancer patient advocate network), "it is very clear that people volunteer their time, their effort and the[ir] bodies into clinical trials so that we can get better results. They are hoping better results for themselves, but if not, certainly for other people" (Collyar, 2013). However, many participants and their advocates also have concerns about increased sharing of individual participant data in particular. They are concerned that data sharing will lead to privacy breaches or that their data will be used for a purpose (or by individuals or organizations) that they do not sanction (IOM, 2009). If concerns about data sharing make participants less willing to enroll in clinical trials, the benefits gained by the public from clinical trials will be reduced.

Informed Consent

Informed consent is required when individuals volunteer to participate in a clinical trial. It often is the primary vehicle for both informing potential subjects about the risks and benefits of a trial and documenting their agreement to participate (see Box 3-2). The informed consent process entails having research participants sign a document that describes the study, including the potential risks and benefits, and the participants' rights and responsibilities. It usually involves a conversation with an investigator about the study as well (CIOMS, 2002).

Sharing clinical trial data was not envisioned for many of the trials for which the data have already been collected. Consent forms for these legacy trials may be silent with respect to data sharing, expressly disallow any sharing, limit sharing to specific entities or uses, allow open sharing, or be uninterpretable or internally inconsistent (O'Rourke and Forster,

---

BOX 3-2
Overview of Informed Consent Laws

Informed consent is fundamental to the ethical conduct of clinical trials, and regulations governing human clinical trials both in the United States and internationally typically require the informed consent of research participants. This is particularly the case when the trial is testing an intervention that may place the subjects at some risk (EMA, 2014a; FDA, 2014; HHS, 2014b).

Concern has been raised that informed consent forms for research often are filled with legal or technical language and are difficult for subjects to understand (Dawson and Kass, 2005; O'Rourke and Forster, 2014). Informed consent processes also focus on the individual and frequently fail to take community norms into account; in some developing countries, for example, individuals defer to or rely on the views of family members or community leaders (Benatar, 2002; Dawson and Kass, 2005; Molyneux et al., 2005).

When research involves identifiable data on individuals, regulations allow a waiver of informed consent processes if the research poses no more than minimal risk to the data subjects and could not practicably be conducted without the waiver* and, when appropriate, if individuals are provided with additional information after participation (HHS, 2014a). Some cluster randomized trials and some large simple trials may qualify for a waiver of informed consent.

---

* 45 CFR § 164.512(i)(2)(ii) (2006).

2014). Problems associated with consent for data sharing for legacy trials may be compounded because different sites in a multisite clinical trial may have altered the consent forms in accordance with local values and Research Ethics Committee requirements.

For most prospective trials, however, the informed consent process provides an opportunity to obtain participants' approval for planned data sharing and to be transparent about potential future data sharing. Although the initial consent process is unlikely to provide full details of future data sharing, investigators and sponsors can explain what data will and will not be shared with the individual participant during and after the trial, as well as under what conditions data might be shared beyond the investigators' organization or research institution. The consent process also provides a good opportunity to educate participants on the benefits and risks of data sharing so they can factor these into their decision to participate.

Debate exists among researchers and participant representatives about whether consent for data sharing should be a condition of trial participation, or whether consent forms should include a separate provision allowing participants to opt out of subsequent data sharing while still being able to participate in a trial (called "compound consent") (Bierer, 2014). On the one hand, the argument for including data sharing as a condition of trial participation (i.e., not allowing choice) is that if data from some participants are not shared, differences between the original and shared data sets will lead to discrepancies between analyses carried out by the primary team and by secondary users and inhibit the ability to reproduce analyses and conduct meta-analyses. This is a concern not only for investigators wishing to perform reanalyses or meta-analyses but also for participants who want their shared data to be of the greatest value. On the other hand, there is an argument to be made for allowing people to participate in a clinical trial without sharing their data. Under compound consent, people need not choose between sharing data they are uncomfortable with releasing and not enrolling. If large numbers of people from a specific demographic, cultural, or ethnic/racial group do not participate in clinical trials, the results will not apply to that group, weakening the evidence base for clinical decisions for the group. Proponents of compound consent argue that at least initially data sharing needs to be approached cautiously (particularly with sensitive conditions and populations that are vulnerable with respect to a particular clinical trial) so as to strengthen trust among participants. This issue requires further consideration in the context of specific clinical trials.

Concerns About Privacy

Clinical trial participants have concerns about their privacy being breached during data sharing (i.e., information about them being made public or released to individuals or organizations that could cause them harm). Participants can be vulnerable to privacy breaches in many ways. Some breaches may cause tangible harms, such as stigma or discrimination directed at persons identified as having sensitive conditions (e.g., mental illness, HIV infection, and other sexually transmitted infections), being at risk for such conditions, or engaging in illegal or stigmatized activities (e.g., use of alcohol or injection drugs, commercial sex work, or certain reproductive practices). Often such vulnerable persons have suffered discrimination in the past (Corbie-Smith et al., 1999). Those who are vulnerable because of these medical conditions often are also vulnerable because they are poor, poorly educated, and politically powerless (Benatar, 2002). The level of stigma and discrimination varies by culture and country, a fact that needs to be kept in mind because clinical trials are increasingly conducted in nations and communities around the world.

The committee examined the current landscape of international privacy protection laws to see how they provide protection against privacy breaches and whether they would offer sufficient protection in an environment of increased transparency of clinical trial data.

International laws protecting personal data—commonly referred to as data protection laws—regulate the collection and use of personal data and are commonly based on fair information practices (Privacy International, 2014). In general, fair information practices help ensure that data are collected only for specified and legitimate purposes, that individuals are informed about data collection, that data are kept secure and accurate, and that appropriate remedies exist should data be breached (Privacy International, 2014). In the case of personal health data, a variety of approaches to protection are taken across jurisdictions (see Box 3-3).

Data protection laws often apply only to identifiable data. For example, European data protection laws cover only information that relates directly or indirectly to an identified or identifiable individual (Retzer

---

BOX 3-3
International Protections for Health Data

In Europe, protections for sensitive data—typically defined as including data on health or medical conditions—commonly require the consent of the subject prior to data access, use, or disclosure; however, there are public policy exceptions (Retzer et al., 2011). When data are used for scientific purposes, for example, most European countries exempt those activities from some or all of the data protection obligations.

Countries often impose various additional requirements on the use of health data. Italy and Austria have security measures specific to the health sector: Italy requires researchers to follow the data protection authority's guidelines, whereas Austria requires encoding of health data. Belgium requires data anonymization and approval from the data protection authority. Ireland, Poland, Slovakia, and the United Kingdom mandate that use of the data not adversely affect individuals. Germany permits secondary use of data for research purposes "if the scientific interest significantly outweighs the individual's interests." Finland and the Netherlands impose no additional safeguards for such secondary use (Retzer et al., 2011).

Failure to comply with these data protection laws can jeopardize a clinical research project. Although not all laws are actively enforced, violations can lead to administrative and criminal penalties, and in some cases even to imprisonment (Retzer et al., 2011).

Although data protection laws are proliferating globally, not all countries have enacted them. In the United States, for example, laws govern research uses of health data in some contexts but not universally (IOM, 2009). Many countries in Asia have considered data protection laws but have failed to implement them or, where they have been implemented, regulators lack adequate powers to enforce them (Privacy International, 2014).

et al., 2011). In the United States, HIPAA and the Common Rule apply only to identifiable data. As discussed in Chapter 5, however, there are no uniform international standards for determining when data have been sufficiently anonymized or de-identified to be exempt from regulatory requirements. Similarly, pseudonymized data—data for which personal identifiers have been replaced with a pseudonym or code—are subject to less onerous restrictions in some European countries (and under HIPAA in the United States), but other countries apply the full range of data protection requirements even to such data (Retzer et al., 2011).

As big data analytics becomes more widespread, even data that have been de-identified may lead to violations of privacy. "Big data" is characterized by the quantity and scope of data that can be analyzed, as well as the large scale of the analysis. Combining rich data from various sources into a data set increases the likelihood of being able to re-identify individuals in the data set or determine whether they belong to a subgroup with certain characteristics (Barocas and Nissenbaum, 2014).

Concerns About Unsanctioned Uses of Data

For participants from vulnerable populations who historically were victims of unethical research, the possibility that if data sharing becomes obligatory their data will be used for purposes or by individuals or organizations they do not sanction (IOM, 2009) may be a particular concern. The history of human subjects research is sullied by several scandals in which vulnerable participants were enrolled in trials without their knowledge or ethically valid consent. In the United States, these scandals included the Tuskegee Syphilis Study, drug clinical trials carried out on prisoners, and research on institutionalized persons with mental disabilities or psychiatric illnesses. Many participants in these unethical trials were poor, poorly educated, or members of racial and cultural groups that suffer discrimination.

In the African American community, the Tuskegee study and other examples of unethical research have led to ongoing mistrust in research generally. Partly because of such mistrust, fewer African Americans than Caucasians enroll in clinical research. In turn, this low participation rate results in a weaker evidence base to guide the clinical care of this population, potentially contributing to health disparities in the United States (Corbie-Smith et al., 1999).

Internationally, violations of informed consent in clinical research involving vulnerable populations have created mistrust toward research sponsored or directed by entities from wealthy developed countries. Recent examples include unethical research on sexually transmitted infections in Guatemala and alleged violations of consent in HIV prevention trials of pre-exposure prophylaxis with tenofovir (Singh and Mills, 2005).

Although this topic has not received extensive empirical study, this evidence of mistrust suggests that certain vulnerable populations—those that have been the victims of unethical research, are disadvantaged socially or economically, or have been discriminated against—might also mistrust sharing of clinical trial data. This possibility might be addressed, strengthening engagement in clinical trials, if representatives of such vulnerable populations were included in the design and implementation of trials and if effective ways of helping participants understand the benefits of data sharing and protecting the subjects of trials were developed.

Research Ethics Committees

Research Ethics Committees are tasked with reviewing, revising, and approving clinical investigations involving humans, with the goal of protecting research participants and ensuring they are treated ethically as a result of their participation. The committees pay close attention to the informed consent process for a particular study (EUREC, 2014; WHO, 2009).

As noted, in the United States, Research Ethics Committees are called IRBs.[1] Testimony provided during the course of this study revealed that currently IRBs generally do not approve informed consent documents that require sharing of individual participant data, citing their charge to protect participants and minimize the harms of research participation (Bierer, 2014). Many countries follow the International Conference on Harmonization's (ICH's) Guideline for Good Clinical Practice (GCP) (ICH E6), which is similar to the U.S. Food and Drug Administration's (FDA's) regulations on IRBs and consent (O'Rourke and Forster, 2014).

FDA regulation 21 CFR Section 50.25(c), which requires disclosure to prospective trial participants that trial results will be posted on ClinicalTrials.gov, includes mandated consent language specifying that

---

[1] A uniform U.S. federal policy for the protection of human subjects (i.e., the Common Rule) applies to proposed research involving human subjects funded by federal departments and agencies that have adopted the Common Rule. Under this framework, research institutions formally file a commitment (i.e., Federalwide Assurance, or FWA) with the federal government to protect participants in federally funded research at their institution by adhering to the Common Rule requirements. IRBs are responsible for implementing these protections at the institutional level and reviewing each proposed research study protocol and the associated informed consent document to ensure compliance with federal rules, institutional policies, and community expectations. IRB members are not associated with the proposed research they review. One academic institution may have multiple IRBs organized by areas of expertise (e.g., biomedical and nonbiomedical research).

only summary results (i.e., no individual participant data) will be posted publicly on that site. This regulatory provision also requires that informed consent forms include statements about the "extent, if any, to which confidentiality of records identifying the individual will be maintained." This language might be interpreted in different ways. One interpretation is that data sharing, even of individual participant data, is not prohibited. On the other hand, some might suggest that because ClinicalTrials.gov is the only data sharing platform mentioned in the regulation and only summary data are to be shared there, sharing of individual participant data in any form is precluded or at least discouraged.

Research Ethics Committees play an important role in protecting research participants and giving due consideration to the interests and values of communities. For example, there is always some level of risk that individual participant data, even if de-identified, could be used to re-identify a research participant, particularly if other auxiliary information were linked with the clinical trial data set (Dwork, 2014). In addition, using auxiliary information, it may be possible to infer or learn information about individuals in a research data set—for example, whether they have a sensitive condition such as alcoholism or mental illness—even without specifically re-identifying them (Dwork, 2014). Chapter 5 examines these privacy challenges in greater detail, as well as appropriate protections and controls that reduce these risks.

Research Ethics Committees can establish policies that allow and promote responsible sharing of individual participant data in the clinical trials they review. To this end, they can ensure that investigators discuss with research participants during the informed consent process both the prospective benefits and the risks, including privacy risks, of sharing clinical trial data. When reviewing trials, Research Ethics Committees also can ensure that the risks of data sharing are minimized and that they are acceptable in light of the anticipated benefits.

Data Monitoring Committees

DMCs/DSMBs have broad responsibilities for monitoring data quality and assessing the risk/benefit ratio during the course of participant recruitment and follow-up (Ellenberg et al., 2002). Initially, the DMC reviews the trial protocol to gain familiarity with the details but generally not to approve it. The DMC also must review the draft DMC Charter carefully in order to execute it as requested by the sponsor and/or the investigators, and make suggested modifications as necessary before final approval. During the conduct of the trial, the DMC typically reviews a detailed report on interim data by intervention arm, usually unblinded to intervention assignment. This review encompasses recruitment progress, baseline data describing the participants' characteristics, comparison of baseline data, concomitant medications or interventions, adverse event data, serious adverse events, primary outcome data, secondary outcome data, and a small list of prespecified subgroups. In addition, DMCs typically request additional analyses motivated by trends in interim data. Interim DMC reports are strictly confidential until the trial is completed. Throughout the conduct of the trail, DMCs are on the alert for signals regarding inadequacies in data integrity and data quality and may ask for specific follow-up reports to clarify or rectify these inadequacies. DMCs usually complete their work with the last participant's last visit and may be asked by the sponsor and investigators to share their view or interpretation of the results when the data files are absolutely complete and locked down. However, their role is not to review or approve papers presenting final results, although their input is often solicited.

DMCs indirectly facilitate data sharing because they commonly ask the trial's data management and biostatistics teams to modify their presentation of data in interim reports so as to make the data clearer and more comprehensible. The DMCs' directions likely lead to improvements in data organization and presentation that are helpful not only to the clinical trial team but also to other investigators who later analyze shared data sets.

Although DMCs are likely to be strongly in favor of data sharing, they are not in a position to enforce that practice any more than they can enforce registration of trials on ClinicalTrials.gov and completion of the uploading of summary results. To give DMCs any responsibility for enforcing data sharing would substantially increase their responsibilities and require them to remain operational for some time beyond completion of a trial.

Disease Advocacy Organizations

Disease advocacy organizations are groups of individuals with a common condition or disease that share resources and knowledge to support clinical research, patient education, and clinical care. These organizations are active in the United States (e.g., American Cancer Society, American Heart Association, National Kidney Foundation) and are becoming more common around the world, including in developing countries (Landy et al., 2012). Traditionally, disease advocacy organizations have been involved primarily in promoting and facilitating participation in clinical trials and raising money to fund research. More recently, their roles have expanded to encompass

- collaborating with investigators on the study design and review of clinical trial protocols;

- developing and managing clinical trial networks;
- incorporating into clinical trials data collected directly by participants, such as from personal devices or sensors, as well as reports of participant-centered outcomes; and
- creating online platforms for patient engagement, such as Patients-LikeMe, Chronology, and CureTogether (American Cancer Society, 2014; CFF, 2013, 2014; Davidson, 2010; Greenwald, 2013; JDRF, 2014; Marcus, 2012; Olivas, 2014).

Furthermore, disease advocacy organizations, through online networks, have acted as a conduit for the expression of participant frustrations regarding the lack of data sharing by investigators. In many online forums, participants often express frustration about the lack of communication from investigators at the conclusion of a clinical trial (Terry and Terry, 2011). A recent study in the cancer community (Ramers-Verhoeven et al., 2014) reinforces these expressions of participant frustration. According to the authors,

> Unfortunately, this feeling of being special in many cases vanished when participation was over. Although all participants were appreciative of the care they received during the trial, there was a very clear sense of feeling that they were no longer a priority when the trial ended. "You are extremely well informed, but once you come off the trial there is not one letter. Nothing. . . . This is the major problem I had with it." (French respondent/patient)

Many participants also expressed frustration at never being told the results of the clinical trial in which they participated:

> The clinical trial experience was similar to how I had imagined it, but I was surprised that I didn't get more information about it all as it progressed and when I was withdrawn. (UK respondent/participant)

> Will the results of the clinical trial be provided? That's what preoccupied me the most. (Japanese respondent/participant)

Disease advocacy organizations are uniquely positioned to address these frustrations—both as a conduit for the expression of concerns and as a potential partner with investigators to create frameworks for continual engagement with trial participants.

An increasing number of patient groups have responded to this frustration by bypassing traditional investigator- or company-initiated clinical trials and organizing themselves to conduct their own trials of experimental agents. For example amyotrophic lateral sclerosis (ALS) patients have banded together to develop homemade versions of an experimental agent and test it on themselves (Marcus, 2012). When acting in this capacity, disease advocacy organizations share many of the same concerns, roles, and responsibilities as those of other nonprofit funders and sponsors of clinical trials with regard to data sharing.

Whether through direct financial support (either alone or as part of a funding syndicate) or other forms of assistance (e.g., participant recruitment, clinical research networks), disease advocacy organizations make significant contributions to the development and execution of clinical trials. These efforts give these organizations an opportunity to influence policies and strategies so as to encourage responsible sharing of clinical trial data.

FUNDERS AND SPONSORS

Both funders and sponsors of clinical trials have significant leverage to set standards and to encourage data sharing for the trials they fund. When considering data sharing, however, it is important to consider the context for each clinical trial in terms of the remit of the organization that has funded the work and the type of organization or institution that is the sponsor of the trial.

Public and nonprofit organizations (e.g., the U.S. National Institutes of Health [NIH], The Wellcome Trust, The Bill & Melinda Gates Foundation, the European Clinical Trial Development Platform, and disease advocacy organizations such as the ALS Association) often will support clinical trials by providing a research grant to a university or other research organization, such as a hospital or charity. The recipient organization is required to take on the role of sponsor or may delegate this role to an appropriate organization or group that has the capacity to act as sponsor. The trial sponsor is defined by ICH GCP as the organization that has specific responsibilities for trial conduct, such as ensuring that the trial is scientifically robust, that its conduct and procedures comply with safety and ethical standards, and that participants will be compensated for any harm that may result from their participation (ICH, 1996). Sponsors also are required to ensure that the trial is listed on a recognized clinical trial registry. Alternatively, a private company (e.g., a pharmaceutical or device company) may directly sponsor a clinical trial for one of its products. Contract research organizations also may work with private companies and research institutions/universities to conduct clinical trials.

Public and Nonprofit Funders

U.S. National Institutes of Health

In the United States, NIH is by far the largest public funder of clinical trials. Currently, NIH supports more than 3,000 open trials (10 percent of all open trials registered on ClinicalTrials.gov), and the agency has expressed support for ensuring that data from every trial are made public to improve the reproducibility of research results and ultimately facilitate their use to improve health (Hudson, 2013). Currently, however, the results of only 46 percent of NIH-funded trials are published within 30 months of trial completion (Ross et al., 2012). As the primary funder of translational and clinical science, NIH has been a crucial force behind major innovations designed to transform and restructure research. First, during the Human Genome Project, NIH was a key driver of researchers' sharing of genome sequencing data soon after they discovered the sequence so that other scientists could benefit from this knowledge to make further discoveries (*NIH issues genomic data sharing policy*, 2014). The U.S. Department of Health and Human Services' (HHS's) regulation on "intangible property" generated through federal awards (which is part of a comprehensive set of HHS administrative rules on awards) states that the federal government has the right to

1. Obtain, reproduce, publish, or otherwise use the data first produced under an award;
2. Authorize others to receive, reproduce, publish or otherwise use such data for Federal purposes.[2]

In line with this regulation, NIH on numerous occasions has adopted policies requiring investigators working on large-scale genome projects to deposit the data they have generated.[3,4]

Second, to promote broader dissemination of the results of the trials it sponsors, NIH requires investigators applying for new funding to link

---

[2] 34 CFR § 74.36 (c)(1-2).

[3] Of interest, patent law may somewhat constrain public release of publicly funded data. Were public funders to mandate data sharing on an extremely compressed time schedule (for example, within 24 hours, as was done with the effort surrounding the NIH-funded Human Genome Project), grantees could argue that such rapid public release interfered with their ability to file patent applications, in violation of the Bayh–Dole Act of 1980, which allows recipients of federal funding broad discretion to patent products of federally funded research. Indeed, although they never brought legal action based on these concerns, certain university technology transfer offices associated with the Human Genome Project did note tensions between immediate data release and patenting.

[4] See, e.g., Contreras (2011) and Eisenberg and Rai (2006).

the publications in their biosketch to the ID number in PubMed Central or similar platforms for sharing articles (NIH, 2014c). Most recently, in November 2014, HHS proposed a rule to clarify and extend the requirements of the Food and Drug Administration Amendments Act of 2007 (FDAAA). The FDAAA originally required that summary-level results of trials of FDA-approved products (including demographic and other baseline participant characteristics, primary and secondary outcomes, and adverse events) be shared on the ClinicalTrials.gov registry within 12 months of study completion. The proposed rule extends the requirement to register and share summary-level results so that it covers trials of unapproved products. Also in November 2014, NIH proposed a draft policy to require registration and summary results reporting of all interventional clinical trials (i.e., surgical and behavioral trials, phase 1 trials) funded by NIH (Hudson and Collins, 2014). To facilitate such reporting of results, ClinicalTrials.gov is increasing one-on-one staff support. Failure to comply with these requirements could result in civil penalties of up to $10,000 per day (assessed by the FDA) and withholding of funding for federally funded trials (Hudson and Collins, 2014). NIH also is taking timely reporting of clinical trial results into account during the review of subsequent funding applications.

Third, through the Clinical and Translational Science Awards (CTSA), NIH has provided funding and leadership to promote team-oriented scientific research and collaborative research among different institutions and research teams (NIH, 2014a).

Finally, the recent *NIH Genomic Data Sharing Policy* sets forth the responsibilities of NIH-funded researchers for sharing genomic data (including clinical trial data) and, notably, "encourages researchers to get consent from participants for future unspecified use of their genomic data" (NIH, 2014b).

NIH could be a driver for the sharing of clinical trial data by making it a requirement in the grant approval process and funding stipulations. Currently, NIH requires grantees to have a plan for data sharing if they request direct costs of $500,000 or more in any budget year, but it does not require data sharing, monitor whether data are shared as planned, or expressly allow a line item for expenses due to data sharing activities (NIH, 2003).

NIH's experience with the legal and policy justification for requirements to share publicly funded genomic data has implications for the sharing of clinical trial data. In the context of human genome data, NIH has sometimes implemented controlled access to accommodate concerns about participant privacy and informed consent.[5] However, the

---

[5] For a recent articulation of the NIH approach to addressing issues of informed consent and privacy for human genome data, see Final NIH Genomic Data Sharing Policy, 78 F.R. 51345, August 27, 2014.

requirement that investigators must deposit data free from claims of trade secrecy/commercially confidential information has not changed. This experience with policies on genomic data could inform policies that NIH and other agencies adopt with respect to publicly funded clinical trial data.

Resolution of the issue of whether and how NIH might enforce data deposition requirements against violators similarly could be informed by the experience with genomic data. For its policies regarding genomic data deposition, NIH generally has refrained from articulating legal enforcement mechanisms. But NIH's most recent genomic data sharing policy does refer to potential sanctions under 45 CFR Section 74.62,[6] which addresses enforcement of the terms and conditions of a grant. Such sanctions include withholding of future research awards and even suspension of an entire institution from receipt of federal funding.

The Wellcome Trust

The Wellcome Trust is a charitable foundation based in the United Kingdom that provides funding for research in the United Kingdom and low- and middle-income countries (The Wellcome Trust, 2014a). The foundation supports increased transparency and sharing of clinical trial data from the research it funds by (1) requiring a data management and data sharing plan for all applications for funding, regardless of whether the investigation is taking place in a resource-poor country or the United Kingdom; (2) requiring any research papers published in peer-reviewed journals to be made available through PubMed Central (PMC) and Europe PubMed Central (Europe PMC) within 6 months of publication and providing funding to cover open access charges; and (3) requiring authors and publishers that receive open access payments to license research papers to be freely copied and reused with proper attribution to the original authors, using the Creative Commons Attribution license (CC-BY) (The Wellcome Trust, 2014b).

In addition, the foundation supports a number of major initiatives that promote data sharing, such as MalariaGEN—the Malaria Genomic Epidemiology Network, a community established in 2005 comprising more than 20 countries and 100 researchers. MalariaGEN serves as the main driver of collaborative research and genomic data sharing for malaria research, both of which play a crucial role in researchers' efforts to work to develop and improve tools for controlling this disease (MalariaGen, 2014a). MalariaGEN receives funding from a variety of nonprofit sources,

---

[6] Ibid.

including The Wellcome Trust, the Foundation for the National Institutes of Health, and The Bill & Melinda Gates Foundation (MalariaGen, 2014b).

The Bill & Melinda Gates Foundation

The Bill & Melinda Gates Foundation is a global foundation that supports clinical research and other projects in resource-poor countries. It has joined the International Aid Transparency Initiative (IATI), which works to improve the transparency of aid, development, and humanitarian resources by establishing a common standard for the publication of aid information and providing an online repository for all raw data published to the IATI standard. In March 2014, the Gates Foundation began publishing open data on its development activities in accordance with IATI standards (Aid Transparency Index, 2014).

Starting in January 2015, the Gates Foundation will require grantees to make publications, and the underlying data sets, available for free immediately upon publication and with no restrictions on use. The foundation will pay open access fees for publication. The foundation is allowing a phase-in period: Until 2017, open access to publications and to underlying data may be delayed for 12 months (The Bill & Melinda Gates Foundation, 2014; Van Noorden, 2014).

Industry Sponsors

In the past, the culture of clinical research in industry did not include proactively sharing clinical trial data. There are several reasons for this culture, including concerns about incorrect or conflicting analyses generated by secondary users; concerns about participant privacy; and the desire to allow participating researchers and investigators the unique opportunity to publish data from trials in which they participated, which is important for their careers. Moreover, clinical research generated in support of marketing applications generally was considered to be commercially confidential information. Sponsors spend significant time and effort in developing drugs, clinical and regulatory strategies, and clinical research protocols and analysis plans. These plans and documents may include considerations based on confidential interactions with regulatory authorities and internal scientific expertise and on strategic ideas. Data gathered from studies often are used in the development of subsequent studies or products and are part of the institutional knowledge base in research and development (R&D) units within companies. Access to this information could give competitors a significant competitive advantage. Thus, sharing clinical trial data could shorten the time between the marketing of a first-in-class product and the marketing of similar products.

This interval, a key driver of return on investment for R&D, has already decreased significantly over time (Lanthier et al., 2013). Further decreases could discourage future investment in new product development.

Appendix C provides additional legal analysis, conducted by the committee, of industry intellectual property concerns. This legal analysis focuses on small molecules and biologics. Of course, clinical trial data also are generated in medical device trials. With medical devices, however, issues regarding data exclusivity, even in jurisdictions like the United States, are less clear-cut. Indeed, according to a submission to this committee from the trade group AdvaMed, release of data associated with receiving FDA clearance through the expensive premarket approval process could facilitate market entry for competitors using the so-called 510(k) pathway for approval (AdvaMed, 2013).[7] Under the 510(k) pathway, an applicant must prove that its device is "substantially equivalent" to a device already on the market. Proving substantial equivalence requires showing that the new device has the same intended use and technological characteristics as the predicate.

In the past, secondary users requesting access to individual participant data or study reports from industry-sponsored studies would approach individual investigators and/or authors of study manuscripts to request access, just as in academia. Many times, if both parties agreed, secondary users requesting access could be asked, for example, to share hypotheses and data analysis plans and/or sign confidentiality agreements, and access would be granted. Some companies had procedures and review committees for external proposals (Rosenblatt, 2014), while others did not.

Independent researchers who have obtained clinical study reports (CSRs)[8] and individual participant data from industry-sponsored trials have identified significant problems with underreporting of negative results and serious adverse events and with failure to publish results of negative trials for widely prescribed therapies and a vaccine (Doshi et al., 2013). These claims, however, have been disputed by sponsors. In several

---

[7] In contrast to AdvaMed's point about data exclusivity, its arguments about the relative weakness of medical device patents or the purported exemption of medical devices from the FDAAA appear to lack foundation.

[8] A CSR is an "integrated full report of an individual study of any therapeutic, prophylactic or diagnostic agent . . . conducted in patients. The clinical and statistical description, presentation, and analyses are integrated into a single report incorporating tables and figures into the main text of the report or at the end of the text, with appendices containing such information as the protocol, sample case report forms, investigator-related information, information related to the test drugs/investigational products including active control/comparators, technical statistical documentation, related publications, patient data listings, and technical statistical details such as derivations, computations, analyses, and computer output" (FDA, 1996, p. 1).

cases, the ensuing scientific and public debate has led to changes in labeling and marketing of drugs, legal settlements, and further clinical trials to address contested clinical hypotheses (see Table 3-1). The results of these additional trials have shown a more complex and nuanced picture than did either the original clinical trial results or the first independent analyses. This back-and-forth debate is part of the scientific method, which leads to ongoing clarification of scientific issues. Although complex and sometimes confusing to the public, this process illustrates how scientific knowledge generally progresses through debate, new data and analyses, and further debate.

Cases in which requests for access by independent investigators were repeatedly denied or delayed have sparked calls for a more systematic and transparent approach to the sharing of industry clinical trial data. In addition, as discussed in the section below on regulatory agencies, the European Medicines Agency (EMA) has generated a great deal of discussion on its mandate to share clinical trial data after marketing approval (EMA, 2013). In parallel with these discussions, recent HIPAA guidance has led to increased comfort with sharing de-identified clinical trial data for scientifically important analyses (HHS, 2012). Thus, over the past several years, the culture in industry has been changing, so that, as noted in Chapter 1, industry now is often leading data sharing initiatives. Several new initiatives launched by pharmaceutical companies and two device companies have significantly changed the paradigm for sharing of clinical trial data (see Appendix D) (Krumholz et al., 2014). In addition, in 2013, the Pharmaceutical Research and Manufacturers of America (PhRMA) and the European Federation of Pharmaceutical Industries and Associations (EFPIA) announced a commitment from all of their member companies to develop a process for and commit to sharing clinical trial data (PhRMA and EFPIA, 2013).

Currently, the costs of sharing clinical trial data (see Box 3-4) are borne by trial sponsors that agree to share the data. A substantial portion of this cost is for redacting commercially confidential information and participant identifiers from the data manually—for example, handwritten notes in CSRs that identify participants or reveal a company's strategy for future research or for interactions with regulators (Shoulson, 2014).

Small companies that account for a significant proportion of new therapeutic discoveries have stated that they currently do not have the revenue to support sharing clinical trial data. In 2012, 42 percent of new drug approvals were for emerging sponsors (FDASIA, 2013). There are precedents for reducing fees for small companies. For example, when small companies seek drug approval from the FDA, they have reduced application fees (FDA, 2011b, p. 9). Sharing clinical trial data may be an

TABLE 3-1 Examples of Effects of Independent Analyses Carried Out on Clinical Trial Data

	Concerns Raised by Independent Analyses of Clinical Trial Data	Effects
Oseltamivir	• Trials with 60 percent of patient data not reported • Full study reports inaccessible for 29 percent of trials • Missing modules for 16 of 17 available full study reports • Discrepancies between published articles and full study reports • Independent analysis showed that oseltamivir did not necessarily reduce hospital admissions and pulmonary complications in patients with influenza and that it had unclear harms; this analysis was contested (Chan et al., 2014)	• Public and scientific debate about the decision to stockpile oseltamivir as part of pandemic preparedness (Godlee, 2009) • Further reanalyses of existing clinical trial data carried out by additional investigators, with conflicting conclusions (Cochrane Neuraminidase Inhibitors Review Team, 2011; Hernán and Lipsitch, 2011a,b; Michiels et al., 2013)
Rosiglitazone	• Independent meta-analysis of 56 rosiglitazone trials, which included 36 unreported trials for which data were obtained from the sponsor's trial registry, showed significantly increased risk of myocardial infarction (Nissen and Wolski, 2007); the methodology of this meta-analysis was subsequently challenged (Diamond et al., 2007)	• In 2010 the U.S. Food and Drug Administration (FDA) restricted prescribing of rosiglitazone to patients with type 2 diabetes who cannot control their diabetes on other medications • In 2013 the FDA removed prescribing restrictions based on reanalysis of data carried out by an independent scientist (Tucker, 2013)
Gabapentin	• Selective outcomes reporting for trials for off-label uses, with 8 of 20 trials not published; in 5 of 8 published trials reporting a significant advantage for gabapentin, primary endpoint in publication differed from that described in protocol (Vedula et al., 2009)	• In 2004, manufacturer agreed to plead guilty and pay $430 million in fines to settle civil and criminal charges regarding the illegal marketing of gabapentin for off-label purposes (DOJ, 2004)

continued

TABLE 3-1 Continued

	Concerns Raised by Independent Analyses of Clinical Trial Data	Effects
Selective Serotonin Reuptake Inhibitors (SSRIs)	• The U.K. Medical and Health Products Regulatory Agency, after requesting unpublished clinical trial data and reviewing all data, concluded in 2003 that the risks of SSRIs for treatment of major depression in children and adolescents outweighed the benefits (except for fluoxetine) (MHRA, 2003) • In 2004, the FDA issued a black-box warning that antidepressants increase suicidality in children and adolescents; this decision was controversial (Brent, 2004; Newman, 2004) • A 2006, the FDA's meta-analysis of clinical trial data submitted to it showed that use of antidepressants in adolescents was associated with a mild increase in suicidality (Hammad et al., 2006); this publication was criticized by a professor with many contracts with industry • Independent review in 2008 showed that 94 percent of publications from clinical trials of antidepressants had positive results, although 51 percent of all trials submitted to the FDA had positive results (Turner et al., 2008); this analysis was contested by the sponsor • A meta-analysis using longitudinal data and depressive symptoms concluded in 2014 found no significant effects of fluoxetine and venlafaxine treatment on suicidal thoughts and behavior in youth (Gibbons et al., 2012)	• In 2012 the manufacturer pleaded guilty to marketing paroxetine to treat patients under age 18, which was not an FDA-approved indication; the manufacturer also paid $3 billion in penalties to settle allegations, among others, that it "misreported that a clinical trial of Paxil demonstrated efficacy in the treatment of depression in patients under age 18, when the study failed to demonstrate efficacy," and that it did not make available data from two other studies in which Paxil also failed to demonstrate efficacy (DOJ, 2012) • A study using health claims data showed that after the FDA issued its black-box warning in 2003, use of antidepressants among youth decreased by 31 percent; during the same period, suicide attempts involving overdoses of psychotropic drugs increased by 22 percent in adolescents (Lu et al., 2014), and there was no change in completed suicides In 2002, about 900,000 prescriptions (costing $55 million) were written for children with mood disorders in the United States for a drug with potential harms and poor evidence of efficacy (Chan et al., 2014)

TABLE 3-1 Continued

	Concerns Raised by Independent Analyses of Clinical Trial Data	Effects
Rofecoxib	• Sponsor's internal meta-analysis of two trials showing increased mortality in Alzheimer's disease not reported; 2-year delay in reporting of the results to regulators (Psaty and Kronmal, 2008) • Selective exclusion of placebo-controlled trials from three reported meta-analyses conducted by the sponsor, which showed no overall increase in cardiovascular events; subsequent independent meta-analysis that included all trials (made available through litigation) showed an increase in cardiovascular events • Inappropriate analysis of short-term cardiovascular harms in clinical trials of the drug (Lagakos, 2006)	• Manufacturer voluntarily withdrew the drug from the market in 2004 • Manufacturer agreed to create a \$4.85 billion fund to settle a product liability class action suit • A 2014 meta-analysis showed that nonselective nonsteroidal anti-inflammatory agents diclofenac and possibly ibuprofen increased major vascular events similarly to selective COX-2 inhibitors such as rofecoxib; naproxen is associated with less vascular risk (Coxib and Traditional NSAID Trialists' [CNT's] Collaboration, 2013)

analogous situation in which small companies should not pay the same costs as large companies.

REGULATORY AGENCIES

Submission of clinical trial data to regulatory authorities to gain approval for a new product or indication is an important consideration in the sharing of clinical trial data. Although health authorities exist around the world,[9] this section focuses primarily on the EMA and the FDA because many other countries worldwide rely on those agencies' review of products instead of conducting their own.

The EMA has been a pioneer in the sharing of clinical trial data; its

---

[9] It is important to note that regulatory agencies in different jurisdictions differ in the types of data they hold and in what authority they have to provide access to data submitted to them or to other parties.

BOX 3-4
Costs of Sharing Clinical Trial Data

Costs associated with current data sharing activities among private sponsors of clinical trials may include the following:

- Protections for privacy, including de-identification of data*
- Redaction of documents
- Setting up databases/participating in data sharing sites (e.g., SAS®)
- Setting up and maintaining websites/portals
- Payments for review panel/steering committee as required
- Payments for third-party administrator
- Solicitation of external experts
- Due diligence assessments—finding data, getting data in the correct format, working with partners to assess data sets, etc.
- Compliance and auditing efforts—registry and publication
- Creation of lay summaries/synopses for posting on external sites (over and above ClinicalTrial.gov requirements)
- Work to create templates for informed consent forms, clinical study reports, etc. to allow for greater data sharing
- Data sharing coordinators—independent roles assigned to manage the intake and fulfillment of requests

---

* The committee was unable to find estimates of the costs associated with anonymizing or de-identifying health data in the published literature. However, the authors of the commissioned paper on de-identification (see Appendix B), both of whom are external consultants who de-identify health data sets, estimate that costs for de-identifying a particular data set can range from $10,000 to $100,000, depending on the amount of effort required. When the work to de-identify data sets goes from being episodic to more routine or ongoing, it may make sense to develop in-house expertise. A de-identification course offered by Privacy Analytics, for example, costs about $2,000 per person. Developing the capacity to automate the de-identification of data sets could cost between $100,000 and $500,000, but these costs would be spread over a number of data sets and years.

---

plan for sharing data submitted to it and its engagement with stakeholders and the public on the issue have stimulated international discussions of data sharing. In the United States, the FDA plays a special role in the review of submitted applications. It obtains the entire database of studies conducted on products submitted for approval: protocols and all amendments, data analysis plans, case report form, summary data, and individual participant data (FDA, 2011a). In addition to a comprehensive review, the FDA conducts its own analyses and produces its own summaries. The EMA also conducts its own extensive reviews of submitted applications (although it does not usually obtain individual participant data), as do agencies in several other countries, most notably the Pharmaceuticals and Medical Devices Agency (Japan) and the China Food and Drug Administration.

It is important to keep in mind that only a small proportion of all clinical trial data is submitted to regulatory authorities. Most academic and publicly funded trials do not have a regulatory goal, and indeed many industry trials will not automatically generate data that are submitted in a regulatory file or for other reasons are ever submitted to an authority. Therefore, although there may be benefit in regulatory agencies' release of the data that have been submitted to them, which are the basis for regulatory decisions, these data do not represent all the clinical trial data that are being generated internationally.

European Medicines Agency (EMA)

As noted, the EMA has been a key promoter of greater transparency in sharing of clinical trial data. From pharmaceutical and device companies, the EMA receives detailed CSR and selected individual participant data that are used in making decisions to approve or reject products for marketing authorization.

The EMA's policy[10] on sharing the data it receives has evolved over the last 4 years, beginning in November 2010 when it began to release CSRs and other documents on a case-by-case basis in response to a formal freedom-of-information request (EMA, 2014c). Then, in June 2013, the EMA published a draft policy proposing to publish proactively both CSRs and de-identified individual participant data at the time of regulatory decisions (EMA, 2013; Wathion and EMA, 2014). In that document, the EMA noted that CSRs do not contain commercially confidential information and therefore could be released with no redactions. The draft policy received more than 1,000 comments from more than 150 organizations (EMA, 2014d). According to the EMA, the comments were centered on three main issues: (1) protection of patient privacy, (2) whether information contained in CSRs could be considered commercially confidential and be used by competitors for commercial advantage, and (3) the legality and enforceability of the data sharing agreement between the EMA and data users. The draft policy also faced legal challenges from pharmaceutical companies AbbVie and Intermune (Adams, 2014; Mansell, 2014).

In October 2014, after extensive deliberations and discussions with industry sponsors, academic researchers, journals, patient representa-

---

[10] The policy relates to clinical trial data submitted under the centralized procedure after the "effective" date. The policy does not relate to legacy data submitted under arbitration/ referral procedures or the centralized procedure.

tives, and others, the EMA finally approved a policy to make available CSRs redacted for commercially confidential information, protocols, and documentation of statistical methods after a regulatory decision to either grant or refuse marketing authorization has been made (EMA, 2014e). Any member of the public may view this information online after registering and agreeing to terms of use. Persons who provide identifying information, including their passport or ID card number, may download and save these data. Downloaded data will have a watermark to emphasize that they may not be used for commercial purposes (EMA, 2014b). The policy applies to products submitted for approval after January 1, 2015, with the data likely to be released around July 2016. The EMA plans to make individual participant data available at a later date after further consultation and discussion; the agency acknowledges that such sharing would need to be consistent with the European Union regulations protecting individual privacy.

U.S. Food and Drug Administration (FDA)

The FDA is currently examining the possibility of releasing "masked" nonsummary data—nonsummary data from which information has been removed so that the data will not identify any specific product or application.[11] In response, various commentators have urged that "masking" is likely to be ineffective (AdvaMed, 2013; Gaffney, 2013). Absent further detail regarding how masking will be accomplished, it is difficult to parse these arguments. Furthermore, critics have objected that effective masking of products would limit the usefulness of the data for secondary analyses of individual clinical trials and meta-analyses.

The power of U.S. regulatory agencies over data submitted by clinical trial sponsors is governed by two statutes: the Freedom of Information Act[12] (FOIA), which addresses disclosure in response to citizen requests; and the Trade Secrets Act[13] (TSA), which addresses the limits of affirmative disclosure by the government. In the case of the FDA in particular, a relevant regulation that essentially mirrors the constraints of these two statutes is 21 CFR 20.61(c). This regulation provides that "data and information submitted or divulged to the Food and Drug Administration which fall within the definitions of a trade secret or confidential commercial or financial information are not available for public disclosure." Moreover, these statutes, together with case law interpreting them, generally prohibit regulatory agencies such as the FDA from releasing

---

[11] 68 Fed. Reg. 3342, June 4, 2013.
[12] 5 U.S.C. § 552.
[13] 18 U.S.C. § 1905 (1982).

information that is likely "to cause substantial harm to the competitive position of the person from whom the information was obtained." Courts have, however, required that those who might allege competitive harm make arguments that go beyond the "conclusory and generalized."[14] For practical purposes, this means that any regulatory steps the FDA might take in the direction of making nonsummary clinical data publicly available would have to take into account (as the EMA has) redaction of information regarding potential new uses, as well as restrictions against copying full data sets for purposes of seeking marketing approval in other jurisdictions.

One important open question is the extent to which the FDA may have the authority to issue regulations that override the ordinary constraints of the TSA. The TSA does allow agencies to disclose trade secrets/commercially confidential information to the extent that such disclosure is "authorized by law."[15] Moreover, under standard principles of administrative law, substantive regulations that the FDA (or any agency) has authority to promulgate constitute "law." Further, some legal scholars have argued that the FDA potentially has the power to disclose trade secrets for public health reasons, citing the provision in the Hatch-Waxman Act stating that the FDA is supposed to release clinical trial data after Hatch-Waxman data exclusivity expires, absent "extraordinary circumstances."[16]

Section 301(j) of the Food, Drug, and Cosmetic Act (FDCA) does specifically prohibit the FDA from releasing to the public information "concerning any method or process which as a trade secret is entitled to protection."[17] Thus, the FDA presumably would not have the authority to issue regulations that disclosed this specific subcategory of trade secrets. However, under section 501(i) of the FDCA,[18] the FDA does have expansive authority to impose on regulated parties "other conditions" that "relat[e] to the protection of the public health." Moreover, in January 2001, the FDA did rely in part on this authority to propose disclosure rules with respect to clinical data concerning human gene therapy.[19] The proposed FDA rules invoked section 505(i) in the context of arguing that "several significant public health goals" would be served through greater disclosure of data. Although these proposed rules were never finalized, they

---

[14] 5 U.S.C. § 552(b)(4).

[15] 18 U.S.C. § 1905 (1982) (emphasis added).

[16] Drug Price Competition and Patent Term Restoration Act, Public Law 98-417, 98th Cong. (September 24, 1984).

[17] 21 U.S.C. § 331(j) (1982).

[18] 21 U.S.C. § 355(i).

[19] See FDA "Proposed Rule on Availability for Public Disclosure and Submission to FDA for Public Disclosure of Certain Data and Information Related to Human Gene Therapy or Xenotransplantation," 66 Fed. Reg. 4692 (2001).

represent an important precedent to consider in thinking through questions of the FDA power in the context of disclosure of clinical trial data.

INVESTIGATORS

Two types of scientific researchers are vitally involved in sharing clinical trial data: (1) the researchers who are key figures in the clinical trial design and at the participant interface, and (2) the researchers who analyze data collected by projects and processes—such as clinical trials, disease registries, and clinical care—in which they were not involved. In this report, the term *trialist* is used to refer specifically to researchers who design and conduct clinical trials, while *investigators* is used for all researchers. Among investigators, the term *secondary users* refers to investigators who use clinical trial data for purposes including reanalyses, novel analyses, and meta-analyses but were not involved in generating the primary data.

Clinical Trialists

Traditionally, trialists are people whose careers are built on conducting clinical trials that provide the evidence base needed for the high-quality practice of medicine. Because trialists have expertise in the condition to be studied by a trial, in the science of designing and conducting trials, or both, they are able to frame the research questions, study the key variables, perform state-of-the-art outcome measurements pertinent to the study question, and determine how best to gather that information. They may be based in academia; in the pharmaceutical, biotechnology, or device industries; in clinical practice; in contract research organizations (CROs); or in nonprofit organizations. In recent years, patients and disease advocates also have increasingly been involved in the design and conduct of trials out of personal interest and not as a career.

Trialists play the key roles in trial design, participant recruitment, and data accrual. Often, the success or failure of a clinical trial hinges on specific aspects of the trial design. Knowledge of how to design trials is thus a critical skill; successful trialists have the experience and expertise to create a design that is simple enough to be practical, comprehensive enough to be informative, and rigorous enough for results to be convincing (Anturane Reinfarction Trial Policy Committee, 1982; Anturane Reinfarction Trial Research Group, 1980; Baron et al., 2008; Bresalier et al., 2005; Canner, 1991; The Coronary Drug Project Research Group, 1980; May et al., 1981; Nissen, 2006; Temple and Pledger, 1980; Thackray et al., 2000; Wedel et al., 2001).

Once a trial has been designed, trialists identify eligible participants, train members of the trial team, organize recruitment, obtain informed consent, and either gather the key outcome data themselves or arrange to have the data gathered by others. For trialists based in CROs or clinical practice, participant recruitment and enrollment may be their only role in the trial. Finally, it is trialists who have the understanding and expertise to interpret the trial data and give them clinical meaning. Thus, without motivated and knowledgeable trialists, the clinical trial process would come to a halt.

Clinical trials are the most rigorous approach to assessing the efficacy and safety of an intervention. Thus, clinical trialists play an essential role in developing the evidence base on which clinical care rests. However, being a successful clinical trialist is a long and arduous career path. To attract talented young people to clinical investigation, a clear career path and rewards for this path are needed. Because most clinical trials are carried out in a time frame of years, if not decades, within one's career, an investigator may participate in a relatively small number of trials and lead only a handful of them. In contrast, basic science investigators, epidemiologists, health services researchers, and other types of scientists may complete many studies in the time it takes to perform one clinical trial.

Because of the time and skill set needed to design a trial, enroll the participants, and accrue and interpret the data, many trialists view the data gathered in a trial as their intellectual property, even if it technically "belongs" to a third party (Royal Society, 2012). Typically, trialists intend to carry out and publish a number of secondary analyses of the collected data. Often the prospect of such secondary analyses helps academic senior clinical trialists recruit trainees and junior faculty members to their research group. Because academic and industrial success depends on published output, and because only a small fraction of the accrued data is published in the primary report of a trial, many academics have been reticent to share data. A principal concern is that others will use the data to publish findings in a data set—and gain the accompanying recognition and academic prestige—before those who labored to design the trial and gather the data have had the opportunity to fully examine and analyze the data.

Clinical trialists also may be concerned that third parties who do not fully understand the subtleties of the trial design and data accrual may draw erroneous conclusions that could cloud or even vitiate the published findings. Thus, trialists want to protect their data from misuse by others. In addition to the potential career benefits of this more restricted approach, many trialists believe it is important and feel a responsibility to limit data access both to protect the research participants from having their data misused and, more broadly, to protect the public from misinterpretation of the data based on flawed analyses by nonexperts. Clinical trialists also fear that responding to invalid challenges to their publications will consume large amounts of time and effort, taking them away from their own work (Wallentin et al., 2014).

Because it takes decades to create seasoned clinical trialists and people at the outset of their careers make choices for the future based in part on the possibility of long-term success, data sharing may be a disincentive to choosing a career as a clinical trialist. Indeed, many trialists may view people who use their data for structured reviews and meta-analyses as "parasites" on the system and as antagonists to the medical progress resulting from their work (Reidpath and Allotey, 2001; Share alike, 2014). Thus, there is a cultural gap that needs to be bridged. This bridge will best be built when trialists see the value to them in sharing data. For example, trialists' examination of a data set accrued by others may help in designing future trials or interpreting data gathered by others. Funders can accelerate this process by providing tangible rewards to trialists for data sharing activities.

Finally, clinical trialists rely on third parties (e.g., industry, public funding entities, private charities) to fund their work. Therefore, they respond to priorities and direction from these organizations. Trialists are concerned that if data sharing becomes an unfunded mandate, the costs of sharing will reduce the funding available for new grants, which in turn would result in fewer new trials. This concern is particularly cogent for trialists working in low-resource settings such as those affected by neglected global diseases, where funding for new clinical trials is already scarce. According to a 2013 World Health Organization (WHO) report (WHO, 2013), unless there is more research, there will be no real improvements in public health in the world's poorest regions. The report emphasizes that these regions "need to be the generators and not the passive recipients of data" (The Global Health Network, 2014; WHO, 2013). However, data sharing also could potentially increase the long-term return on grants by catalyzing secondary data analyses and helping to avoid future research that is redundant or based on an unpromising approach. Furthermore, making clinical trial data shareable could make future clinical trials more efficient in the long run because new research could build on secondary analyses of the shared data. New models for funding the sharing of clinical trial data may alleviate some concerns if the costs of sharing are spread more equitably among the various stakeholders.

Secondary Users

Only a small minority of clinical investigators are trialists conducting interventional trials (Nussenblatt and Meinert, 2010). Other researchers conduct observational studies (e.g., disease registries, cohort studies) or secondary analyses of existing data from such sources as electronic health records, administrative data, and clinical trials. Meta-analysts are the investigators most interested in sharing clinical trial data, for they analyze and synthesize results from multiple trials to arrive at the overall findings from the evidence base (Stewart and Tierney, 2002). Meta-analysts are critical for advancing summary understanding of a body of research, and meta-analytic results are highly valuable for informing the design of new clinical trials. Currently, relatively few investigators analyze publicly available results of clinical trials for new hypotheses and findings, simply because trial results currently are not widely shared, but this type of investigator is likely to be more prevalent if responsible data sharing becomes more widespread. Trialists, of course, can also be involved in these other types of clinical research.

Clinical investigators who do not conduct trials themselves may generate numerous publications by analyzing preexisting data sets in less time than it takes clinical trialists to generate even their initial results (IOM, 2010). However, just because data are accessible does not mean that they are usable. Data are usable if an investigator can search and retrieve them, can make sense of them, and can analyze them within a single trial or combine them across many trials. Given the large volume of data anticipated to become available from the sharing of clinical trial data, the data will have to be in a computable form amenable to automated methods of search, analysis, and visualization (the committee discusses this challenge further in Chapter 6).

In contrast with the foregoing disincentives for investigators to share data, the incentives for investigators to share data are almost universally regarded as insufficient (EAGDA, 2014; Tenopir et al., 2011). At least four parties—research institutions and universities, research funders, biomedical journals, and professional societies—could provide meaningful incentives for investigators to share data.

RESEARCH INSTITUTIONS AND UNIVERSITIES

Universities can influence data sharing activities through infrastructure support, incentives, training, and scientific review.

Infrastructure Support

Academic centers typically provide infrastructure in support of investigators who conduct clinical trials and generate new data. This infrastructure can consist of data managers, research coordinators, biostatistical and informatics support, and other clinical trial coordinating center expertise. By contrast, academic centers provide comparatively sparse support for data curation, archiving, and sharing. High-quality data curation and management are required to prepare for data sharing, so that investigators must both recognize this need and have appropriately skilled personnel available to them. However, the level of such support varies widely among institutions, as can investigators' recognition of how much of this support may be necessary. Academic centers also often provide insufficient recognition of the time, effort, and value of sharing clinical trial data (Bonham, 2014; Dickersin, 2013; IOM, 2013). Further, few universities have transitioned to being "digital enterprises" (Bourne, 2014) that manage their digital assets to full advantage, although the NIH CTSA program's continuing emphasis on informatics has substantially improved clinical research informatics capacity at CTSA institutions (Kahn and Weng, 2012) and through common tools such as i2b2 (i2b2, 2014). For sharing of clinical trial data in particular, institutions continue to face challenges, including supporting faculty in sharing data or ensuring that trials are registered on ClinicalTrials.gov as required (Hudson and Collins, 2014). Better overall support of the clinical trials enterprise within most institutions is needed to support the kinds of data structuring and documentation that will be needed for data sharing.

Incentives

In the eyes of performance review and promotion committees, the primary criteria for academic success rest on publications, funding, leadership, and teaching. Data sharing is not an activity that receives attention from promotion committees, and there is insufficient recognition of the intellectual effort involved in designing, accruing, curating, and completing a clinical trial data set. In this way, the lack of incentives for sharing clinical trial data is analogous to the recognized dearth of incentives for team science within university settings (Chan et al., 2014; NRC, 2012). Positive examples of promotion committees' acknowledging the important contributions of investigators in creating high-quality, widely used data sets and sharing them with others are currently lacking. Appropriate recognition of data sharing activities in the promotion process would provide incentives for sharing data and obtaining maximal value from completed trials. Other promotion-related incentives for data sharing would exist if promotion committees took into account secondary publications by others based on clinical trial data produced and shared by their faculty.

Training

Most of the workforce that would be involved in activities related to the sharing of clinical trial data are trained in universities. Currently, there is little or no training within traditional clinical research education in the procedures and structures needed to share data. The development of such modules, either online or in classroom settings, could be instrumental in helping to move the field of data sharing forward.

Scientific Review

Many academic institutions perform some form of internal scientific review for studies that are not reviewed externally or that fall within certain areas in which internal review is required (e.g., cancer studies in cancer centers designated by the National Cancer Institute). Including an assessment of data sharing plans in such reviews, together with trial registration and results reporting, would both serve as an incentive to create such plans and potentially provide valuable technical guidance in how to do so in that institution.

JOURNALS

Biomedical journals serve as an intermediary between investigators who gather data and write research reports and readers, including clinicians, clinician-scientists, scientists, and laypeople. Journals play an essential role in providing peer review, evaluating research claims for scientific accuracy, and preparing reports for publication in a clear and lucid fashion. They provide a measure of assurance that the claims made by authors have validity and value. In this role as an intermediary between author-investigators and readers, journals want to be sure that the ideas reported under their imprimatur are correct. Journals often are perceived as the arbiters of the scientific and societal value of research in that their decision whether to publish submitted research results determines whether that research reaches an audience. The trialists who conducted the research also have a great interest in the publication decisions of journals, which are the gatekeepers for the academic credit and prestige that accompany being a lead author on research published in a high-impact journal.

The core goal of biomedical journals is to connect people (e.g., physicians, other researchers, patients, policy makers) with valid and important scientific research to improve scientific knowledge, patient care, and health outcomes. This goal is aligned with responsible sharing of clinical trial data. Broad sharing of clinical trial data also would advance the interests of journals in helping to ensure that published research findings are reproducible (Collins and Tabak, 2014).

Although responsible sharing of clinical trial data is consistent with the goals of biomedical journals, journals in general cannot take on data sharing responsibilities that are beyond their scope of work and resources.

It is not feasible for journals to assume the responsibilities entailed in serving as the repository of data for the studies they publish, adjudicating who will have access to the data, and negotiating interactions between authors of primary research reports and investigators whose secondary analyses reach different conclusions. Biomedical journals can, however, leverage their role as evaluators and publishers of research results, implementers of academic standards, and gatekeepers of academic credit and prestige to create and enforce policies that require sharing of clinical trial data (IOM, 2013; Laine et al., 2007).

Biomedical journals have an important role to play in advancing the creation of an environment in which sharing of clinical trial data is a standard and an expectation for publication in the scientific literature. Journals could require and enforce data sharing as a condition of submission and publication, with the goal of increasing the transparency and validity of clinical trial results they publish. Biomedical journals previously have played important roles in setting and enforcing important standards for clinical research. In 2004, for example, member journals of the International Committee of Medical Journal Editors (ICMJE) adopted a position that they would publish only clinical trials that had been registered in an appropriate, publicly accessible database prior to the enrollment of the first participant in the study (De Angelis et al., 2004). There was some initial pushback from the research community, but when the date for trial registration arrived on September 13, 2005, there was a spike in new trial registrations at ClinicalTrials.gov, the largest ICMJE-compliant website, as academic and industrial researchers rushed to bring their trials into compliance with this mandate (Zarin, 2013). Similarly, journals could provide leadership in setting minimal requirements for data sharing that would have a great impact on clinical trial investigators and sponsors. The *Annals of Internal Medicine*, the *British Medical Journal*, and the family of journals belonging to the Public Library of Science (PLoS) have already promulgated positions that they will publish only articles whose authors indicate willingness to share data (*Annals of Internal Medicine*) or agree to share data (*British Medical Journal*, PLoS) (Godlee and Groves, 2012; Laine et al., 2007; Silva, 2014). The challenge with these statements is that the specifics of what data will be shared, with whom, and by what means have not been clearly delineated. As recommended in this report, these details are key to the success of any data sharing program.

In addition, medical journals could help address challenges to responsible sharing of clinical trial data, particularly concerns about the usefulness and validity of secondary analyses of shared data. Journals could require authors of papers using shared clinical trial data sets to agree to make the analytic data set supporting their findings, tables, and figures available, similar to requirements for authors of primary analyses of clinical trial data. In addition, journals might require authors submitting secondary analyses for publication to explain how their analytic approach differs from that of the primary analysis. Such an explanation would help reviewers and editors of submitted manuscripts and readers of published articles assess the validity of the secondary analyses and compare them with the primary analysis by the clinical trial team. Moreover, this requirement would discourage secondary analyses based on scientifically invalid analysis plans—for example, because they entail carrying out multiple analyses using statistically inappropriate methods.

PROFESSIONAL SOCIETIES

Physicians' professional societies can play a role in setting standards and establishing norms for data sharing. Most societies have an official journal (e.g., the American Medical Association's *Journal of the American Medical Association*, the American College of Physicians' *Annals of Internal Medicine*, and the American Heart Association's *Circulation*), and investigators commonly present abstracts of clinical trials at the societies' annual meetings. "Late-breaking" abstracts of clinical trials often attract considerable press coverage, as occurred with the recent clinical trial of the use of ezetimibe plus simvastatin in patients with acute coronary syndrome (Kolata, 2014; Peck, 2014; Vaczek, 2014). Moreover, professional societies often convene committees to develop evidence-based clinical practice guidelines, consistent with their mission to improve the evidence base upon which members make clinical decisions for patients.

Professional societies could require that authors in their official journals follow the recommendations in this report for responsible sharing of clinical trial data and that investigators submitting and presenting abstracts at their meetings agree to do so when they publish their clinical trial findings. Members of professional societies commonly take the lead in designing and carrying out clinical trials in their specialty. At annual meetings, professional societies could hold workshops on the sharing of clinical trial data. In these ways, professional societies could set expectations for responsible sharing of clinical trial data in their professional codes for members. Finally, professional organizations could help develop common data elements for clinical trials in their specialty and advocate for the use of those data elements in clinical trials.

RECOMMENDATION

The committee concluded that although no one stakeholder alone can achieve the benefits of the sharing of clinical trial data and minimize its risks, all stakeholders have a role and responsibility in responsible sharing of clinical trial data.

Recommendation 1: Stakeholders in clinical trials should foster a culture in which data sharing is the expected norm, and should commit to responsible strategies aimed at maximizing the benefits, minimizing the risks, and overcoming the challenges of sharing clinical trial data for all parties.

Funders and sponsors should
- promote the development of a sustainable infrastructure and mechanism by which data can be shared, in accordance with the terms and conditions of grants and contracts;
- provide funding to investigators for sharing of clinical trial data as a line item in grants and contracts;
- include prior data sharing as a measure of impact when deciding about future funding;
- include and enforce requirements in the terms and conditions of grants and contracts that investigators will make clinical trial data available for sharing under the conditions recommended in this report; and
- fund and promote the development and adoption of common data elements.

Disease advocacy organizations should
- require data sharing plans as part of protocol reviews and criteria for funding grants;
- provide guidance and educational programs on data sharing for clinical trial participants;
- require data sharing plans as a condition for promoting clinical trials to their constituents; and
- contribute funding to enable data sharing.

Regulatory and research oversight bodies should
- work with industry and other stakeholders to develop and harmonize new clinical study report (CSR) templates that do not include commercially confidential information or personally identifiable data;

- work with regulatory authorities around the world to harmonize requirements and practices to support the responsible sharing of clinical trial data; and
- issue clear guidance that the sharing of clinical trial data is expected and that the role of Research Ethics Committees or Institutional Review Boards (IRBs) is to encourage and facilitate the responsible and ethical conduct of data sharing through the adoption of protections such as those recommended by this committee and the emerging best practices of clinical trial data sharing initiatives.

Research Ethics Committees or IRBs should

- provide guidance for clinical trialists and templates for informed consent for participants that enable responsible data sharing;
- consider data sharing plans when assessing the benefits and risks of clinical trials; and
- adopt protections for participants as recommended by this committee and the emerging best practices of clinical trial data sharing initiatives.

Investigators and sponsors should

- design clinical trials and manage trial data with the expectation that data will be shared;
- adopt common data elements in new clinical trial protocols unless there is a compelling scientific reason not to do so;
- explain to participants during the informed consent process
  - what data will (and will not) be shared with the individual participants during and after the trial,
  - the potential risks to privacy associated with the collection and sharing of data during and after the trial and a summary of the types of protections employed to mitigate this risk, and
  - under what conditions the trial data may be shared (with regulators, investigators, etc.) beyond the trial team; and
- make clinical trial data available at the times and under the conditions recommended in this report.

Research institutions and universities should

- ensure that investigators from their institutions share data from clinical trials in accordance with the recommendations in this report and the terms and conditions of grants and contracts;
- promote the development of a sustainable infrastructure and mechanisms for data sharing;
- make sharing of clinical trial data a consideration in promotion of faculty members and assessment of programs; and

- provide training for data science and quantitative scientists to facilitate sharing and analysis of clinical trial data.

Journals should
- require authors of both primary and secondary analyses of clinical trial data to
  - document that they have submitted a data sharing plan at a site that shares data with and meets the data requirements of the World Health Organization's International Clinical Trials Registry Platform before enrolling participants, and
  - commit to releasing the analytic data set underlying published analyses, tables, figures, and results no later than the times specified in this report;
- require that submitted manuscripts using existing data sets from clinical trials, in whole or in part, cite these data appropriately; and
- require that any published secondary analyses provide the data and metadata at the same level as in the original publication.

Membership and professional societies should
- establish policies that members should participate in sharing clinical trial data as part of their professional responsibilities;
- require as a condition of submitting abstracts to a meeting of the society and manuscripts to the journal of the society that clinical trial data will be shared in accordance with the recommendations in this report; and
- collaborate on and promote the development and use of common data elements relevant to their members.

REFERENCES

Adams, B. 2014. *Intermune drops EMA lawsuit over data release.* http://www.pharmafile.com/news/187640/intermune-drops-ema-lawsuit-over-data-release (accessed October 27, 2014).

AdvaMed. 2013. *Re: Docket no. FDA-2013-N-0271: Availability of masked and de-identified non-summary safety and efficacy data; request for comments; notice.* http://advamed.org/res.download/346 (accessed December 8, 2014).

Aid Transparency Index. 2014. *The Bill and Melinda Gates Foundation.* http://ati.publishwhatyoufund.org/donor/gates (accessed November 25, 2014).

American Cancer Society. 2014. *American Cancer Society clinical trials matching service.* http://www.cancer.org/treatment/treatmentsandsideeffects/clinicaltrials/app/clinical-trials-matching-service (accessed October 15, 2014).

Anturane Reinfarction Trial Policy Committee. 1982. The Anturane Reinfarction Trial: Re-evaluation of outcome. *New England Journal of Medicine* 306(16):1005-1008.

Anturane Reinfarction Trial Research Group. 1980. Sulfinpyrazone in the prevention of sudden death after myocardial infarction. The Anturane Reinfarction Trial Research Group. *New England Journal of Medicine* 302(5):250-256.

Barocas, S., and H. Nissenbaum. 2014. Big data's end run around anonymity and consent. In *Privacy, big data, and the public good: Frameworks for engagement*, edited by J. Lane, V. Stodden, S. Bender, and H. Nissenbaum. New York: Cambridge University Press. Pp. 44-75.

Baron, J. A., R. S. Sandler, R. S. Bresalier, A. Lanas, D. G. Morton, R. Riddell, E. R. Iverson, and D. L. DeMets. 2008. Cardiovascular events associated with rofecoxib: Final analysis of the approve trial. *Lancet* 372(9651):1756-1764.

Benatar, S. R. 2002. Reflections and recommendations on research ethics in developing countries. *Social Science & Medicine* 54(7):1131-1141.

Bierer, B. E. 2014. *Guiding principles for clinical trial data sharing*. Paper presented at IOM Committee on Strategies for Responsible Sharing of Clinical Trial Data: Meeting Two, February 3-4, Washington, DC.

The Bill & Melinda Gates Foundation. 2014. *Open access policy*. http://www.gatesfoundation. org/how-we-work/general-information/open-access-policy (accessed December 10, 2014).

Bonham, A. 2014. *Cultural and financial incentives for data sharing: Recognition and promotion*. Paper presented at IOM Committee on Strategies for Responsible Sharing of Clinical Trial Data: Meeting Two, February 3-4, Washington, DC.

Bourne, P. E. 2014. What big data means to me. *Journal of the American Medical Informatics Association* 21(2):194.

Brent, D. A. 2004. Antidepressants and pediatric depression—the risk of doing nothing. *New England Journal of Medicine* 351(16):1598-1601.

Bresalier, R. S., R. S. Sandler, H. Quan, J. A. Bolognese, B. Oxenius, K. Horgan, C. Lines, R. Riddell, D. Morton, A. Lanas, M. A. Konstam, and J. A. Baron. 2005. Cardiovascular events associated with rofecoxib in a colorectal adenoma chemoprevention trial. *New England Journal of Medicine* 352(11):1092-1102.

Canner, P. L. 1991. Covariate adjustment of treatment effects in clinical trials. *Controlled Clinical Trials* 12(3):359-366.

CFF (Cystic Fibrosis Foundation). 2013. *TDN protocol review process*. http://www.cff.org/ research/TDN/WorkingWithTDN/ProtocolReview (accessed October 15, 2014).

CFF. 2014. *Therapeutics development centers*. http://www.cff.org/research/TDN/Therapeutics DevelopmentCenters (accessed October 15, 2014).

Chan, A. W., F. J. Song, A. Vickers, T. Jefferson, K. Dickersin, P. C. Gotzsche, H. M. Krumholz, D. Ghersi, and H. B. van der Worp. 2014. Increasing value and reducing waste: Addressing inaccessible research. *Lancet* 383(9913):257-266.

CIOMS (Council for International Organizations of Medical Sciences). 2002. *International ethical guidelines for biomedical research involving human subjects*. Geneva: CIOMS.

Cochrane Neuraminidase Inhibitors Review Team. 2011. Does oseltamivir really reduce complications of influenza? *Clinical Infectious Diseases: An Official Publication of the Infectious Diseases Society of America* 53(12):1302-1303.

Collins, F. S., and L. A. Tabak. 2014. Policy: NIH plans to enhance reproducibility. *Nature* 505(7485):612-613.

Collyar, D. 2013. *What patients want from clinical trials—results from data!* Paper presented at IOM Committee on Strategies for Responsible Sharing of Clinical Trial Data: Meeting One, October 22-23, Washington, DC.

Contreras, J. 2011. Bermuda's legacy: Policy, patents, and the design of the genome commons. *Minnesota Journal of Law, Science & Technology* 12:61-125.

Corbie-Smith, G., S. B. Thomas, M. V. Williams, and S. Moody-Ayers. 1999. Attitudes and beliefs of African Americans toward participation in medical research. *Journal of General Internal Medicine* 14(9):537-546.

The Coronary Drug Project Research Group. 1980. Influence of adherence to treatment and response of cholesterol on mortality in the coronary drug project. *New England Journal of Medicine* 303(18):1038-1041.

Coxib and Traditional NSAID Trialists' (CNT's) Collaboration. 2013. Vascular and upper gastrointestinal effects of non-steroidal anti-inflammatory drugs: Meta-analyses of individual participant data from randomised trials. *Lancet* 382(9894):769-779.

Davidson, M. 2010. *Help today, help tomorrow is goal of MDA's Duchenne Clinical Research Network.* http://quest.mda.org/article/help-today-help-tomorrow-goal-mdas-duchenne-clinical-research-network (accessed October 15, 2014).

Dawson, L., and N. E. Kass. 2005. Views of US researchers about informed consent in international collaborative research. *Social Science & Medicine* 61(6):1211-1222.

De Angelis, C., J. M. Drazen, F. A. Frizelle, C. Haug, J. Hoey, R. Horton, S. Kotzin, C. Laine, A. Marusic, A. J. Overbeke, T. V. Schroeder, H. C. Sox, and M. B. Van Der Weyden. 2004. Clinical trial registration: A statement from the International Committee of Medical Journal Editors. *Canadian Medical Association Journal* 171(6):606-607.

Diamond, G. A., L. Bax, and S. Kaul. 2007. Uncertain effects of rosiglitazone on the risk for myocardial infarction and cardiovascular death. *Annals of Internal Medicine* 147(8):578-581.

Dickersin, K. 2013. *Principles of responsible data sharing.* Paper presented at IOM Committee on Strategies for Responsible Sharing of Clinical Trial Data: Meeting One, October 22-23, Washington, DC.

DOJ (U.S. Department of Justice). 2004. *Warner-Lambert to pay $430 million to resolve criminal and civil health care liability relating to off-label promotion.* Washington, DC: DOJ.

DOJ. 2012. *GlaxoSmithKline to plead guilty and pay $3 billion to resolve fraud allegations and failure to report safety data.* http://www.justice.gov/opa/pr/glaxosmithkline-plead-guilty-and-pay-3-billion-resolve-fraud-allegations-and-failure-report (accessed December 8, 2014).

Doshi, P., K. Dickersin, D. Healy, S. S. Vedula, and T. Jefferson. 2013. Restoring invisible and abandoned trials: A call for people to publish the findings. *British Medical Journal* 346:f2865.

Dwork, C. 2014. Differential privacy: A cryptographic approach to private data analysis. In *Privacy, big data, and the public good,* edited by J. Lane, V. Stodden, S. Bender, and H. Nissenbaum. New York: Cambridge University Press. Pp. 296-322.

EAGDA (Expert Advisory Group on Data Access). 2014. *Establishing incentives and changing cultures to support data access.* http://www.wellcome.ac.uk/stellent/groups/corporatesite/@msh_peda/documents/web_document/wtp056495.pdf (accessed December 16, 2014).

Eisenberg, R., and A. Rai. 2006. Harnessing and sharing the benefits of state sponsored research. *Berkeley Technology Law Journal* 21:1187-1213.

Ellenberg, S. S., T. R. Fleming, and D. L. DeMets. 2002. *Data monitoring committees in clinical trials: A practical perspective.* West Sussex, England: John Wiley & Sons.

EMA (European Medicines Agency). 2013. *Publication and access to clinical-trial data.* http://www.ema.europa.eu/docs/en_GB/document_library/Other/2013/06/WC500144730.pdf (accessed October 15, 2014).

EMA. 2014a. *Clinical trials in human medicines.* http://www.ema.europa.eu/ema/index.jsp?curl=pages/special_topics/general/general_content_000489.jsp&mid=WC0b01ac058060676f (accessed October 17, 2014).

EMA. 2014b. *European Medicines Agency policy on publication of clinical data for medicinal products for human use.* http://www.ema.europa.eu/docs/en_GB/document_library/Other/2014/10/WC500174796.pdf (accessed October 27, 2014).

EMA. 2014c. *Finalisation of the EMA policy on publication of and access to clinical trial data—targeted consultation with key stakeholders in May 2014.* http://www.ema.europa.eu/docs/en_GB/document_library/Report/2014/09/WC500174226.pdf (accessed October 17, 2014).

EMA. 2014d. *Publication and access to clinical data: An inclusive development process.* http://www.ema.europa.eu/ema/index.jsp?curl=pages/special_topics/general/general_content_000556.jsp (accessed October 24, 2014).

EMA. 2014e. *Release of data from clinical trials.* http://www.ema.europa.eu/ema/index.jsp?curl=pages/special_topics/general/general_content_000555.jsp&mid=WC0b01ac0580607bfa (accessed October 14, 2014).

EUREC (European Network of Research Ethics Committees). 2014. *European Network of Research Ethics Committees—EUREC.* http://www.eurecnet.org/index.html (accessed December 8, 2014).

FDA (U.S. Food and Drug Administration). 1996. *Guideline for industry: Structure and content of clinical study reports.* http://www.fda.gov/downloads/drugs/guidancecompliance regulatoryinformation/guidances/ucm073113.pdf (accessed October 17, 2014).

FDA. 2011a. *Detailed description of clinical trials database.* http://www.fda.gov/AboutFDA/CentersOffices/OfficeofMedicalProductsandTobacco/CDRH/CDRHTransparency/ucm208389.htm (accessed October 29, 2014).

FDA. 2011b. *Guidance for industry: User fee waivers, reductions, and refunds for drug and biological products.* http://www.fda.gov/downloads/Drugs/GuidanceComplianceRegulatory Information/Guidances/ucm079298.pdf (accessed October 24, 2014).

FDA. 2014. *A guide to informed consent—information sheet.* http://www.fda.gov/Regulatory Information/Guidances/ucm126431.htm (accessed October 17, 2014).

FDASIA (Food and Drug Administration Safety and Innovation Act). 2013. *Small business report to Congress.* http://www.fda.gov/downloads/RegulatoryInformation/Legislation/FederalFoodDrugandCosmeticActFDCAct/SignificantAmendments totheFDCAct/FDASIA/UCM360058.pdf (accessed October 18, 2014).

Gaffney, A. 2013. *Device, pharmaceutical industries say FDA proposal to release trial data illegal.* http://www.raps.org/focus-online/news/news-article-view/article/4248/device-pharmaceutical-industries-say-fda-proposal-to-release-trial-data-illegal.aspx (accessed October 29, 2014).

Gibbons, R. D., C. H. Brown, K. Hur, J. M. Davis, and J. J. Mann. 2012. Suicidal thoughts and behavior with antidepressant treatment: Reanalysis of the randomized placebo-controlled studies of fluoxetine and venlafaxine. *Archives of General Psychiatry* 69(6):580-587.

The Global Health Network. 2014. *About The Global Health Network.* https://tghn.org/about (accessed December 11, 2014).

Godlee, F. 2009. We want raw data, now. *British Medical Journal* 339:b5405.

Godlee, F., and T. Groves. 2012. The new *BMJ* policy on sharing data from drug and device trials. *British Medical Journal* 345:e7888.

Greenwald, T. 2013. *Patients take control of their health care online.* http://www.technology review.com/news/518886/patients-take-control-of-their-health-care-online (accessed October 15, 2014).

Hammad, T. A., T. Laughren, and J. Racoosin. 2006. Suicidality in pediatric patients treated with antidepressant drugs. *Archives of General Psychiatry* 63(3):332-339.

Hernán, M. A., and M. Lipsitch. 2011a. Oseltamivir and risk of lower respiratory tract complications in patients with flu symptoms: A meta-analysis of eleven randomized clinical trials. *Clinical Infectious Diseases* 53(3):277-279.

Hernán, M. A., and M. Lipsitch. 2011b. Reply to Cochrane Neuraminidase Inhibitors Review Team. *Clinical Infectious Diseases: An Official Publication of the Infectious Diseases Society of America* 53(12):1303-1304.

Hesterlee, S. 2013. *Research participant perspectives.* Paper read at IOM Committee on Strategies for Responsible Sharing of Clinical Trial Data: Meeting One, October 22-23, Washington, DC.

HHS (U.S. Department of Health and Human Services). 2012. *Guidance regarding methods for de-identification of protected health information in accordance with the Health Insurance Portability and Accountability Act (HIPAA) Privacy Rule.* http://www.hhs.gov/ocr/privacy/hipaa/understanding/coveredentities/De-identification/guidance.html (accessed October 15, 2014).

HHS. 2014a. *Federal policy for the protection of human subjects ("Common Rule").* http://www.hhs.gov/ohrp/humansubjects/commonrule (accessed October 17, 2014).

HHS. 2014b. *Informed consent.* http://www.hhs.gov/ohrp/policy/consent (accessed October 17, 2014).

Hudson, K. 2013. *Strategies for responsible sharing of clinical trial data: NIH perspective.* Paper presented at IOM Committee on Strategies for Responsible Sharing of Clinical Trial Data: Meeting One, October 22-23, Washington, DC.

Hudson, K. L., and F. S. Collins. 2014. Sharing and reporting the results of clinical trials. *Journal of the American Medical Association.* http://dx.doi.org/10.1001/jama.2014.10716 (accessed December 10, 2014).

i2b2 (Informatics for Integrating Biology and the Bedside). 2014. *About us.* https://www.i2b2.org/about/index.html (accessed December 8, 2014).

ICH (International Conference on Harmonisation of Technical Requirements for Registration of Pharmaceuticals for Human Use). 1996. *Guideline for good clinical practice E6(R1).* http://www.ich.org/fileadmin/Public_Web_Site/ICH_Products/Guidelines/Efficacy/E6/E6_R1_Guideline.pdf (accessed December 16, 2014).

IOM (Institute of Medicine). 2009. *Beyond the HIPAA Privacy Rule: Enhancing privacy, improving health through research.* Washington, DC: The National Academies Press.

IOM. 2010. *Transforming clinical research in the United States: Challenges and opportunities: Workshop summary.* Washington, DC: The National Academies Press.

IOM. 2013. *Sharing clinical research data: Workshop summary.* Washington, DC: The National Academies Press.

JDRF (Juvenile Diabetes Research Foundation). 2014. *To find a cure, JDRF needs people with type 1 diabetes to consider participation in human clinical trials of experimental new therapies.* https://trials.jdrf.org/patient (accessed October 15, 2014).

Kahn, M. G., and C. Weng. 2012. Clinical research informatics: A conceptual perspective. *Journal of the American Medical Informatics Association* 19(e1):e36-e42.

Kolata, G. 2014. Study finds alternative to anti-cholesterol drug. *The New York Times,* http://www.nytimes.com/2014/11/18/health/study-finds-alternative-to-statins-in-preventing-heart-attacks-and-strokes.html?_r=1 (accessed December 8, 2014).

Krumholz, H. M., C. P. Gross, K. L. Blount, J. D. Ritchie, B. Hodshon, R. Lehman, and J. S. Ross. 2014. Sea change in open science and data sharing: Leadership by industry. *Circulation: Cardiovascular Quality and Outcomes* 7(4):499-504.

Lagakos, S. W. 2006. Time-to-event analyses for long-term treatments—the APPROVe trial. *New England Journal of Medicine* 355(2):113-117.

Laine, C., S. N. Goodman, M. E. Griswold, and H. C. Sox. 2007. Reproducible research: Moving toward research the public can really trust. *Annals of Internal Medicine* 146(6):450-453.

Landy, D. C., M. A. Brinich, M. E. Colten, E. J. Horn, S. F. Terry, and R. R. Sharp. 2012. How disease advocacy organizations participate in clinical research: A survey of genetic organizations. *Genetics in Medicine* 14(2):223-228.

Lanthier, M., K. L. Miller, C. Nardinelli, and J. Woodcock. 2013. An improved approach to measuring drug innovation finds steady rates of first-in-class pharmaceuticals, 1987-2011. *Health Affairs (Millwood)* 32(8):1433-1439.

Lu, C. Y., F. Zhang, M. D. Lakoma, J. M. Madden, D. Rusinak, R. B. Penfold, G. Simon, B. K. Ahmedani, G. Clarke, E. M. Hunkeler, B. Waitzfelder, A. Owen-Smith, M. A. Raebel, R. Rossom, K. J. Coleman, L. A. Copeland, and S. B. Soumerai. 2014. Changes in antidepressant use by young people and suicidal behavior after FDA warnings and media coverage: Quasi-experimental study. *British Medical Journal* 348:g3596.

MalariaGen. 2014a. *About the malaria genomic epidemiology network.* http://www.malariagen. net/about (accessed December 10, 2014).

MalariaGen. 2014b. *Funding.* http://www.malariagen.net/about/funding (accessed November 25, 2014).

Mansell, P. 2014. *AbbVie strikes compromise with EMA on data disclosure.* http://www. pharmatimes.com/article/14-04-08/AbbVie_strikes_compromise_with_EMA_on_ data_disclosure.aspx (accessed May 22, 2014).

Marcus, A. D. 2012. *Frustrated ALS patients concoct their own drug.* http://online.wsj.com/ news/articles/SB10001424052702304818404577345953943484054 (accessed October 15, 2014).

May, G. S., D. L. DeMets, L. M. Friedman, C. Furberg, and E. Passamani. 1981. The randomized clinical trial: Bias in analysis. *Circulation* 64(4):669-673.

MHRA (Medicines and Healthcare Products Regulatory Agency). 2003. *Safety review of antidepressants used by children completed.* http://www.mhra.gov.uk/PrintPreview/ PressReleaseSP/CON002045 (accessed December 8, 2013).

Michiels, B., K. Van Puyenbroeck, V. Verhoeven, E. Vermeire, and S. Coenen. 2013. The value of neuraminidase inhibitors for the prevention and treatment of seasonal influenza: A systematic review of systematic reviews. *PLoS ONE* 8(4):e60348.

Molyneux, C. S., N. Peshu, and K. Marsh. 2005. Trust and informed consent: Insights from community members on the Kenyan coast. *Social Science & Medicine* 61(7):1463-1473.

Newman, T. B. 2004. A black-box warning for antidepressants in children? *New England Journal of Medicine* 351(16):1595-1598.

NIH (U.S. National Institutes of Health). 2003. *Final NIH statement on sharing research data.* http://grants1.nih.gov/grants/guide/notice-files/NOT-OD-03-032.html (accessed October 14, 2014).

NIH. 2014a. *Clinical and translational science awards.* http://www.ncats.nih.gov/research/ cts/ctsa/ctsa.html (accessed October 24, 2014).

NIH. 2014b. *NIH issues finalized policy on genomic data sharing.* http://www.nih.gov/news/ health/aug2014/od-27.htm (accessed October 14, 2014).

NIH. 2014c. *Public access policy.* http://publicaccess.nih.gov (accessed October 24, 2014).

NIH issues genomic data sharing policy. 2014. *Nature Biotechnology* 32(10):966-966.

Nissen, S. E. 2006. Adverse cardiovascular effects of rofecoxib. *New England Journal of Medicine* 355(2):203-205.

Nissen, S. E., and K. Wolski. 2007. Effect of rosiglitazone on the risk of myocardial infarction and death from cardiovascular causes. *New England Journal of Medicine* 356(24):2457-2471.

NRC (National Research Council). 2012. *For attribution—developing data attribution and citation practices and standards: Summary of an international workshop.* Washington, DC: The National Academies Press.

Nussenblatt, R. B., and C. L. Meinert. 2010. The status of clinical trials: Cause for concern. *Journal of Translational Medicine* 8:65.

Olivas, R. 2014. *International consortium provides $2m funding for phase 1 clinical trial of ReveraGen DMD drug.* http://mda.org/media/press-releases/international-consortium-provides-2m-funding-phase-1-clinical-trial-reveragen (accessed October 15, 2014).

O'Rourke, P. P., and D. Forster. 2014. *Considerations of informed consent in the discussion of clinical trial data sharing—domestic issues.* Paper presented at IOM Committee on Strategies for Responsible Sharing of Clinical Trial Data: Meeting Two, February 3-4, Washington, DC.

Peck, P. 2014. AHA: Improve-it proves ezetimibe benefit. *MedPage Today,* www.medpage today.com/MeetingCoverage/AHA/48637 (accessed December 8, 2014).

PhRMA (Pharmaceutical Research and Manufacturers of America) and EFPIA (European Federation of Pharmaceutical Industries and Associations). 2013. *Principles for responsible clinical trial data sharing: Our commitment to patients and researchers.* http://www.phrma.org/sites/default/files/pdf/PhRMAPrinciplesForResponsibleClinicalTrial DataSharing.pdf (accessed October 16, 2014).

Privacy International. 2014. *The state of privacy.* https://www.privacyinternational.org/sites/privacyinternational.org/files/file-downloads/state-of-privacy_2014.pdf (accessed October 17, 2014).

Psaty, B. M., and R. A. Kronmal. 2008. Reporting mortality findings in trials of rofecoxib for Alzheimer disease or cognitive impairment: A case study based on documents from rofecoxib litigation. *Journal of the American Medical Association* 299(15):1813-1817.

Ramers-Verhoeven, C. W., F. Perrone, and K. Oliver. 2014. Exploratory research into cancer patients' attitudes to clinical trials. *Ecancermedicalscience* 8:432.

Reidpath, D. D., and P. A. Allotey. 2001. Data sharing in medical research: An empirical investigation. *Bioethics* 15(2):125-134.

Retzer, K., J. Lopatowska, and C. Rich. 2011. *Navigating the sea of data protection in European clinical research.* http://media.mofo.com/files/Uploads/Images/111201-Data-Privacy-SRC.pdf (accessed October 31, 2014).

Rosenblatt, M. 2014. Cultural and Financial Incentives for Data Sharing—Recognition and Promotion. Discussion Panel at IOM Committee on Strategies for Responsible Sharing of Clinical Trial Data: Meeting Two, February 3-4, Washington, DC.

Ross, J. S., T. Tse, D. A. Zarin, H. Xu, L. Zhou, and H. M. Krumholz. 2012. Publication of NIH funded trials registered in ClinicalTrials.gov: Cross sectional analysis. *British Medical Journal* 344:d7292.

Royal Society. 2012. *Science as an open enterprise.* London: Royal Society.

Share alike. 2014. *Nature* 507(7491):140-140.

Shoulson, I. 2014. *Cultural and financial incentives for data sharing: Recognition and promotion.* Paper presented at IOM Committee on Strategies for Responsible Sharing of Clinical Trial Data: Meeting Two, February 3-4, Washington, DC.

Silva, L. 2014. PLOS' new data policy: Public access to data. *The PLoS ONE Community Blog,* http://blogs.plos.org/everyone/2014/02/24/plos-new-data-policy-public-access-data-2 (accessed October 29, 2014).

Singh, J. A., and E. J. Mills. 2005. The abandoned trials of pre-exposure prophylaxis for HIV: What went wrong? *PLoS Medicine* 2(9):e234.

Stewart, L. A., and J. F. Tierney. 2002. To IPD or not to IPD?: Advantages and disadvantages of systematic reviews using individual patient data. *Evaluation & the Health Professions* 25(1):76-97.

Temple, R., and G. W. Pledger. 1980. The FDA's critique of the anturane reinfarction trial. *New England Journal of Medicine* 303(25):1488-1492.

Tenopir, C., S. Allard, K. Douglass, A. U. Aydinoglu, L. Wu, E. Read, M. Manoff, and M. Frame. 2011. Data sharing by scientists: Practices and perceptions. *PLoS ONE* 6(6):e21101.

Terry, S. F., and P. F. Terry. 2011. Power to the people: Participant ownership of clinical trial data. *Science Translational Medicine* 3(69):69cm63.

Thackray, S., K. Witte, A. L. Clark, and J. G. Cleland. 2000. Clinical trials update: OPTIME-CHF, PRAISE-2, ALL-HAT. *European Journal of Heart Failure* 2(2):209-212.

Tucker, M. E. 2013. FDA panel advises easing restrictions on rosiglitazone. *British Medical Journal* 346:f3769.

Turner, E. H., A. M. Matthews, E. Linardatos, R. A. Tell, and R. Rosenthal. 2008. Selective publication of antidepressant trials and its influence on apparent efficacy. *New England Journal of Medicine* 358(3):252-260.

Vaczek, D. 2014. Merck's IMPROVE-IT trial hits big, supports wider Zetia use. *Medical Marketing & Media*, http://www.mmm-online.com/mercks-improve-it-trial-hits-big-supports-wider-zetia-use/article/383761 (accessed December 8, 2014).

Van Noorden, R. 2014. Gates Foundation announces world's strongest policy on open access research. *Nature News Blog*, http://blogs.nature.com/news/2014/11/gates-foundation-announces-worlds-strongest-policy-on-open-access-research.html (accessed November 25, 2014).

Vedula, S. S., L. Bero, R. W. Scherer, and K. Dickersin. 2009. Outcome reporting in industry-sponsored trials of gabapentin for off-label use. *New England Journal of Medicine* 361(20):1963-1971.

Wallentin, L., R. C. Becker, C. P. Cannon, C. Held, A. Himmelmann, S. Husted, S. K. James, H. S. Katus, K. W. Mahaffey, K. S. Pieper, R. F. Storey, P. G. Steg, and R. A. Harrington. 2014. Review of the accumulated PLATO documentation supports reliable and consistent superiority of ticagrelor over clopidogrel in patients with acute coronary syndrome. Commentary on: DiNicolantonio JJ, Tomek A, Inactivations, deletions, non-adjudications, and downgrades of clinical endpoints on ticagrelor: Serious concerns over the reliability of the PLATO trial, International Journal of Cardiology, 2013. *International Journal of Cardiology* 170(3):E59-E62.

Wathion, N., and EMA. 2014. *Finalisation of EMA policy on publication of and access to clinical trial data.* http://www.eucope.org/en/files/2014/05/2014-05-Finalisation-of-EMA-policy-on-CT-data-Mtgs-with-stakeholders.pdf (accessed December 16, 2014).

Wedel, H., D. DeMets, P. Deedwania, B. Fagerberg, S. Goldstein, S. Gottlieb, A. Hjalmarson, J. Kjekshus, F. Waagstein, and J. Wikstrand. 2001. Challenges of subgroup analyses in multinational clinical trials: Experiences from the MERIT-HF trial. *American Heart Journal* 142(3):502-511.

The Wellcome Trust. 2014a. *Funding.* http://www.wellcome.ac.uk/Funding/index.htm (accessed December 10, 2014).

The Wellcome Trust. 2014b. *Open access policy.* http://www.wellcome.ac.uk/About-us/Policy/Policy-and-position-statements/WTD002766.htm (accessed November 25, 2014).

WHO (World Health Organization). 2009. *Casebook on ethical issues in international health research.* http://whqlibdoc.who.int/publications/2009/9789241547727_eng.pdf (accessed December 8, 2014).

WHO. 2013. *Research for universal health coverage: World health report 2013.* Geneva: WHO.

Zarin, D. A. 2013. *Trial transparency.* Paper presented at IOM Committee on Strategies for Responsible Sharing of Clinical Trial Data: Meeting One, October 22-23, Washington, DC.

4

The Clinical Trial Life Cycle
and When to Share Data

During the course of a clinical trial, different types of data are collected, transformed into analyzable data sets to address specific research questions, and used to generate various publications and reports for different audiences (Drazen, 2002).

Publication in peer-reviewed scientific journals is currently the primary method for sharing clinical trial data with the scientific and medical communities, as well as the public (often through media coverage of published findings). These publications, however, contain only a small subset of the data collected, produced, and analyzed in the course of a trial (Doshi et al., 2013; Zarin, 2013).

Clinical trial sponsors seeking regulatory approval from authorities such as the U.S. Food and Administration (FDA) and the European Medicines Agency (EMA) must submit detailed clinical study reports (CSRs) and individual participant data, which form the basis for the marketing application for a product. In trials that are not part of a regulatory submission, detailed CSRs may or may not be prepared (Doshi et al., 2012; Teden, 2013).

Beyond the selected clinical trial data that are disclosed in journal publications, individual participant data and metadata (i.e., "data about the data") have not been shared routinely with the broader scientific community or the public. As stated in previous chapters, however, an increasing number of organizations are taking the initiative to share their data more actively, and the committee believes the time is right to make recommendations for responsible sharing of clinical trial data that will increase the availability and usefulness of the data while mitigating the risks outlined in Chapter 2. The committee acknowledges that no single body or authority in the global clinical trials ecosystem has the power to enforce the recommendation offered at the end of this chapter on what data to share and when. Moreover, the committee recognizes that no single solution will fit all clinical trials, and there will be exceptions to any proposed recommendations. The risks and benefits of sharing data may vary depending on the context and purpose of a trial and/or the particular type of data to be shared. Thus, there will be instances when it is reasonable for data to be shared either sooner or later than would generally be expected. The committee interpreted its charge as helping to establish professional standards and set expectations for responsible sharing of clinical trial data, together with requirements to be imposed by supporting organizations such as funders, medical journals, and professional societies, rather than suggesting new laws and regulations.

Many discussions of the sharing of clinical trial data to date have failed to specify which of the many clinical trial data elements or data sets might be shared at different time points in the life cycle of a trial. To address this shortcoming, this chapter briefly describes the major stages of the clinical trial life cycle and then offers specific definitions and descriptions of the individual participant data, metadata, and summary data that are generated at each stage. It then examines the benefits and risks associated with sharing the various types of data generated and presents the committee's recommendation for when to share specific data packages in common scenarios such as after publication or regulatory application, as well as the case of sharing data with participants themselves.

THE CLINICAL TRIAL LIFE CYCLE

Data are generated at nearly every stage of the clinical trial life cycle, from the initial protocol and statistical analysis plan prepared prior to registration, to the collection of baseline participant data at participant enrollment, to the analysis of the analyzable data set. To help frame the discussion of what data should be shared at what times, the committee conceptualized the clinical trial life cycle as consisting of five major stages (see Figure 4-1):

1. **Trial design and registration:** Clinical trials are carefully designed; the protocol[1] for conducting the trial and the statistical analysis

---

[1] The protocol is approved by a Research Ethics Committee (in the United States, an Institutional Review Board [IRB]) and explained to participants through the informed consent process.

plan (SAP) detailing the planned data analyses are developed well before the first participant is enrolled. The protocol and the SAP constitute some of the most important metadata of the trial. During the course of a trial, the protocols and the SAP generally undergo amendments, which should be explicitly documented within the protocol and the SAP. Since 2004, the International Committee of Medical Journal Editors (ICMJE) has required that all trials be registered prior to participant enrollment as a condition for consideration of publication (De Angelis et al., 2004). In 2006, the World Health Organization's (WHO's) International Clinical Trials Registry Platform identified a set of 20 data elements for all trials to include in registration. These 20 elements, along with narrative summaries of the protocol, make up the registration elements in Figure 4-1 (Sim et al., 2006).

2. **Participant enrollment:** Clinical trial data originate from patients and healthy volunteers who participate in studies. Raw data are collected between the time of first participant enrollment and study completion. During the course of the trial, the raw data are abstracted, coded, and transcribed. After participant activities have ended, the data are cleaned into an analyzable data set. Both the raw data and the analyzable data set are individual participant data.

3. **Study completion:** For the purposes of this report, study completion is defined as either "the study has concluded normally; participants are no longer being examined or treated," or the study has been terminated;[2] "recruiting or enrolling participants has halted prematurely and will not resume; participants are no longer being examined or treated" (ClinicalTrials.gov, 2012).[3] Although study completion is often referred to as "last participant's last visit" (European Union Clinical Trials Register, 2011), study completion may in fact include measurements that occur without face-to-face interaction between participants and investigators (e.g., data may be collected remotely using sensors or from medical records or reports by patients, or an endpoint such as death may occur after the last visit). After study completion, investigators and/or sponsors clean the data, derive additional variables, adjudicate endpoints, lock

---

[2] A study may be completed prematurely for various reasons: a Data Monitoring Committee/Data and Safety Monitoring Board may recommend termination to the sponsor on the basis of interim monitoring for ethical and scientific reasons, or the sponsor may decide to terminate the study for ethical, scientific, or business reasons.

[3] "STUDY COMPLETION DATE: The date that the final data for a clinical study were collected because the last study participant has made the final visit to the study location (that is, 'last subject, last visit'). The estimated study completion date is the date that researchers think will be the completion date for the study" (ClinicalTrials.gov, 2012).

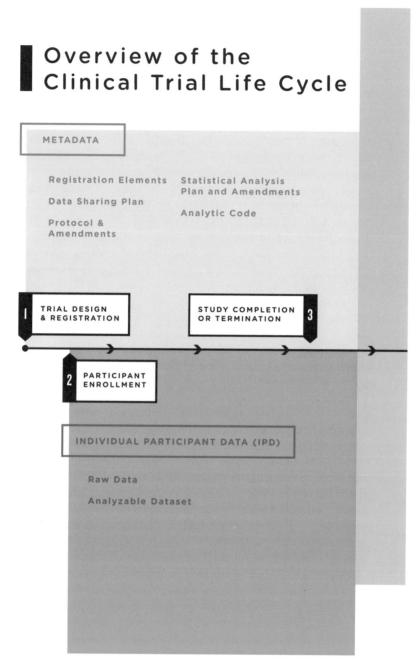

FIGURE 4-1 Overview of the clinical trial life cycle.

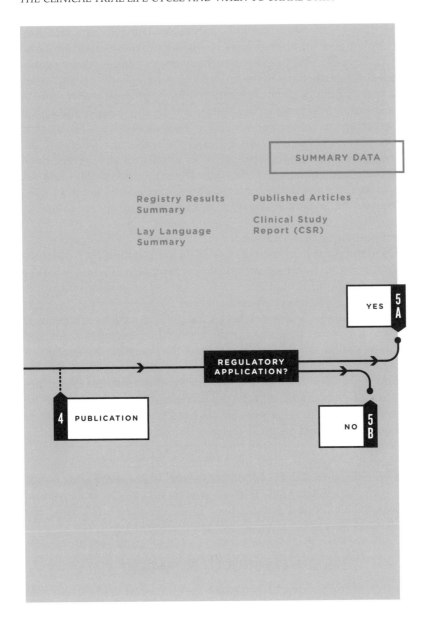

the data set to create the full analyzable data set, carry out pre-specified and additional analyses using software programs (the analytic code), and prepare manuscripts for publication. Investigators also can use parts of the analyzable data set to prepare analyses for presentations, data exploration, and hypothesis generation. A biostatistics best practice is to freeze a copy of whatever data were used in an analysis so the results can be repeated later if necessary. It is also desirable to store the analytic code that generated the results (i.e., the computer program), especially for any derived data.

4. **Publication:** A subset of the data from the analyzable data set is used to generate the tables, figures, and results for published articles. Publication may occur at any time during the course of the clinical trial life cycle, although it most often occurs after study completion. Several publications may result from one trial.

5. **Regulatory application:** Clinical trials are required by regulatory authorities in countries around the world before a new medical product can be brought to market, or before a new indication, formulation, or target population can be approved for an intervention already on the market (ICH, 1995). Analyses prespecified in the SAP form the basis for the CSR, which includes a detailed analysis of the study efficacy data and the complete adverse event data. After a product's introduction, additional clinical trials are commonly conducted by both industry and academia to further define the product's efficacy and safety. Clinical trials also are used to study interventions that do not involve regulated medical products, such as surgical techniques, behavioral interventions, means of improving disease management practice, or changes to a health care system (Califf, 2013).[4] Thus, as the committee examined what clinical trial data should be shared and when, it was useful to consider clinical trials in these two broad categories: (5a) those intended to support a regulatory application[5] and (5b) those not intended to support a regulatory application.

WHAT DATA SHOULD BE SHARED

This section further describes each of the above forms of clinical trial data and presents the committee's analysis of the benefits and risks of sharing each.

---

[4] As noted in Chapter 1, the scope of this study is limited to interventional clinical trials, as defined in Box 1-1.

[5] Whether or not the product or indication ultimately receives regulatory approval, is abandoned by the sponsor, or licensed to another entity.

Individual Participant Data

Raw Data

Raw data (sometimes called source data) are observations about individual participants used by the investigators. These data may be collected specifically for the study protocol or as part of routine care. At the source, these data may be in the form of measurements of participant characteristics such as weight, blood pressure, or heart rate and may be associated with the baseline (or initial) visit or subsequent follow-up visits. Raw data may also include a baseline description of the participant's medical history, physical exam information, clinical laboratory results (e.g., serum lipid values, hemoglobin levels), whole exome or genome sequences, imaging results (e.g., X-ray, magnetic resonance imaging [MRI]), procedure results (e.g., electroencephalogram [EKG], endoscopy), or self-reported data (e.g., symptoms, quality of life). Some data are derived or calculated from raw data (e.g., change in weight from baseline). Other data must be abstracted (i.e., interpreted) according to rules set forth in the protocol—for example, reading the X-ray for tumor size or evaluating the electrocardiogram (ECG) for evidence of a heart attack. Depending on the study under consideration, demographics, clinical outcome data, and other appropriate raw data are entered into case report forms. Some observations (e.g., imaging studies) are interpreted by study investigators—a process referred to as abstraction—and are entered into case report forms as transcribed narrative data or as coded data according to study guidelines (e.g., men may be coded as "1" and women as "0"). Abstracted data may also include assessments by clinical study staff or adjudication committees to determine whether specific clinical endpoints or adverse events (e.g., heart attack, cardiac death) meet protocol-specified criteria. In addition to physiologic and clinical measurements, other types of health data are increasingly being collected in clinical trials, including quantified sensor data (e.g., readings from remote monitoring devices, including smartphone apps), consumer genomics data (e.g., 23andMe), and participant-reported outcomes (e.g., PatientsLikeMe).

After collection, as well as derivation, assessment, abstraction, or adjudication as appropriate, data must be entered into an organized data management system (i.e., database) for further evaluation and processing. Data typically undergo a process of cleaning, quality assurance, and quality control to detect inconsistent, incomplete, or inaccurate entries, and to confirm that the data were collected and evaluated according to the protocol and match the source data. This process of data transcription continues over the course of the trial as data are collected and afterward.

The argument for sharing raw data is that raw data most closely reflect the study observations. The analyzable data set, by contrast, is the result of many decisions made by clinical trialists, as explained above. If there are errors, flaws, or biases in the processing of raw data, such problems will not necessarily be identified in the analyzable data set. Examples of the value of raw data include the detection of serious errors or biases as well as fraud uncovered by detailed and intense audits of raw data conducted by central statistical centers when inconsistencies or anomalies have been noted in analyzable data sets (Fisher et al., 1995; Soran et al., 2006; Temple and Pledger, 1980). Secondary researchers who have questions about the original analyses may therefore want the raw data to verify how the analytic data set was derived or to test alternative ways of deriving the variables in that data set. In other cases, sharing raw data can be extremely beneficial for additional research. For instance, the Alzheimer Disease Neuroimaging Initiative (ADNI) has published a number of important secondary analyses of a shared raw data set of images among a group of neuroscience investigators (ADNI, 2014; Bradshaw et al., 2013; Casanova et al., 2013; Haight et al., 2013).

However, there are strong arguments against sharing raw data routinely. Raw data sets are large and complex, include potentially sensitive individual participant data, and are not needed for most secondary analyses of shared clinical trial data. For example, raw data from MRI and computed tomography (CT) scans or genome sequences may be very large, require extensive documentation, and carry inherent privacy risks. The effort and cost of sharing such data routinely might better be spent on improved quality control and independent oversight of the data processing carried out during the course of a trial such that the analyzable data set can be shared with high levels of confidence in its integrity. These quality control processes should be documented and made available along with the analytic data set. If questions remained, investigators, sponsors, regulatory agencies, or external researchers could request "for cause" audits on a case-by-case basis.

Conclusion: For most trials sharing raw data would be overly burdensome and impractical; on a case-by-case basis, however, it would be beneficial to share raw data in response to reasonable requests.

Analyzable Data Set

Typically, after data have been entered in computerized form, new variables are generated mathematically to serve as the basis for later analyses. These variables are sometimes called "derived" variables. For example, patient age may not be entered directly but calculated by subtracting the birth date from the date of a given clinic visit, or "treatment response" may be entered as a mathematical comparison of lesion sizes recorded from two images. After the trial has been declared complete and the editing and cleaning process is done, the data are moved into an analyzable data file and locked (i.e., no further changes may be made). If the study is blinded (or masked), the treatment code file is typically merged with the analyzable data file after the latter has been locked, and the data are unblinded to the investigators. Some or all of this now-unblinded analyzable data set is then used for data analyses.[6] It is called analyzable rather than analyzed because a very large percentage of it is never used. The final cleaned and locked analyzable data set consists of various components (participant characteristics and primary outcome, prespecified secondary and tertiary outcomes, adverse event data, and exploratory data). A statistical analysis may involve a composite outcome using any of the various components. In addition, when data are missing, values may be imputed using this data set. Results are derived from data in the cleaned and locked analyzable data set, which have undergone statistical analysis.

The full analyzable data set is generally the most useful set of data to share from a trial, with large and likely important benefits to science and society. First, in most trials, as noted, large portions of the full analyzable data set are never analyzed and published. Sharing these data may increase the scientific return on the funder's investment in the trial and the benefits to the public and future patients. Second, sharing the full analyzable data set allows other investigators to reproduce the original analyses and carry out alternative, scientifically valid analyses of the primary study aim. Such additional analyses help determine how robust the original analyses are. Third, meta-analytic syntheses of the results of similar trials increase the statistical power for detecting effects and maximize the evidentiary value of the clinical trial knowledge base. Finally, sharing analyzable data allows for further scientific discovery through additional secondary analyses, as well as the conduct of exploratory research to general hypotheses for additional studies.

Sharing the full analyzable data set also poses risks, as described in Chapter 2. One risk is invalid secondary analyses and use of statistical techniques that are not scientifically accepted. A particular concern is that a secondary user will carry out multiple statistical analyses on a complex data set without adjusting for the increased likelihood that one association will be found to be significant at a p level of 0.05 by chance alone. A second concern is that the clinical trial team often plans to publish a series of secondary analyses, particularly in large clinical trials. Often junior members of the team who are assigned to be lead author on one of these

---

[6] Best practice is to conduct the analyses on blinded data with dummy codes representing treatment arms.

secondary analyses regard this authorship as a key opportunity for career advancement and a quid pro quo for the effort they put into working on the trial. The clinical trialists may fear that sharing the full analyzable data set will give other investigators who did not contribute to the conduct of the study an opportunity to publish additional analyses before the members of the study team have done so. A third risk is that the more detailed the information is in a data set, the easier it is to re-identify an individual in that data set, particularly if "side information" is included (Dwork, 2014). For some situations in which the risk of identification is judged to be too high—for example, with sensitive health conditions or when harm may come to identified participants—sharing may not be advisable. Finally, the risk of re-identification of trial participants increases as the scope of data on each person and the number of participants increase. Using "big data" analytic techniques on de-identified data, researchers may re-identify participants by combining additional information, or they may determine whether an individual about whom they have independent information is a participant in the study and draw inferences about him or her, as discussed in Chapter 3.

> **Conclusion:** *Sharing the analyzable data set would benefit science and public health by allowing reanalysis, meta-analysis, and scientific discovery through hypothesis generation.*

> **Conclusion:** *The risks of sharing individual participant data are significant and need to be mitigated in most cases through appropriate controls. In certain circumstances, the risks or burdens may be so great that sharing is not feasible or requires enhanced privacy protections.*

Metadata and Additional Documentation

To use clinical trial data (e.g., to perform the primary analysis or carry out confirmatory or exploratory analyses), researchers need metadata (i.e., "data about the data") and additional documentation beyond the individual participant data described above. Currently the trial registration data set of 20 items identified by WHO is publicly available for most trials (WHO, 2014). This data set includes the trial and investigator identification information, names of sponsors and funders, study type, participant enrollment information, and primary and secondary outcomes. These 20 items, however, are a small subset of the metadata and additional documentation developed for clinical trials, which include the data sharing plan, protocol and all amendments, the SAP and all amendments, analytic code, and other documents described in Box 4-1 and in the following pages.

BOX 4-1
Metadata and Additional Documentation

- Data sharing plan
- Clinical trial registration number and data set (available through Clinical Trials.gov and other World Health Organization [WHO] registries)
- Full trial protocol (e.g., all outcomes, study structure), including first version, final version, and all amendments
- Manual of operations describing how a trial is conducted (e.g., assay method) and standard operating procedures, including names of parties involved, specifically
  - names of persons on the clinical trial team, trial sponsor team, data management team, and data analysis team; and
  - names of members of the steering committee, Clinical Events Committee (CEC, which adjudicates endpoints), and Data and Safety Monitoring Board (DSMB)/Data Monitoring Committee (DMC), as well as committee charters
- Details of study execution (e.g., participant flow, deviations from protocol)
- Case report templates describing what measurements will be made and at what timepoints during the trial, as defined in the protocol
- Informed consent templates describing what participants agreed to, what hypotheses were included, and for what additional purposes participants' data may be used
- Full statistical analysis plan (SAP), which includes all amendments and all documentation for additional work processes (including codes, software, and audit of the statistical workflow)
- Analytic code describing the clinical and statistical choices made during the clinical trial

---

Data Sharing Plan

The data sharing plan describes what specific types of data will be shared at various time points and how to seek access to the data. According to the U.S. National Institutes of Health (NIH):

> The precise content of the data-sharing plan will vary, depending on the data being collected and how the investigator is planning to share the data. Applicants who are planning to share data may wish to describe briefly the expected schedule for data sharing, the format of the final data set, the documentation to be provided, whether or not any analytic tools also will be provided, whether or not a data-sharing agreement will be required and, if so, a brief description of such an agreement (including the criteria for deciding who can receive the data and whether or not any conditions will be placed on their use), and the mode of data sharing (e.g., under their own auspices by mailing a disk or posting

data on their institutional or personal website, through a data archive or enclave). (NIH, 2003)

Sharing the data sharing plan publicly before the first participant is enrolled allows the public, Research Ethics Committee, and potential participants to know what the sponsor and investigator are planning to do. As noted in Chapter 3 and Box 4-1, the data sharing plan should be discussed during the informed consent process. Disclosure of the data sharing plan also helps identify cases in which the sponsor changed its plan for data sharing after the trial began.

To be useful to potential secondary users of a clinical trial data set, the data sharing plan needs to be publicly available and readily accessible. One means of accomplishing this goal is to make data sharing plans a 21st element in the WHO trial registration data set.

In the interests of full transparency, the data sharing plan should include a comprehensive justification for any intent not to share data. In some situations, an exception to sharing the analyzable data set may be appropriate, or additional controls over access may be required. This may occur, for example, because of exceptional privacy risks. Such exceptions to usual data sharing plans should be made publicly available.

Trial Protocol

The trial protocol provides the overall experimental design. It describes the rationale for the trial, the eligibility and exclusion criteria for participants, the primary and secondary hypotheses and the corresponding primary and secondary outcome measures, the methods used to identify and adjudicate adverse events, and other measures intended for use in evaluating the intervention, as well as a full description of the entire study and all interventions and tests and how they are to be administered. A SAP should also be part of the protocol. When registering a trial, investigators and sponsors must provide both a brief summary and a detailed description of the protocol (see Box 4-2).

Over the life of a clinical trial, the protocol usually is modified a number of times. All amendments to the initial protocol should be dated and saved. To replicate or reproduce a study, other investigators need the version of the protocol in effect when the first participant was enrolled, as well as all modifications and the full protocol version in force when the data set was locked (and before unblinding). This should be the final protocol, as revisions made after the data set has been locked and unblinded are fraught with bias.

Sharing of protocols promotes protocol quality improvement efforts (e.g., Standard Protocol Items: Recommendations for Interventional Trials

---

BOX 4-2
Required Descriptions of Trial Protocols

According to ClinicalTrials.gov, the following descriptions of the protocol for a trial are required:

Brief Summary
Definition: Short description of the protocol intended for the lay public. Include a brief statement of the study hypothesis. (Limit: 5,000 characters)

Example: The purpose of this study is to determine whether prednisone, methotrexate, and cyclophosphamide are effective in the treatment of rapidly progressive hearing loss in both ears due to autoimmune inner ear disease.

Detailed Description
Definition: Extended description of the protocol, including more technical information (as compared to the Brief Summary) if desired. Do not include the entire protocol; do not duplicate information recorded in other data elements, such as eligibility criteria or outcome measures. (Limit: 32,000 characters)

SOURCE: ClinicalTrials.gov, 2012.

[SPIRIT]) (Chan et al., 2013), complements trial registration in identifying trials that were initiated, allows future auditing of data sharing, facilitates meta-analyses and systematic reviews, promotes greater standardization of protocol elements (e.g., interventions, outcomes), and may help reduce unnecessary duplication of studies. The full protocol with all amendments (see Figure 4-1) should be shared to help other investigators understand the original analysis, replicate or reproduce the study, and carry out additional analyses.

Statistical Analysis Plan

A SAP also is prespecified before the start of a trial. It may be amended during the trial while the data are blinded but is finalized before the analysis is completed and the data are unblinded. The SAP drives the primary analyses of the analyzable data set. It describes the analyses to be conducted and the statistical methods to be used, as determined by the protocol. The SAP includes, for example, plans for analysis of baseline descriptive data and adherence to the intervention, prespecified primary and secondary outcomes, definitions of adverse and serious adverse events, and comparison of these outcomes across interventions for prespecified subgroups. These SAP-defined analyses are often extensive and can result in several dozen tables and figures.

For many clinical trials, the SAP-defined analyses may not use all of the data available in the analyzable data set. Moreover, as discussed earlier, publications of clinical trials in peer-reviewed journals generally draw on only part of the analyzable data set. Supplemental data often are collected to permit exploration of ancillary questions not directly related to the primary purpose of the protocol, and researchers may conduct exploratory and post hoc analyses not defined in the SAP to answer additional questions.

The full SAP describes how each data element was analyzed, what specific statistical method was used for each analysis, and how adjustments were made for testing multiple variables. The full SAP includes all amendments and all documentation for additional work processes from earlier versions. If some analysis methods require critical assumptions, data users will need to understand how those assumptions were verified.

Sharing the SAP enables additional scientific discoveries by allowing other investigators to carry out alternative or additional analyses to test the robustness of published findings, such as post hoc subgroup analyses or composite endpoints; to compare outcomes from other trials; to plan meta-analyses; and to carry out exploratory studies to generate new hypotheses. In addition, sharing the SAP allows other investigators to replicate or reproduce the original analysis. Reproducibility of results is discussed in more detail below.

Analytic Code

The analyzable data set from a clinical trial is transformed into scientific results through an analytic process that involves many steps and many clinical and statistical choices. These choices include but are not limited to which and how many analyses to conduct, which variables to include in an analysis, which statistical procedures to use, and whether and how to adjust analyses statistically for confounders. Some of these choices are detailed in the study's SAP, while other choices are necessarily made during the process of data analysis. Regardless, these choices are reflected in the statistical programming code used to produce the study results. Another researcher attempting to reproduce the findings of a trial will need access to the statistical programming code, as well as the version of the software used.

To promote overall scientific validity and trust in the clinical research enterprise, there has been an increasing focus on ensuring the reproducibility of research (Collins and Tabak, 2014; IOM, 2014; Jasny, 2011). Reproduction requires access to the original analytic code, which reflects the investigators' clinical and statistical choices, detailed earlier, that may not have been included in any data analysis plan or publication. Access to the analytic code also allows for verification of the correctness of the code and should be coincident with the availability of the data. Recent examples of coding errors in widely quoted economic reports have come to light because independent researchers had access to the data and the analytic code (Giles, 2014; Krugman, 2013). In a highly publicized example, external scientists raised concerns about the validity of gene-expression tests that were used to assign treatment arms in three NIH-sponsored cancer clinical trials. The study team did not respond to requests by external scientists to obtain the analytic code for the studies presenting the tests; when external biostatisticians obtained access, they identified serious errors (IOM, 2012). Arguably, had the analytic code and full analytic data set of the publications been shared, serious harms to participants in the cancer clinical trials—including misclassification of patients as being at low or high risk of recurrence—could have been averted. Such examples illustrate the importance of demonstrating statistical reproducibility. Sharing of the analytic code along with the analytic data set also aligns with the principles of transparency and accountability that underlie effective sharing of clinical trial data. At the same time, licensing models for reproducible research are needed to protect the rights of investigators over their code and associated products (IOM, 2012; Laine et al., 2007; Sandve et al., 2013; Stodden, 2009, 2013).

> **Conclusion:** *The clinical trial protocol, the SAP, amendments, and other metadata need to be shared along with the analyzable data set so that secondary investigators can plan and carry out analyses rigorously and efficiently.*

Thus, a "full data package"—which the committee defines as the full analyzable data set, the full protocol (including first version, final version, and all amendments), the SAP (including all amendments and all documentation for additional work processes), and the analytic code—will allow for the majority of secondary analyses that other investigators may wish to carry out, including systematic reviews and meta-analyses of individual participant data.

Summary Data

Box 4-3 lists some of the documents that are that are commonly generated from analysis of the data from a clinical trial. These include publications describing the primary and major secondary outcomes specified

---

BOX 4-3
Documents Based on Analysis of Clinical Trial Data

- Publications (including those in peer-reviewed scientific journals)
- Summaries of results for registries (e.g., for ClinicalTrials.gov)
- Lay-language summaries
- Clinical study reports (CSRs)
  - Full CSR, with or without appendixes
  - CSR synopsis (executive summary)
  - Redacted CSR
  - Abbreviated CSR

---

in the protocol, summaries for registries, lay summaries, and CSRs for regulators.

Publications

Several scientific journal publications are commonly derived from the prespecified analyses driven by the SAP and from post hoc analyses. Typically, a primary publication will address the primary and possibly the leading secondary outcome measures specified in the protocol. The primary publication will also include the baseline measures to demonstrate the comparability of participants in the different intervention arms and comparisons across the intervention arms of any adverse events of major interest or frequency. Subsequent journal publications may address in greater detail a specific aspect of the primary analysis that was not included in the primary publication or analyze outcomes in particular prespecified subgroups of participants. Each journal publication is supported by a specific analytic data set corresponding exclusively to the data used to generate the tables and figures in the publication (which will be a subset of the full analyzable data set). A snapshot of each analytic data subset is typically stored in a separate set of data files to document the data used for each journal publication.

The committee appreciates that many clinical trialists plan to publish a number of papers from the data collected during a trial, particularly a long and complex trial. Other important secondary analyses may become apparent only after the trial team has become familiar with the data. As noted earlier, particularly for junior members of the clinical trial team, the prospect of being lead author on a secondary analysis is viewed as their fair professional reward for their work in planning and carrying out the trial. Understandably, these investigators might feel distressed and demoralized by the possibility that other investigators who did not put effort into collecting the data would gain priority in publishing secondary analyses on the basis of shared data. On this issue, the committee shares the view of a previous National Research Council committee (addressing the more general context of life science research):

> Community standards for sharing publication-related data and materials should flow from the general principle that the publication of scientific information is intended to move science forward. More specifically, the act of publishing is a quid pro quo in which authors receive credit and acknowledgment in exchange for disclosure of their scientific findings. An author's obligation is not only to release data and materials to enable others to verify or replicate published findings (as journals already implicitly or explicitly require) but also to provide them in a form on which other scientists can build with further research. All members of the scientific community—whether working in academia, government, or a commercial enterprise—have equal responsibility for upholding community standards as participants in the publication system, and all should be equally able to derive benefits from it. (NRC, 2003, p. 4)

The committee agrees that sharing the analytic data set supporting a publication is an integral part of the process of communicating results through publication. Once a study finding has been published, the scientific process is best served by allowing other investigators to reproduce the findings and carry out additional analyses to test the robustness of the published conclusions. Robust conclusions increase confidence in the validity of the publication's findings. For example, repeating the prespecified analysis and obtaining identical results will provide evidence that the results of the study, given the approach taken to data collection and analysis, are accurate. If alternative analyses addressing the research questions in the publication also yield the same findings, the reported findings can be considered robust. By contrast, if the published results do not hold when analytic approaches other than the prespecified approach are used, the report's findings may need to be qualified, modified, or discussed further. In this case, readers of the publication will have reason to be cautious in applying the reported results to clinical practice or the design of future trials. Access to data that allow replication of the published results can therefore benefit the public by strengthening the evidence base on which physicians draw when making clinical recommendations.

Turning to what data should be shared after publication of a manuscript, the committee advocates sharing all the data that are needed to support the results reported in a manuscript, including those presented in tables, figures, and supplementary material. The committee refers to this as the "post-publication data package," which consists of the analytic data set and metadata, including the protocol, the SAP, and analytic code, supporting published results.

> **Conclusion:** *It is beneficial to share the analytic data set and appropriate metadata supporting published results.*

Results Summary for Registries and Lay-Language Summary

Many clinical trials are subject to a requirement that their results be reported to one or more registries, in formats specified by the particular registry. These summaries, which are publicly available on the registry website, are generally limited to major outcomes and adverse events.[7] As mentioned in Chapter 3, the Food and Drug Administration Amendments Act of 2007 (FDAAA) requires results of trials of FDA-regulated products to be reported to ClinicalTrials.gov within 12 months of study completion. However, a 2012 study found that the results of 30 percent of 400 clinical trials had neither been published nor reported on ClinicalTrials.gov 4 years after study completion (Saito and Gill, 2014). Following this study and others showing a similar dearth of reporting of results for registered trials, the U.S. Department of Health and Human Services (HHS) has proposed a new rule requiring that results of trials of unapproved products be reported to ClinicalTrials.gov within 12 months of study completion. NIH has also proposed a draft policy calling for all NIH-funded trials not subject to the FDAAA (e.g., trials of surgical or behavioral interventions and phase 1 trials) to also be reported to ClinicalTrials.gov within 12 months of study completion (Hudson and Collins, 2014). In support of this proposed rule, Drs. Hudson and Collins state in an editorial in the *Journal of the American Medical Association (JAMA)*,

> When research involves human volunteers who agree to participate in clinical trials to test new drugs, devices, or other interventions, this principle of data sharing properly assumes the role of an ethical man-

---

[7] Adverse events are "unfavorable changes in health, including abnormal laboratory findings, that occur in trial participants during the clinical trial or within a specified period following the trial" (ClinicalTrials.gov, 2014). Generally, two types of adverse event data sets are generated at the conclusion of a trial, described as follows by ClinicalTrials.gov:

> Serious Adverse Events: A table of all anticipated and unanticipated serious adverse events, grouped by organ system, with number and frequency of such events in each arm of the clinical trial.

> Other (Not Including Serious) Adverse Events: A table of anticipated and unanticipated events (not included in the serious adverse event table) that exceed a frequency threshold within any arm of the clinical trial, grouped by organ system, with number and frequency of such events in each arm of the clinical trial.

date. These participants are often informed that such research might not benefit them directly, but may affect the lives of others. If the clinical research community fails to share what is learned, allowing data to remain unpublished or unreported, researchers are reneging on the promise to clinical trial participants, are wasting time and resources, and are jeopardizing public trust. (Hudson and Collins, 2014)

The committee strongly endorses this reasoning and agrees that public reporting of clinical trial results is an ethical mandate. As noted above, although sharing of clinical trial results has been a requirement, not all investigators and sponsors have fulfilled it. In conjunction with the proposed new requirement, NIH recently announced a multipronged approach to increasing the reporting of public summaries of clinical trial results (NIH, 2014). As a positive incentive, ClinicalTrials.gov is increasing one-to-one support for the posting of these summaries. As an enforcement mechanism, NIH will begin to withhold funds from grantees who do not comply and will take reporting of results into account when reviewing future grant applications (Kaiser, 2014). The committee appreciates that, in a similar manner, adoption of recommendations for sharing clinical trial data (beyond public posting of summary results) may well face challenges in implementation and acceptance. The committee notes that, in support of the requirement to post summary results, ICMJE has modified its statement on registration of clinical trials to make clear that reporting summary results in tabular form in a registry or with a 500-word descriptive abstract is not considered prior publication (ICMJE, 2014).

Additionally, clinical trial participants are interested in knowing the aggregate results of the trial in lay language. A lay-language summary is a brief, nontechnical overview written for the general public and trial participants. Lay summaries of the clinical trial protocol are often required by Research Ethics Committees to assist their nonscientist members in the protocol review and approval process. Sponsors or investigators commonly prepare lay-language press releases after publishing articles or making presentations at professional meetings. However, sending lay-language summaries of clinical trial results to participants is uncommon (Getz et al., 2012). A recent study suggests that trial participants would value such summaries and that providing them is feasible (Getz et al., 2012).

As a matter of public transparency and respect for participants, the committee supports publicly sharing summaries of results for registries and lay-language summaries with participants after publication of an article, presentation at a professional meeting, issuance of a press release, or disclosure to the Securities and Exchange Commission, or no later than 1 year after completion of the trial.

Clinical Study Report

When a clinical trial is submitted to regulatory agencies as part of an application for marketing approval of an intervention or new indication, the trial sponsors usually submit a detailed CSR. Specifications for CSRs have been defined by the International Conference on Harmonisation (ICH) and adopted by the FDA, the EMA, and the Japanese Ministry of Health, Labor, and Welfare in an effort to simplify the application process for new interventions globally (ICH, 1995). According to the FDA guidance, the CSR is an

> integrated full report of an individual study of any therapeutic, prophylactic or diagnostic agent ... conducted in patients. The clinical and statistical description, presentation, and analyses are integrated into a single report incorporating tables and figures into the main text of the report or at the end of the text, with appendices containing such information as the protocol, sample case report forms, investigator-related information, information related to the test drugs/investigational products including active control/comparators, technical statistical documentation, related publications, patient data listings, and technical statistical details such as derivations, computations, analyses, and computer output. (FDA, 1996, p. 1)

Although a CSR contains mainly summary data and summary tables and graphs, it also usually contains considerable additional information (often thousands of pages), including, as described in the definition above, numerous large appendixes. Supplemental information can include detailed narratives describing individual participants. In some instances, the CSR and/or its appendixes may include identifiable participant information, commercially confidential information, or other protected health information or intellectual property. Currently sensitive information about sponsor strategy or manufacturing may be contained in the background, rationale, and interpretation sections of a CSR because the investigators and sponsor did not anticipate that anyone other than the sponsor, regulatory authorities, and the investigative team would have access to the CSR. A CSR synopsis (i.e., executive summary) is sometimes drafted to accompany a full CSR. Some of the supporting clinical trials included in a regulatory submission do not directly contribute to the evaluation of the effectiveness of the intervention; for these studies, sponsors may be permitted to submit an abbreviated CSR (FDA, 1999). CSRs need to be carefully reviewed and manually redacted of any personally identifiable and commercially confidential information before they are shared with persons other than regulatory authorities.

Sharing CSRs, which provide far more information than is contained in published articles, allows other investigators to carry out meta-analyses and systematic reviews that combine data from a number of trials. Because a large proportion of clinical trial data is never published, critical reviews and meta-analyses that do not draw on unpublished data in CSRs may be biased (Doshi et al., 2013). Furthermore, there can be discrepancies between published results and CSRs (Doshi and Jefferson, 2013; Jefferson et al., 2014), so access to CSRs allows other investigators to correct errors or understand discrepancies in the published literature. In addition, sharing CSRs allows other investigators to gain new insights by analyzing the spectrum of data, including data on efficacy and safety, among different subgroups of patients. Therefore, a "post-regulatory data package" will consist of the full data package, including the full analyzable data set, the full protocol (including the initial and final versions and all amendments), the SAP (including all amendments and all documentation for additional work processes), the analytic code, and the CSR (redacted for commercially or personal confidential information).

Conclusion: *Sharing the CSR will benefit science and public health by allowing a better understanding of regulatory decisions and facilitating use of the analyzable data set.*

Conclusion: *CSRs may contain sensitive information, including participant identifiers and commercially confidential information. The risks of sharing CSRs are significant and may need to be mitigated in most cases through appropriate controls.*

Legacy Trials

The benefit of sharing data from legacy trials (i.e., trials initiated before this report was issued) is similar to the benefit of sharing data from future trials: Other researchers can reproduce the original findings and carry out secondary analyses and meta-analyses, and this additional knowledge benefits the public and patients. Many treatment decisions are based on evidence from past clinical trials, and thus the potential benefits from sharing those data should not be ignored.

However, sharing data from legacy clinical trials also presents particular risks and challenges, which need to be balanced against the potential benefits. One concern is the higher cost of preparing the data for sharing relative to future trials. Data collected during older trials may not be as easily redacted for sensitive information; for example, CSRs can contain commercially confidential information about further analyses, studies, or strategies for regulatory approval or data or narratives that allow participants to be identified. Such CSRs may need to be redacted by hand to remove commercially confidential information[8] and identifiable participant information—a laborious and expensive process. In contrast, future clinical trials can design CSRs to exclude such sensitive information prospectively.

A second concern is that after a trial has been completed staff who are most familiar with the data set generally move on to other research projects or organizations and therefore are not available to answer questions about the data set from secondary users. Even if the staff can be located and are available, they may have forgotten key features of the data set. Staff turnover and loss of familiarity are an issue after the conclusion of any clinical trial, but the problem becomes more serious as the time since study completion becomes longer.

A third challenge is the marked variability in how consent forms for older clinical trials address data sharing (O'Rourke and Forster, 2014). Some consent forms expressly exclude the type of data sharing that is being considered here, while others may be ambiguous or silent on the matter. Although it is legally acceptable to share the trial data without the consent of the trial participants (for example, if the data have been de-identified), Research Ethics Committees may or may not allow data sharing that is contrary to the consent form even if the data are de-identified. Moreover, in a multisite trial, consent forms from different sites may differ. If data from only some sites are available for sharing, secondary analyses will be carried out on a different data set from that used by the original clinical trialists, and inconsistencies between secondary and original analyses will result.

Finally, the results of some completed trials may be viewed as having little scientific or clinical import, for example, because the trial was poorly designed, the intervention was not approved, or if approved is not widely used in clinical care. For such legacy trials, the costs and effort of data sharing may better be spent on creating infrastructure and processes for data sharing for future clinical trials, when data collection can be designed with data sharing in mind. However, the committee believes great benefit would be gained from sharing data from legacy trials that continue to influence decisions about clinical care, and sponsors and investigators are encouraged to make every effort to share those data when requested to do so.

Conclusion: *Sponsors and principal investigators will decide, on a case-by-case basis, whether they will share data from clinical trials initi-*

---

[8] Some companies have committed to sharing CSRs without redaction for CCI; for example, GlaxoSmithKline has committed to posting CSRs from the year 2000 forward on its multi-sponsor data request system.

ated before the recommendations in this report are implemented. They are strongly urged to do so for major and significant clinical trials whose findings influence decisions about clinical care.

WHEN DATA PACKAGES SHOULD BE SHARED

As discussed previously, vast amounts of data from clinical trials currently are never made public or shared beyond the original investigator team or company, although, as noted in previous chapters, this situation is beginning to change. This section presents the committee's findings and conclusions regarding when the various types of clinical trial data detailed above should be shared. As noted earlier, the committee acknowledges that currently no single body or authority is capable of enforcing its recommendations for all stakeholders; rather, the committee interpreted its charge as helping to establish professional standards and set expectations for responsible sharing of clinical trial data. Given the complexities of the issues surrounding data sharing, the committee found it helpful to separate the consideration of *when* data should be shared from that of *how* they should be shared. This chapter focuses on the former question; the terms, conditions, and operational strategies for how data should be shared—including whether data should be made available to the public or access should be controlled in some manner—are discussed in detail in Chapter 5.

The committee appreciates the wide variation in clinical trials with regard to the clinical conditions and interventions studied, trial designs, and populations of participants. Given this variation, the recommendations regarding the timing for sharing specific types of data detailed at the end of this chapter need to be implemented with discretion and a willingness to consider exceptions to general rules. Justifiable exceptions should be permitted, particularly when there are compelling public health reasons for doing so. The committee believes that agreement regarding common exceptions will develop over time.

The committee expects that standards for responsible sharing of clinical trial data will evolve. The implementation of data sharing will require new infrastructure and will be facilitated by changes in how clinical trials are carried out and analyzed, as well as changes in the culture of the clinical trials enterprise. As this occurs, the committee expects that data will be shared in a more timely manner than as currently recommended, particularly with respect to the analytic data set supporting a publication.

Finally, the committee hopes that the evolution of responsible sharing of clinical trial data will be guided by evidence. There are many unknowns, opportunities, and controversies entailed in sharing clinical trial data that could be clarified with empirical data. For example, it is not yet known what actual benefits will flow from sharing clinical trial data and what adverse consequences will occur. Comparisons of different approaches to implementing data sharing will be enlightening, helping to identify challenges, ways of overcoming them, and best practices that could be more widely adopted. It would be desirable for stakeholders in clinical trials to convene after some experience with sharing clinical trial data has been gained, perhaps in 3 to 5 years, so they can reconsider, based on evidence, the timing of data sharing and the conditions under which various types of data should be shared.

In deliberating on when the various types of clinical trial data should be shared, the committee found it helpful to summarize the benefits and concerns, discussed in detail in Chapter 3, associated with the timing of data sharing from the perspectives of key stakeholders:

- *Benefit patients and future research participants.* An essential step in science is verification and replication of investigators' claims. Once investigators have published their findings, as responsible scientists they should allow other researchers to subject those findings to scrutiny. Allowing timely verification and reproduction serves the public good by preventing other researchers or clinicians from building on findings whose validity cannot be established and by preventing patients from receiving recommendations for clinical care that are based on invalid information. Moreover, sharing clinical trial data benefits patients by allowing other investigators to carry out additional analyses that provide valid scientific information about the effectiveness and safety of the study intervention. In addition, sharing clinical trial data prevents participants in future research from being placed at unwarranted risk because the benefits of an intervention are smaller or the risks greater than claimed in a publication. Furthermore, sharing clinical trial data may increase public trust in the scientific and clinical trials ecosystem.

- *Protect the professional interests of clinical trialists in gaining fair professional rewards for their intellectual effort and time by giving them reasonable time to analyze and publish data from a trial they have planned and carried out.* In the long run, this protection of the interests of trialists will benefit the public and future patients by creating incentives for investigators to carry out clinical trials; conversely, failure to allow clinical trialists time to publish their findings will discourage investigators from proposing and conducting trials.

- *Protect the commercial interests of the sponsors in gaining regulatory approval for a product or indication they have developed and tested, so that they can gain fair financial rewards for their investment of financial and intellectual capital.* If a sponsor shares extensive data before a product gains regulatory approval, follow-on developers may gain commercial and strategic advantages. In addition, as a matter of fairness, other companies should not use shared clinical trial data as the predominant basis for their own regulatory submissions— for example, seeking approval for a generic version of the product in a country that does not recognize data exclusivity. In the long run, such incentives to sponsors will benefit the public and future patients by incentivizing investors and companies to develop new medical products and bring basic science discoveries to patients; failure to do so will discourage investments in health care innovation and product development that would ultimately benefit future patients.

- *Allow other researchers to access the data in order to reproduce the results of a published trial, synthesize results across trials, and carry out additional or exploratory analyses.* Such secondary uses of the data will increase the benefits to society and future patients in terms of knowledge gained from the clinical trial and the contributions of the trial participants.

Policies regarding responsible sharing of specific clinical trial data at particular times in the life cycle of a clinical trial need to balance these countervailing goals and interests. To strike a reasonable balance, the committee proposes releasing specific types of clinical trial data "packages" at different timepoints in the life of a clinical trial (see Figure 4-2).

As discussed below, the committee determined that most clinical trial data should not be shared routinely before study completion. Sharing data before this time would jeopardize the integrity of the clinical trial process and risk the scientific validity of the results. As a matter of fairness, clinical trialists should have a moratorium that lasts long enough for them to gain fair professional rewards from their effort by publishing their work. Similarly, sponsors should have a "quiet period" of a reasonable length to allow for the regulatory process of seeking approval for a new product or indication. Giving too much weight to the interests of secondary users and competitor sponsors in gaining access to data would in the long run present strong disincentives for clinical trialists to design and carry out future trials and for sponsors and their investors to develop and test new products and indications.

Notwithstanding this general presumption that clinical trial data should not be shared before the conclusion of a trial, and allowing for a reasonable moratorium and quiet period, the committee recognizes that exceptions to this presumption are justified. For example, as discussed in more detail below, once a clinical trialist and sponsor publish the results

Clinical Trial Life Cycle: When to Share Data

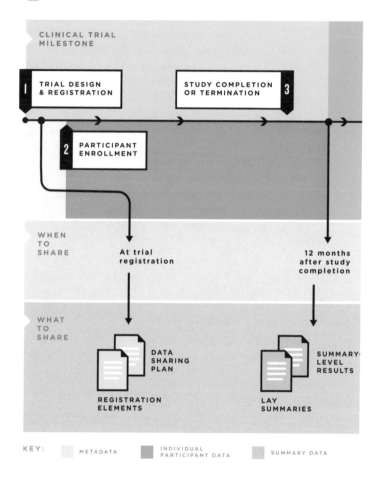

FIGURE 4-2 The clinical trial life cycle: When to share data.
NOTES: Full data package = the full analyzable data set, full protocol (including initial version, final version, and all amendments), full statistical analysis plan (including all amendments and all documentation for additional work processes), and analytic code. Post-publication data package = a subset of the full data package supporting the findings, tables, and figures in the publication. Post-regulatory

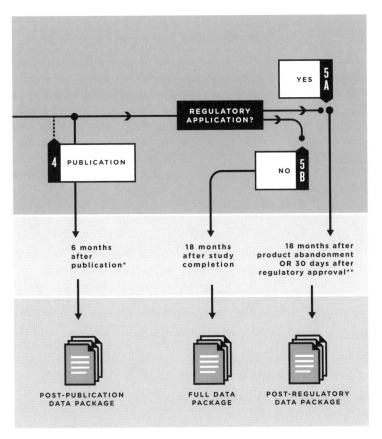

YES **5 A**

REGULATORY APPLICATION?

4 PUBLICATION

NO **5 B**

6 months after publication*

18 months after study completion

18 months after product abandonment OR 30 days after regulatory approval**

POST-PUBLICATION DATA PACKAGE

FULL DATA PACKAGE

POST-REGULATORY DATA PACKAGE

* No later than 6 months after publication applies to all studies, whether intended or not intended to support regulatory applications and regardless of publication timing relative to study completion, though publication is most likely to occur after study completion.
** Sharing the post-regulatory data package should occur 30 days after approval or 18 months after study completion, whichever is later; 18 months after abandonment of the product or indication. This applies to all studies intended and to support regulatory applications, even if abandonment occurs prior to actual regulatory application.

data package = the full data package plus the clinical study report (redacted for commercially or personal confidential information). Legacy trials: For trials initiated prior to the publication of these recommendations, sponsors and principal investigators should decide on a case-by-case basis whether to share data from the completed trials. They are strongly urged to do so for major and significant clinical trials whose findings will influence decisions about clinical care.

of a clinical trial, the goal of allowing verification and replication of a public claim regarding the study intervention takes on additional importance and changes how the countervailing goals described above should be balanced.

Publication

As noted earlier, a publication from a clinical trial is a public statement and discussion about the findings of a trial. Rapid publication commonly occurs with findings that are considered highly important scientifically or clinically. Thus, clinical trialists may publish the results of a trial shortly after its completion. For some trials, trialists may publish the primary trial endpoints despite ongoing longer-term participant follow-up; in this case, the last participant's last visit may not occur for some time, and hence the full analyzable data set may not be complete at the time of the original publication. Regardless, once a study finding has been published, the scientific process is best served by allowing other investigators to reproduce the findings and carry out additional analyses to test the robustness of the published conclusions. Unless other investigators can reproduce the findings, claims could be made that might mislead other researchers working on similar products or create an impression among clinicians that a drug is safer or more effective than it really is. Even if a drug is not yet on the market, the "buzz" anticipating approval might set the stage for overly enthusiastic adoption.

As discussed previously, the committee appreciates that many clinical trialists feel strongly that, having put years of effort into carrying out a clinical trial, it is only fair that they have the opportunity to write a series of papers analyzing data collected during the trial before other investigators have access to the data. Although sharing data after the results of a trial have been published benefits the public and the scientific process, trial investigators face risks that competitors could publish additional trial findings before they can do so. When reporting the primary results of clinical trials, investigators routinely report a variety of participant characteristics. Reporting these characteristics enables readers to assess the types of patients to whom the results apply, and investigators sometimes use such characteristics to adjust analyses for differences among participants across the trial arms. These uses of participant characteristics augment the utility of the primary manuscript. On the one hand, sharing the individual participant analytic data set supporting the results reported in the publication will allow other researchers to scrutinize, verify, and reproduce the conclusions reported to determine their validity and robustness. On the other hand, the analytic data set supporting the publication, if shared, will also enable other investigators to carry out subgroup analyses, or assessments of whether the effects of the intervention differ among different types of patients. Because such prespecified subgroup analyses are often the topic of a second paper planned by the trialists, they have an interest in maintaining a period of exclusive access to these data following publication of the initial manuscript.

The committee was mindful of these countervailing goals of sharing clinical trial data soon after publication and appreciates that the scientific community is divided over when the analytic data set supporting a publication should be shared. It is likely that some trialists believe they need 1 year to carry out secondary analyses they were planning. Moreover, clinical trialists may fear that preparing the analytic data set for sharing immediately upon publication would pose an undue administrative burden. On the other hand, other stakeholders believe that the analytic data set should be shared simultaneously with publication so that others can reproduce the findings and build on discoveries. As noted previously, for example, The Bill & Melinda Gates Foundation recently announced that it will require that "data underlying the published research results be immediately accessible and open" (The Bill & Melinda Gates Foundation, 2014). However, the Gates Foundation will allow a 1-year embargo on this requirement to allow investigators to transition to it (The Bill & Melinda Gates Foundation, 2014).

In an ideal clinical trials ecosystem, the committee would favor sharing of the analytic data set supporting a publication immediately upon publication. However, the committee recognizes that currently many practical constraints and challenges need to be addressed before this can be recommended. For the present, the committee recommends a pragmatic compromise time frame of no later than 6 months after publication, with the expectation that in several years the standard will become sharing simultaneously with publication. The committee believes that at the present time, an expectation of no later than 6 months after publication balances the public health benefits of facilitating rapid reanalysis of reported data with the interests of investigators in maintaining a deserved competitive advantage in generating subsequent manuscripts.

In its deliberations, the committee also considered the possibility that an expectation to share data within 6 months of publication may cause some investigators to delay publication to protect their competitive advantage. The committee believes this is unlikely because investigators are strongly motivated to publish important papers rapidly in order to gain credit and prestige. The committee also noted that for the vast majority of clinical trials, there is a time period in which a manuscript is under review and in press, during which the trial team can work on secondary analyses without competitors having access to any data.

The committee recognizes that, as with any guideline, there will be justifiable exceptions to this 6-month time period; thus, it is not intended to be a hard-and-fast, inflexible rule. Case-by-case exceptions can and should be made with respect to the time period or what data need to be shared for trials that adjust for covariates at baseline and for which sharing the underlying data supporting the adjustments would allow other investigators to carry out subgroup analyses that the clinical trialists had preplanned.

For trials that are likely to have a major clinical, public health, or policy impact, the committee favors sharing the analytic data set sooner than the 6-month window. More rapid sharing will allow the results of important trials to be translated more promptly into improved clinical care, public health, and public policy after other investigators have scrutinized the data. The committee notes that for the majority of trials sharing the analytic data set will not allow other investigators to carry out secondary analyses but only to reproduce the published findings.

One situation that would justify a shorter time period between publishing the primary results and sharing the analytic data set is a publication showing that a drug already marketed is effective for preventing or treating an infection causing a public health crisis, such as pandemic influenza. In such a case, to enable public health officials to plan guidelines and decide whether to stockpile and distribute the drug, it would be desirable to have other investigators analyze data from this pivotal clinical trial to ascertain whether its findings were robust. In this situation, urgent public health considerations should override the clinical trialists' interests in protecting their advantage in carrying out additional analyses. These additional analyses may supplement discussions among government agencies and sponsors around the world as new data are being generated.

Another example of justification for a shorter time period before sharing the analytic data set supporting a publication is a trial comparing standard medical practices or therapeutic targets in wide clinical use with no implications for regulatory approval of products or indications. If a well-designed, adequately powered trial showed that a widely used practice was less effective or less safe than another widely used alternative, and if the differences would have great clinical significance, the trial findings could strongly influence clinical practice. In such a case, shortening the time before clinical trial data are shared would be justified so that other investigators could reproduce the published findings or employ different valid analytic approaches. These additional analyses could establish more rapidly whether the trial findings were sufficiently robust to warrant prompt modifications in clinical practice. Shortening the period before data are shared would be particularly warranted if it were highly unlikely that a second confirmatory trial of the same hypothesis would be carried out.

An example of a high-impact pivotal clinical trial comparing clinical interventions and therapeutic approaches widely used in practice is the ARDSNet studies showing "improved survival with lung protective ventilation and shortened duration of mechanical ventilation with conservative fluid management" (NHLBI ARDS Network, 2010). Additional trials suggested "no role for routine use of corticosteroids, beta agonists, [or] pulmonary artery catheterization." These trials had an important impact on the clinical care of patients with acute respiratory distress syndrome (ARDS). In such a case, the public health interest in major improvements in patient outcomes should override the concerns of the clinical trialists that their advantage in carrying out secondary analyses might be compromised by sharing data on how outcomes were adjusted for covariates.

Trials Not Part of Regulatory Application

As noted previously, the results of many clinical trials remain unpublished long after the trial's completion. Fewer than half (46 percent) of NIH-funded trials are published within 30 months of completion, and a Kaplan-Meier plot of the time to publication shows a continuous curve with no discontinuities (Gordon et al., 2013; Ross et al., 2012) (see Figure 4-3). According to Gordon and colleagues,

> The NHLBI [National Heart, Lung, and Blood Institute], along with other stakeholders in the research enterprise, should seriously examine how best to comprehend and enhance the investment value of smaller trials with surrogate end points and should consider how best to facilitate the rapid publication of all funded randomized trials. (Gordon et al., 2013, p. 1933)

Similarly, Ross and colleagues (2012) found that one-third of trials remained unpublished a median of 51 months after study completion. The authors suggest that

> Steps must be taken to ensure the timely dissemination of publicly funded research so that data from all those who volunteer are available to inform future research and practice. (Ross et al., 2012)

This problem exists not just for publicly funded trials but also for trials funded privately by industry and nonprofit sponsors, and across countries and sizes and phases of trials (Ross et al., 2009). Another study found that 29 percent of completed clinical trials had not been published or posted 4 years after completion (Saito and Gill, 2014). Further, a body of evidence reveals selective publication bias (i.e., publication of posi-

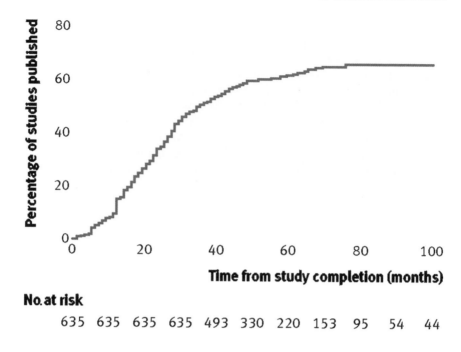

No. at risk
635   635   635   635   493   330   220   153   95   54   44

FIGURE 4-3 Cumulative percentage of studies published in a peer-reviewed biomedical journal indexed by Medline during 100 months after trial completion among all National Institutes of Health (NIH)–funded clinical trials registered in ClinicalTrials.gov.
SOURCE: Reproduced from [*British Medical Journal*, Joseph S. Ross, Tony Tse, Deborah A. Zarin, Hui Xu, Lei Zhou, and Harlan M. Krumholz, 344, d7292, 2012] with permission from BMJ Publishing Group Ltd.

tive results at a higher rate) (Bardy, 1998; Chan et al., 2004; Decullier et al., 2005; Dickersin and Min, 1993; Dickersin et al., 1992; Dwan et al., 2008; Easterbrook et al., 1991; Ioannidis, 1998; Krzyzanowska et al., 2003; Misakian and Bero, 1998; Stern and Simes, 1997; Turner et al., 2008; von Elm et al., 2008).

From these findings, the committee concluded that steps should be taken to encourage timely publication of clinical trial results and sharing of clinical trial data after the study investigators have had a fair opportunity to publish their findings. However, if the clinical trial team does not publish its findings in timely manner, other investigators should have the opportunity to access and analyze the trial data so the public can gain the benefit of knowledge produced by the trial and the contributions of participants who volunteered to participate. It is important that negative as well as positive clinical trial results be made known and the underlying data shared. The committee rejected the option of sharing clinical trial data immediately upon the conclusion of a trial. Instead, the committee concluded that the moratorium discussed above should be provided, for several reasons. First, the primary investigators, who designed the trial, secured funding, implemented trial-related procedures, trouble-shot unexpected problems, and carried out data collection, should be given a fair opportunity to gain the rewards of publication and professional recognition for their intellectual contributions and efforts. Second, the primary investigators have unique insights into the strengths, weaknesses, and idiosyncrasies of the trial's conduct and data, so they may be able to complete the planned analyses in the most rigorous and efficient fashion. Third, without having some competitive advantage in analyzing and publishing the results of a trial to which they devoted years of professional effort, highly trained clinical trialists might shift their careers toward other paths. In its public meetings, the committee heard clinical trialists declare that if other scientists could publish the results of a trial first, the trialists would have strong disincentives for undertaking the arduous process of organizing and conducting trials. If fewer scientists became clinical trialists, the production of clinical trial data would decline and the result in the long run could be fewer new therapies and less evidence for important clinical decisions. Fourth, junior members of a clinical trial team might expect to be first author on a secondary paper from the trial, which would be a major milestone in their careers.

The committee understands that the recommendations presented here apply for the current academic reward system. As discussed previously, fair sharing of clinical trial data necessitates that sharing be valued independently as a duty of scientific citizenship. Thus, as the academic reward system recognizes and affords fair credit for sharing data that enable other investigators to publish findings, the committee anticipates that the calculus for how much total credit can be obtained by sharing data earlier will evolve to favor more rapid sharing.

Conclusion: *Once a clinical trial has been completed, a moratorium before the trial data are shared is generally appropriate to allow the trialists who have planned the trial and generated the data to complete their analyses.*

After concluding that clinical trial data should be shared only after a moratorium following completion of the trial, the committee considered how long that moratorium should be. In addition to balancing the countervailing interests and goals discussed above, the committee weighed the following pragmatic considerations. First, as noted above, the available data on the time to publication after completion of a clinical trial suggest that the percentage of trials published increases continuously over time, with a leveling off between 40 and 60 months after completion. Second, the original investigators in the clinical trial have a head start relative to secondary users that is longer than the moratorium period because, even after obtaining access to clinical trial data, a secondary investigator will require time to become familiar with the data set, to plan and run data analyses, and to prepare a manuscript for submission to a medical journal. Third, changing the incentives and expectations for sharing data and publishing results of clinical trials may change investigator behaviors. If investigators know they will share data at a certain time after completion of a trial, they may alter their planning to attempt to obtain appropriate levels of funding and staffing or arrange to collaborate so as to publish the primary and some secondary analyses within the moratorium period. For junior investigators planning to be lead author in secondary analyses, it will be important to carry out those analyses as soon as possible so that they can be submitted shortly after the primary paper has been accepted.

How long the moratorium after trial completion should be is a matter of judgment. However, establishing a professional standard for the length of a moratorium is important to give all stakeholders in the clinical trials enterprise the same expectations. Sponsors and investigators who decide to release data sooner would be encouraged to do so for the sake of more rapid completion of secondary analyses. Other sponsors and investigators may have justifiable and predictable reasons to delay release beyond the moratorium period recommended here. If such circumstances can be anticipated when the trial is designed, it will be appropriate to include the expected delay as part of the data sharing plan at registration, and to provide the alternative expected time at which data will be shared for the trial.

The committee also recognizes that what stakeholders consider acceptable for a moratorium period may change over time as more experience is gained with sharing clinical trial data, particularly if data are collected prospectively on the outcomes of such a data sharing policy. Such outcomes might include the Kaplan-Meier curves on the percentage and types of trials published as a function of time since trial completion, as well as investigators' willingness to lead or participate in other clinical trials. Taking all these considerations into account, the committee reached the following conclusion regarding the best balance of countervailing interests and goals, recognizing that some stakeholders will advocate a shorter and some a longer moratorium.

Conclusion: *It is reasonable to expect clinical trial data that will not be part of a regulatory application to be available for sharing no later than 18 months after study completion.*

Regulatory Application

This section addresses when the post-regulatory data package should be shared for those clinical trials that are intended to support a regulatory application for a new product or a new indication for a product already marketed. The committee considered when data should be shared for products and indications that are (1) granted regulatory approval or (2) abandoned by the sponsor (either before or after a regulatory submission) and/or licensed to another entity for further development.

Regulatory Approval

Regulatory authorities such as the EMA and the FDA have a more comprehensive view of clinical trial data than do other secondary users of shared data. These two agencies make extensive efforts to understand, challenge, and reanalyze submitted data. In addition, both have mechanisms for asking questions, requesting new analyses or data sets from the trial sponsors, and obtaining external expert advice. Moreover, they have the authority—which they often exercise—to audit sponsors as well as investigational sites. These audits include, for example, announced or unannounced visits to the sponsor to review the accuracy and veracity of the submitted files, interview staff, and test software and systems. Visits to investigational sites allow these agencies to review study documentation and procedures through interviews with study and hospital staff and review of administrative documents and patient and study records. Therefore, the agencies have the benefit of seeing how the data were collected and how they were handled and analyzed by the sponsor and of performing their own independent analysis of the data. They have the unique ability to evaluate individual study data in the context of all other studies conducted on the product, as well as other products—from other sponsors—in the same therapeutic area (especially those with similar mechanisms).

Regulatory authorities have public health responsibilities. The FDA, for example, is charged with "protecting the public health by assuring the safety, efficacy and security of human and veterinary drugs, biological products, medical devices," and "is also responsible for advancing the public health by helping to speed innovations that make medicines more effective, safer and more affordable, and by helping the public get the accurate, science-based information they need to use medicines and foods

to maintain and improve their health" (FDA, 2014). Regulatory authorities also may have fewer conflicts of interest relative to sponsors and
clinical trial investigators, by their very nature. The FDA is firewalled
from the direct financial conflicts of interest that other secondary users of
shared clinical trial data may have through research grants and contracts,
although the FDA does receive funding through user fees. In addition, the
FDA staff are free from the academic need to publish papers to advance
their careers.

Given regulatory agencies' broad perspective on the data, their public health mandate, and their accountability as government agencies, the
committee believes, as noted earlier, that it is beneficial to allow regulators
a "quiet period" as they carry out their review, during which clinical trial
data need not be shared with other secondary users, even beyond the
18-month period after study completion. The committee concludes that
a "post-regulatory data package"—consisting of the CSR (redacted for
commercially or personal confidential information), the full analyzable
data set, the full protocol (including the initial and final versions and all
amendments), the SAP (including all amendments and all documentation
for additional work processes), and the analytic code—should be shared
either 18 months after study completion or 30 days after the FDA and/
or the EMA approval, whichever occurs later. If regulatory approval is
denied and the sponsor continues to pursue approval, the regulatory quiet
period should continue so that competitors will not have the opportunity
to use shared data for their own regulatory submissions even before the
originator has obtained approval. Sponsors should have the opportunity
to resubmit their application or have data and information requested by
the regulatory authority evaluated during a quiet period. As discussed
later, there should also be no disincentive for secondary sponsors that
may want the opportunity to license and repurpose the product even after
initial nonapproval from regulatory authorities (see the discussion below
regarding abandonment).

An important exception to the quiet period arises if a sponsor chooses
to publish a manuscript prior to regulatory approval, as commonly occurs
with important trials and novel therapies. In this case, the sponsor has put
the results out for scientific and medical discussion and therefore should
share the analytic data set supporting the publication—in essence, negat-
ing the quiet period. Once the scientific and medical community has read
a publication with the sponsor's analysis and conclusions, the community
should have the opportunity to scrutinize and reproduce the analysis
and conclusions. Therefore, if the sponsor has elected to publish, the data
supporting the publication—the post-publication data package—should
be shared no later than 6 months after publication even if the product has
not yet been approved.

Conclusion: It is beneficial to allow a "quiet period" while a product or indication is undergoing development for a regulatory application during which the full analyzable data set and metadata need not be shared unless the data are published.

Abandonment

In some cases, a clinical trial (whether terminated early or completed) may be part of a product development program that is abandoned. Products and indications may be abandoned either before or after regulatory submission and for a variety of reasons. Sponsors may decide to abandon products and indications undergoing development for regulatory application for scientific or medical reasons (e.g., a lack of efficacy for the indication of interest or a serious safety issue) or for administrative reasons (e.g., business considerations, drug supply) (Paul and Lewis-Hall, 2013; Psaty and Rennie, 2003). If a product development program is abandoned,

- the sponsor may continue to seek or already have regulatory approval for the product for a different indication, using other clinical trial data; or
- the sponsor may abandon the new product under development for all indications, in which case the sponsor may or may not decide to transfer intellectual property rights to another sponsor, either for-profit or nonprofit, that wants to develop the product.

If the sponsor transfers intellectual property rights to another sponsor, the new sponsor has an interest in having an exclusive period in which to conduct additional trials, seek additional patents, and prepare a regulatory submission (Rai and Rice, 2014). Lack of such an exclusive period would be a disincentive for another sponsor to develop the product and seek regulatory approval. Indeed, because of the potential importance of this approach to developing new therapies, the committee encourages making such decisions to transition abandoned products to other interested parties as expeditiously as possible.

The committee also considered the case in which a sponsor abandons a product or indication and does not transfer the intellectual property rights to develop the product to another sponsor. In such cases, sharing clinical trial data may help other researchers studying and other sponsors developing similar products. The design of trials on these other products may be modified by the results of the abandoned trial, for example, if the results suggest safety or efficacy endpoints. If a sponsor abandons a new indication for a marketed product, sharing the clinical trial data can benefit other researchers, clinicians, and the public. Sharing data on a product approved for other uses will increase general knowledge of the product, including its efficacy and safety profile.

Taking the above considerations into account, the committee reached the following conclusions regarding abandoned trials (whether terminated early or completed) conducted for products or indications intended for regulatory application.

> **Conclusion:** *If a clinical trial has ended and the sponsor abandons development of a new product (and does not transfer rights to develop the product to another sponsor), it is appropriate to share the post-regulatory data package 18 months after the decision has been made definitively to abandon the product and not pursue further development.*

In this case, the 18-month moratorium will allow the trial investigators to analyze the data from the trial and publish their findings. This 18-month moratorium is similar to the moratorium for completed trials, allowing investigators to analyze and publish their work. As with all trial data, the analytic data set supporting a publication should be available no later than 6 months after publication.

> **Conclusion:** *If a product will continue to be developed by the sponsor or if it is transitioned or licensed to a new sponsor that is pursuing development and approval, it is appropriate to share the post-regulatory data package 30 days after regulatory approval of the product or 18 months after study completion, whichever occurs later.*

> **Conclusion:** *If a sponsor will not be seeking regulatory approval of the new indication for a marketed product for which a trial was intended to be part of a regulatory submission, it is appropriate to share the post-regulatory data package 18 months after the decision has been made definitively to abandon the indication.*

Box 4-4 presents three case examples of the timeline for sharing clinical trial data.

Sharing Data with Participants

Clinical trial participants are interested in certain types of trial data, sometimes for purposes other than carrying out secondary analyses. Table 4-1 summarizes these types of data, when they should be shared, and the benefits/risks of sharing them. (Sharing of a summary of clinical trial results with participants was discussed earlier in the chapter.)

The committee next turned to the issue of sharing individual par-

---

BOX 4-4
Case Examples: Timeline for Sharing Clinical Trial Data

Case 1: Trial Not for Regulatory Application

University X conducts a comparative effectiveness trial that is not intended for regulatory approval. The trial starts January 1, 2015, and includes secondary outcomes that are 5 years out, with study completion anticipated January 1, 2020. On July 1, 2018, University X publishes a paper on early outcomes. It should then release the post-publication data package by December 1, 2018. The remainder of the data that constitute the full data package should be released by July 1, 2021.

Case 2: Regulatory Application—Approval

Sponsor Y runs a trial on a drug intended for regulatory approval. The trial is completed on July 1, 2014. Because this is a regulatory trial, the post-regulatory data package should be released 18 months after study completion (December 31, 2015) or 30 days after approval, whichever is later, if the product is approved, or 18 months after product abandonment if the product is abandoned. Sponsor Y publishes an article on the primary outcome of the trial on February 1, 2015. As recommended by the committee, the investigators should then release the post-publication data package no later than August 1, 2015 (6 months after publication). The product is approved on March 1, 2016. The remainder of the data that constitute the post-regulatory data package should be released by April 1, 2016.

Case 3: Regulatory Application—Abandonment

Sponsor Z runs a trial on a drug intended for regulatory approval. The trial is completed on July 1, 2014. Because this is a regulatory trial, the post-regulatory data package should be released 18 months after study completion (December 31, 2015) or 30 days after approval, whichever is later, if the product is approved, or 18 months after product abandonment if the product is abandoned. Although results of the initial phase 2 trial ending on July 1, 2014, are encouraging, final analyses of the phase 3 trials reveal new safety issues, and the product is abandoned on August 31, 2017. Sponsor Z publishes an article on December 1, 2017. Sponsor Z should then release the post-publication data package before June 1, 2018. The remainder of the data that constitute the post-regulatory data package should be released by February 28, 2019.

---

ticipant data with participants. Clinical trial participants are increasingly interested in obtaining their own data gathered during a trial. In accordance with the conceptual framework for this report, the committee considered what individual data might be shared with a clinical trial's participants and at what points during the trial.

Baseline individual data. At baseline, data may be collected from physical examinations; blood tests; and other tests that are routinely available in clinical practice, such as urine analyses, ECGs, and chest X-rays. These data may have implications for participants' own clinical care. For

TABLE 4-1 Timing and Benefits/Risks of Sharing Data with Participants

Type of Data	When Shared	Benefits/Risks
Trial results in lay language	1 year after study completion	Benefit: informing participants of the trial's scientific benefits Benefit: better public understanding of clinical trial results
Individual participants' own results of baseline clinical tests	As discussed during participant enrollment and the informed consent process	Benefit: potential benefit to participants through routine screening
Individual participants' own results of clinical tests obtained during the trial	As discussed during participant enrollment and the informed consent process—typically after study completion	Benefit: potential personal benefit to participants or to inform participation in future research Risk: concern that if results are shared during the trial, the trial could be unblinded and its results potentially biased through differential dropout rates Risk: concern that the clinical significance of innovative tests may be unclear

example, abnormal results for blood pressure or cholesterol may need to be followed up by a participant and his or her physician. If a participant has a chronic condition that requires periodic monitoring with clinical tests, sharing these data can obviate the need for duplicative tests. It is already good clinical trial practice to share such clinically actionable data with participants in real time.

Clinical data collected during the course of the trial. As in the case of baseline individual data, some data collected during a trial come from tests that are routinely available in clinical practice, such as tests ordered to assess endpoints or monitor adverse events. Abnormal findings may require follow-up by the participant and his or her physician in real time—for example, if there is evidence of cancer recurrence. In addition, it may be necessary to modify the dose of a drug, suspend its use, or carry out additional monitoring tests. The nature of the condition being studied and the study intervention will determine the benefits to the patient of sharing data that are widely available in clinical care.

Sharing some of their individual participant data with participants in real time may increase the risk of unblinding the study. For instance, participants may infer which arm of a trial they were assigned to if certain laboratory abnormalities are known to be much more likely in one arm. (Of course, participants may also infer which arm they are in from clinical signs and symptoms, such as a local reaction to an active vaccination or a slower pulse rate from a study drug.) Unblinding may alter participants' behavior, for example, causing higher dropout rates in the control arm compared with the active arm. If such behaviors are widespread and differ between the arms of a trial bias may result, compromising the scientific validity of the trial and thereby undermining the contributions of other participants and the potential benefits of the trial.

Participants are increasingly collaborating to pool their individual clinical trial data and experiences and using the pooled data. For example, participants may share their symptoms and signs, as well as results of laboratory tests obtained as part of or outside the trial. Furthermore, clinical trial participants may pool their individual data to analyze the outcomes of a trial before its prespecified completion. As a result of such interim analyses, participants may decide to drop out of a trial or take additional therapies outside the protocol and its restrictions. Although pooling and analyzing individual data may make sense from the perspective of an individual participant, dropouts and deviations from the protocol may compromise the power of the trial to detect a clinically meaningful difference between the two arms or cause bias in the trial results. As a result, the trial may not fulfill its objective of obtaining valid scientific information about the benefits and risks of the study intervention. Moreover, there is a risk that such interim analyses may be misleading if they do not take into account the variability of outcomes due to chance early in a trial and the need to correct statistical analyses for multiple interim analyses of the data before a trial's prespecified conclusion.

Novel data that may not be clinically interpretable until after the trial is completed. For levels of new biomarkers for the study drug or for innovative tests not yet used in clinical care, individual results may be of uncertain significance and little direct clinical benefit until clinical trial data have been analyzed. For example, a trial may be assessing the predictive power of new biomarkers or the sensitivity of a new imaging technique. However, some participants may want to know their own data even if the clinical significance is unclear, and some clinical trial sponsors and investigators may choose to offer participants such data together with appropriate information about their clinical significance or lack thereof.

The committee believes the appropriateness of sharing individual data collected in the course of a trial is highly dependent on the particular trial, the condition being studied, the study interventions, and the risk of altering adherence to the study protocol and/or unblinding the trial. As noted above, the sponsor and investigators often share standard baseline clinical data from routine laboratory tests with individual participants shortly after the samples have been collected and analyzed. Such sharing increases potential benefits to participants and may incentivize enrollment. Moreover, clinically actionable information clearly should be shared with participants in a timely manner as appropriate as a matter of exercising good clinical trial practice and acting to benefit participants. The protocol should specify what kinds of abnormal follow-up test results would be disclosed and how the study interventions would be modified. Additional disclosures should be made in the case of unexpected serious adverse events that require clinical follow-up.

Clinical trial sponsors and investigators may also benefit from reaching out to disease groups and community groups at various stages of a trial. In addition to strengthening the trial design, the consent process, and recruitment, these groups can help draft lay-language summaries of trial results, disseminate those summaries through their organizations, and provide information and support to trial participants who have received individual participant data. Such outreach and collaboration may also increase public understanding of and trust in the clinical trial process.

> **Conclusion:** *Investigators can help uphold public trust in clinical trials and adhere to current best practices and legal standards by*
> - *explaining to trial participants what data will be shared with them and with other interested parties and when, as part of the informed consent process; and*
> - *as appropriate, making individual participants' own data collected during the course of a trial available to them following study completion and data analysis.*

RECOMMENDATION

Drawing together the considerations detailed above, the committee formulated the following recommendation for what data should be shared after key points in a clinical trial. The committee believes that this recommendation will set as professional standards that clinical trial data should be shared while mitigating associated risks and concerns.

Recommendation 2: Sponsors and investigators should share the various types of clinical trial data no later than the times specified

below. Sponsors and investigators who decide to make data available for sharing before these times are encouraged to do so.

Trial registration:
- The data sharing plan for a clinical trial (i.e., what data will be shared when and under what conditions) should be publicly available at a third-party site that shares data with and meets the data requirements of WHO's International Clinical Trials Registry Platform; this should occur before the first participant is enrolled.

Study completion:
- Summary-level results of clinical trials (including adverse event summaries) should be made publicly available no later than 12 months after study completion.
- Lay summaries of results should be made available to trial participants concurrently with the sharing of summary-level results, no later than 12 months after study completion.
- The full data package (including the full analyzable data set, the full protocol,[9] the full statistical analysis plan, and the analytic code) should be shared no later than 18 months after study completion (unless the trial is in support of a regulatory application).

Publication:
- The post-publication data package (including the subset of the analyzable data set supporting the findings, tables, and figures in the publication and the full protocol, full statistical analysis plan, and analytic code that supports the published results) should be shared no later than 6 months after publication.

Regulatory application:
- For studies of products or new indications that are approved, the post-regulatory data package (including the full analyzable data set and clinical study report redacted for commercially or personal confidential information, together with the full protocol, full statistical analysis plan, and analytic code) should be shared 30 days after regulatory approval or 18 months after study completion, whichever occurs later.
- For studies of new products or new indications for a marketed product that are abandoned, the post-regulatory data package should be shared no later than 18 months after abandonment.

---

[9] Includes the protocol in place at the start of the trial, any modifications, and the final protocol.

However, if the product is licensed to another party for further development, these data need be shared only after publication, approval, or final abandonment.

REFERENCES

ADNI (Alzheimer's Disease Neuroimaging Initiative). 2014. *ADNI publications*. http://www.adni-info.org/scientists/adniscientistshome/adnipublications.aspx (accessed October 29, 2014).

Bardy, A. H. 1998. Bias in reporting clinical trials. *British Journal of Clinical Pharmacology* 46(2):147-150.

The Bill & Melinda Gates Foundation. 2014. *Open access policy*. http://www.gatesfoundation.org/how-we-work/general-information/open-access-policy (accessed December 10, 2014).

Bradshaw, E. M., L. B. Chibnik, B. T. Keenan, L. Ottoboni, T. Raj, A. Tang, L. L. Rosenkrantz, S. Imboywa, M. Lee, A. Von Korff, M. C. Morris, D. A. Evans, K. Johnson, R. A. Sperling, J. A. Schneider, D. A. Bennett, and P. L. De Jager. 2013. CD33 Alzheimer's disease locus: Altered monocyte function and amyloid biology. *Nature Neuroscience* 16(7):848-850.

Califf, R. M. 2013. *Clinical trial data sharing and challenges to data sharing: Current and future*. Paper presented at IOM Committee on Strategies for Responsible Sharing of Clinical Trial Data: Meeting One, October 22-23, Washington, DC.

Casanova, R., F. C. Hsu, K. M. Sink, S. R. Rapp, J. D. Williamson, S. M. Resnick, and M. A. Espeland. 2013. Alzheimer's disease risk assessment using large-scale machine learning methods. *PLoS ONE* 8(11):e77949.

Chan, A. W., K. Krleza-Jeric, I. Schmid, and D. G. Altman. 2004. Outcome reporting bias in randomized trials funded by the Canadian Institutes of Health Research. *Canadian Medical Association Journal* 171(7):735-740.

Chan, A. W., J. M. Tetzlaff, D. G. Altman, K. Dickersin, and D. Moher. 2013. Spirit 2013: New guidance for content of clinical trial protocols. *Lancet* 381(9861):91-92.

ClinicalTrials.gov. 2012. *Glossary of common site terms*. http://clinicaltrials.gov/ct2/about-studies/glossary (accessed October 15, 2014).

ClinicalTrials.gov. 2014. *"Basic results" data element definitions (draft)*. http://prsinfo.clinicaltrials.gov/results_definitions.html#AdverseEvents (accessed October 16, 2014).

Collins, F. S., and L. A. Tabak. 2014. NIH plans to enhance reproducibility. *Nature* 505(7485):612-613.

De Angelis, C., J. M. Drazen, F. A. Frizelle, C. Haug, J. Hoey, R. Horton, S. Kotzin, C. Laine, A. Marusic, A. J. P. M. Overbeke, T. V. Schroeder, H. C. Sox, and M. B. V. D. Weyden. 2004. Clinical trial registration: A statement from the International Committee of Medical Journal Editors. *New England Journal of Medicine* 351(12):1250-1251.

Decullier, E., V. Lheritier, and F. Chapuis. 2005. Fate of biomedical research protocols and publication bias in France: Retrospective cohort study. *British Medical Journal* 331(7507):19.

Dickersin, K., and Y. I. Min. 1993. NIH clinical trials and publication bias. *The Online Journal of Current Clinical Trials* 50.

Dickersin, K., Y. I. Min, and C. L. Meinert. 1992. Factors influencing publication of research results. Follow-up of applications submitted to two institutional review boards. *Journal of the American Medical Association* 267(3):374-378.

Doshi, P., and T. Jefferson. 2013. Clinical study reports of randomised controlled trials: An exploratory review of previously confidential industry reports. *BMJ Open* 3(2):e002496.

Doshi, P., T. Jefferson, and C. Del Mar. 2012. The imperative to share clinical study reports: Recommendations from the Tamiflu experience. *PLoS Medicine* 9(4):e1001201.

Doshi, P., K. Dickersin, D. Healy, S. S. Vedula, and T. Jefferson. 2013. Restoring invisible and abandoned trials: A call for people to publish the findings. *British Medical Journal* 346:f2865.

Drazen, J. M. 2002. Who owns the data in clinical trial? *Science and Engineering Ethics* 8(3):407-411.

Dwan, K., D. G. Altman, J. A. Arnaiz, J. Bloom, A. W. Chan, E. Cronin, E. Decullier, P. J. Easterbrook, E. Von Elm, C. Gamble, D. Ghersi, J. P. A. Ioannidis, J. Simes, and P. R. Williamson. 2008. Systematic review of the empirical evidence of study publication bias and outcome reporting bias. *PLoS ONE* 3(8):e3081.

Dwork, C. 2014. *State of the art of privacy protection.* Paper presented at Big Data Privacy Workshop: Co-hosted by The White House Office of Science and Technology Policy and MIT, March 3, Cambridge, MA.

Easterbrook, P. J., R. Gopalan, J. A. Berlin, and D. R. Matthews. 1991. Publication bias in clinical research. *Lancet* 337(8746):867-872.

European Union Clinical Trials Register. 2011. *Clinical trials.* https://www.clinicaltrials register.eu/ctr-search/trial/2010-020943-10/GB#P (accessed December 9, 2014).

FDA (U.S. Food and Drug Administration). 1996. *Guideline for industry: Structure and content of clinical study reports.* http://www.fda.gov/downloads/drugs/guidancecompliance regulatoryinformation/guidances/ucm073113.pdf (accessed October 17, 2014).

FDA. 1999. *Guidance for industry: Submission of abbreviated reports and synopses in support of marketing applications.* http://www.fda.gov/downloads/Drugs/Guidances/ucm072053.pdf (accessed October 16, 2014).

FDA. 2014. *What we do.* http://www.fda.gov/AboutFDA/WhatWeDo (accessed October 16, 2014).

Fisher, B., S. Anderson, C. K. Redmond, N. Wolmark, D. L. Wickerham, and W. M. Cronin. 1995. Reanalysis and results after 12 years of follow-up in a randomized clinical trial comparing total mastectomy with lumpectomy with or without irradiation in the treatment of breast cancer. *New England Journal of Medicine* 333(22):1456-1461.

Getz, K., Z. Hallinan, D. Simmons, M. J. Brickman, Z. Jumadilova, L. Pauer, M. Wilenzick, and B. Morrison. 2012. Meeting the obligation to communicate clinical trial results to study volunteers. *Expert Review of Clinical Pharmacology* 5(2):149-156.

Giles, C. 2014. Thomas Piketty's exhaustive inequality data turn out to be flawed. *Financial Times,* http://www.ft.com/cms/s/0/c9ce1a54-e281-11e3-89fd-00144feabdc0.html#axzz3GR9NAHW5 (accessed October 17, 2014).

Gordon, D., W. Taddei-Peters, A. Mascette, M. Antman, P. G. Kaufmann, and M. S. Lauer. 2013. Publication of trials funded by the National Heart, Lung, and Blood Institute. *New England Journal of Medicine* 369(20):1926-1934.

Haight, T. J., S. M. Landau, O. Carmichael, C. Schwarz, C. DeCarli, and W. J. Jagust. 2013. Dissociable effects of Alzheimer disease and white matter hyperintensities on brain metabolism. *JAMA Neurology* 70(8):1039-1045.

Hudson, K. L., and F. S. Collins. 2014. Sharing and reporting the results of clinical trials. *Journal of the American Medical Association.* http://dx.doi.org/10.1001/jama.2014.10716 (accessed December 10, 2014).

ICH (International Conference on Harmonisation of Technical Requirements for Registration of Pharmaceuticals for Human Use). 1995. *Structure and content of clinical study reports (E3).* http://www.ich.org/fileadmin/Public_Web_Site/ICH_Products/Guidelines/Efficacy/E3/E3_Guideline.pdf (accessed October 16, 2014).

ICMJE (International Committee of Medical Journal Editors). 2014. *Clinical trials registration.* http://www.icmje.org/about-icmje/faqs/clinical-trials-registration (accessed November 25, 2014).

Ioannidis, J. P. 1998. Effect of the statistical significance of results on the time to completion and publication of randomized efficacy trials. *Journal of the American Medical Association* 279(4):281-286.

IOM (Institute of Medicine). 2012. *Evolution of translational omics: Lessons learned and the path forward.* Washington, DC: The National Academies Press.

IOM. 2014. Workshop on principles and best practices for sharing data from environmental health research, March 19, Washington, DC.

Jasny, B. R. 2011. Again, and again, and again... *Science* 334(6060):1225.

Jefferson, T., M. A. Jones, P. Doshi, C. B. Del Mar, R. Hama, M. J. Thompson, I. Onakpoya, and C. J. Heneghan. 2014. Risk of bias in industry-funded oseltamivir trials: Comparison of core reports versus full clinical study reports. *BMJ Open* 4(9):e005253.

Kaiser, J. 2014. Proposed rules will vastly expand trove of clinical trial data reported in U.S. database. *Science News*, http://news.sciencemag.org/health/2014/11/proposed-rules-will-vastly-expand-trove-clinical-trial-data-reported-u-s-database (accessed December 9, 2014).

Krugman, P. 2013. The Excel depression. *The New York Times*, April 19, 2013, A31.

Krzyzanowska, M. K., M. Pintilie, and I. F. Tannock. 2003. Factors associated with failure to publish large randomized trials presented at an oncology meeting. *Journal of the American Medical Association* 290(4):495-501.

Laine, C., S. N. Goodman, M. E. Griswold, and H. C. Sox. 2007. Reproducible research: Moving toward research the public can really trust. *Annals of Internal Medicine* 146(6):450-453.

Misakian, A. L., and L. A. Bero. 1998. Publication bias and research on passive smoking: Comparison of published and unpublished studies. *Journal of the American Medical Association* 280(3):250-253.

NHLBI ARDS Network (National Heart, Lung, and Blood Institute Acute Respiratory Distress Syndrome Network). 2010. *ARDSNet studies.* http://www.ardsnet.org/clinicians/studies (accessed October 24, 2014).

NIH (U.S. National Institutes of Health). 2003. *NIH data sharing policy and implementation guidance.* http://grants.nih.gov/grants/policy/data_sharing/data_sharing_guidance.htm (accessed December 9, 2014).

NIH. 2014. *HHS and NIH take steps to enhance transparency of clinical trial results.* http://www.nih.gov/news/health/nov2014/od-19.htm (accessed December 9, 2014).

NRC (National Research Council). 2003. *Sharing publication-related data and materials: Responsibilities of authorship in the life sciences.* Washington, DC: The National Academies Press.

O'Rourke, P. P., and D. Forster. 2014. *Considerations of informed consent in the discussion of clinical trial data sharing—domestic issues.* Paper presented at IOM Committee on Strategies for Responsible Sharing of Clinical Trial Data: Meeting Two, February 3-4, Washington, DC.

Paul, S. M., and F. Lewis-Hall. 2013. Drugs in search of diseases. *Science Translational Medicine* 5:186fs118.

Psaty, B. M., and D. Rennie. 2003. Stopping medical research to save money: A broken pact with researchers and patients. *Journal of the American Medical Association* 289(16): 2128-2131.

Rai, A. K., and G. Rice. 2014. Use patents can be useful: The case of rescued drugs. *Science Translational Medicine* 6(248):248fs230.

Ross, J. S., G. K. Mulvey, E. M. Hines, S. E. Nissen, and H. M. Krumholz. 2009. Trial publication after registration in ClinicalTrials.gov: A cross-sectional analysis. *PLoS Medicine/Public Library of Science* 6(9):e1000144.

Ross, J. S., T. Tse, D. A. Zarin, H. Xu, L. Zhou, and H. M. Krumholz. 2012. Publication of NIH funded trials registered in ClinicalTrials.gov: Cross sectional analysis. *British Medical Journal* 344:d7292.

Saito, H., and C. J. Gill. 2014. How frequently do the results from completed US clinical trials enter the public domain? A statistical analysis of the ClinicalTrials.gov database. *PLoS ONE* 9(7):e101826.

Sandve, G. K., A. Nekrutenko, J. Taylor, and E. Hovig. 2013. Ten simple rules for reproducible computational research. *PLOS Computational Biology* 9(10):e1003285.

Sim, I., A. W. Chan, A. M. Gulmezoglu, T. Evans, and T. Pang. 2006. Clinical trial registration: Transparency is the watchword. *Lancet* 367(9523):1631-1633.

Soran, A., L. Nesbitt, E. P. Mamounas, B. Lembersky, J. Bryant, S. Anderson, A. Brown, and M. Passarello. 2006. Centralized medical monitoring in phase III clinical trials: The National Surgical Adjuvant Breast and Bowel Project (NSABP) experience. *Clinical Trials* 3(5):478-485.

Stern, J. M., and R. J. Simes. 1997. Publication bias: Evidence of delayed publication in a cohort study of clinical research projects. *British Medical Journal* 315(7109):640-645.

Stodden, V. 2009. Enabling reproducible research: Licensing for scientific innovation. *International Journal of Communications Law and Policy* 13:1-25.

Stodden, V. 2013. *What scientific idea is ready for retirement?* http://edge.org/annual-question/2014/response/25340 (accessed October 17, 2014).

Teden, P. 2013. *Types of clinical trial data to be shared.* Paper presented at IOM Committee on Strategies for Responsible Sharing of Clinical Trial Data: Meeting One, October 22-23, Washington, DC.

Temple, R., and G. W. Pledger. 1980. The FDA's critique of the Anturane Reinfarction Trial. *New England Journal of Medicine* 303(25):1488-1492.

Turner, E. H., A. M. Matthews, E. Linardatos, R. A. Tell, and R. Rosenthal. 2008. Selective publication of antidepressant trials and its influence on apparent efficacy. *New England Journal of Medicine* 358(3):252-260.

von Elm, E., A. Rollin, A. Blumle, K. Huwiler, M. Witschi, and M. Egger. 2008. Publication and non-publication of clinical trials: Longitudinal study of applications submitted to a Research Ethics Committee. *Swiss Medical Weekly* 138(13-14):197-203.

WHO (World Health Organization). 2014. *WHO data set.* http://www.who.int/ictrp/network/trds/en (accessed December 12, 2014).

Zarin, D. A. 2013. Participant-level data and the new frontier in trial transparency. *New England Journal of Medicine* 369(5):468-469.

5

Access to Clinical Trial Data: Governance

In Chapter 4, the committee offers recommendations for what specific types of data should be shared and at what times during the life of a clinical trial. These recommendations are intended to strike a balance between benefiting the public through timely access to data and allowing investigators and sponsors time to complete planned analyses and obtain regulatory approval. This chapter examines with whom the data are shared and under what conditions. Potential data recipients may seek access to data for a variety of purposes (see Box 5-1), which may present different potential benefits and risks.

As previously stated, data sharing is the practice of making data from scientific research available to other investigators for secondary uses. The term "open access" was first applied to allowing any member of the public with Internet access to read and download for free the full text of articles from scientific journals for unrestricted use. In the context of clinical trial data, "open access" implies unrestricted and free access to data (Krumholz and Peterson, 2014). An example of such open access is the posting of registration information and summary trial results on ClinicalTrials.gov, a public website. In Chapter 4, the committee recommends that sponsors and investigators publicly share their data sharing plans at registration and summary-level results 12 months after study completion (as currently required under the Food and Drug Administration Amendments Act [FDAAA]). In Chapter 4, the committee concludes that the risks of sharing individual participant data and clinical study reports (CSRs) are significant and that these data elements may contain

BOX 5-1
Potential Recipients of Clinical Trial Data

- Researchers seeking to carry out additional analyses or explore new scientific questions
- Attorneys, who may be seeking information for use in litigation*
- Other companies, which may be competitors of the sponsor of the trial
- Consultants, whose clients may include investment and financing companies and research organizations
- Participants in the trial, who are interested in its results
- Journalists writing about a specific treatment or condition or about clinical trials generally
- Disease advocacy groups seeking to provide information to patients, families, and the public or to advance research
- Interested members of the public who wish to know more about the treatment or condition studied
- Research Ethics Committees, Institutional Review Boards, or scientific peer review committees reviewing a new study of the same or a similar intervention to obtain a more comprehensive safety profile of the intervention
- The Data and Safety Monitoring Board/Data Monitoring Committee for another clinical trial, whose decision to recommend continuing or terminating that trial may be informed by the results of a trial that has been completed but not published
- Educators seeking to use a data set for teaching purposes (e.g., in a biostatistics class)

---

* In the European Medicines Agency's (EMA's) experience with sharing clinical trial data, lawyers, other companies, and consultants were the most common data requestors (Rabesandratana, 2013).

---

sensitive data, a risk that in most cases needs to be mitigated through appropriate controls on data access and use. The committee applies the term "controlled access" to any arrangement whereby data sharers place certain restrictions on access to or conditions of use of data. Controlled access includes a range of models, from relatively light controls, such as requiring registration and data use agreements, to more extensive controls, such as review of secondary users' qualifications, research proposals, or data analysis plans.[1] Thus, controlled access can be viewed along a spectrum, from more open to more restrictive models.

---

[1] At the extreme is a closed model in which access is available only to persons in an organization or research network. The committee viewed this model as so restrictive that for purposes of this report it is not discussed in depth.

OPEN ACCESS

The key argument in favor of open access is that removing barriers for those who seek access to data and not placing limitations on how data can be used will promote transparency, reproducibility, and more rapid advancement of new knowledge and discovery. Proponents of open access argue that it is more important to promote this potential for innovation—with the accompanying risk of invalid analyses—than to impose barriers that are too restrictive and impede potential scientific discovery and progress. Proponents argue that barriers to access in the past have led to invalid information in the medical literature, resulting in serious adverse public health consequences (see Table 3-1) (Godlee, 2009). Furthermore, proponents of open access believe that individuals and organizations with bad intentions could easily find ways to overcome the controls instituted by sponsors, and the controls would therefore serve only to slow the rate of scientific discovery and advancement without mitigating risks (Butte, 2014; Eichler, 2013; Wilbanks, 2014). Current proposals for restricted access and conditions of use have been criticized as deeply flawed: ambiguous wording and poorly specified provisions have mired those seeking secondary access in prolonged delays, legal risks, and lawsuits (Goldacre et al., 2014). It is also argued that data derived from research that is publicly funded or publicly subsidized (for example, through tax incentives or support for public universities) should be shared with the public that paid for it.

The committee believes that open access (to the public with no controls) is appropriate and desirable for sharing clinical trial results and that in some cases, no or few controls on sharing other types of clinical trial data may be the preferred approach when all stakeholders involved in a clinical trial (i.e., sponsors, investigators, and participants) are comfortable with this approach and believe the benefits outweigh the risks. For example, the Immune Tolerance Network (ITN) makes data and analytic code underlying ITN-published manuscripts available via the webportal TrialShare after registration and agreement to terms of use (Immune Tolerance Network, 2014). In many cases, however, sponsors, investigators, and/or participants may have concerns about an open access model for certain clinical trial data and wish to place some conditions on data access or use.

Some organizations, such as the European Medicines Agency (EMA) and the U.S. National Institutes of Health (NIH), in its Genomic Data Policy, employ a graded approach to data sharing, placing more controls on sharing data that are considered more sensitive (EMA, 2013; NIH, 2014). For example, the EMA plans to provide public access to redacted CSRs in a nondownloadable format and will provide the CSRs in a downloadable format only to known requesters who commit to using the data for scientific purposes only and to other conditions of use (EMA, 2014a).

The remainder of this chapter analyzes concerns about and the risks of sharing clinical trial data and the controls proposed for addressing them. The final section presents the committee's recommendation on operational strategies for addressing these concerns and mitigating these risks. In general, the committee believes no single approach to access can be recommended at this time for all types of clinical trials.

APPROACHES TO MITIGATING THE RISKS OF DATA SHARING

Various approaches to mitigating the risks of sharing clinical trial data are currently being implemented according to the interests, concerns, and

---

BOX 5-2
Use of Shared Data for Another Company's
Regulatory Submission

Sponsors of clinical trials have serious concerns about competitors copying data packages that lack strong regulatory data protection. If competitors can obtain regulatory approval primarily on the basis of shared data and not their own work, companies and their investors may be reluctant to assume the high costs and risks of developing new therapies and carrying out the clinical trials required for regulatory approval. In the long run, patients and the public would suffer if the development of new therapies declined. These concerns have some empirical basis; the majority of early requests to the European Medicines Agency (EMA) to access clinical trial data were made by drug companies, lawyers, and consultants, not academic investigators (Rabesandratana, 2013).

What types of policies might be implemented to protect data from "unfair commercial use" is a difficult question. Some such policies may have unintended adverse effects on attempts to reanalyze data and merge data from other clinical trials. As of October 2014, the EMA's data release policy included a contractual provision under which data requestors agree not to reuse the data to seek regulatory approval in other jurisdictions (EMA, 2014a). Although this provision is unlikely to pose difficulties for researchers, effective enforcement and sanctions may be difficult to implement. Additionally, only the person or entity that first accesses the data is bound by this contractual provision. If the data become available publicly, those who access the data are under no restrictions. Perhaps in recognition of the relatively limited effectiveness of a contractual provision, the EMA will place watermarks on published clinical report data "to emphasize the prohibition of its use for commercial purposes" (EMA, 2014a). The efficacy of a watermark-based approach remains to be seen. Further, according to its October 2014 statement, the EMA will consider "the nature of the product concerned, the competitive situation of the therapeutic market in question, the approval status in other jurisdictions, resources of the organizations and individuals involved. As stated above, sharing analyzable data sets and the CSRs presents risks. The first risk is to participant privacy. Analyzable data sets and the CSRs contain identifiable data, and participants may be harmed if the data are not adequately de-identified and other appropriate privacy protections are not in place. Second, the CSRs may be used for "unfair commercial purposes," such as wholesale copying of originator data sets for purposes of receiving regulatory approval in jurisdictions with limited regulatory data protection laws (see also Box 5-2). Such use of shared data could harm individual companies, the industry as a whole, and ultimately the public by reducing incentives to develop new therapies. Third, data recipients may perform and disseminate invalid secondary analyses as a result of misunderstanding the analyzable data set and its limitations or performing improper

---

and the novelty of the clinical development" in making determinations regarding redaction (EMA, 2014a).

By not allowing data to be downloaded or copied, the Yale University Open Data Access (YODA) agreement with Johnson & Johnson goes a substantial step further, which may make it more difficult for researchers to aggregate data sets (for example, for meta-analyses) (YODA Project, 2014). Thus, proposals for such limitations should be approached cautiously, or other provisions should be made for providing data sets for meta-analyses. That being said, to the extent that data set providers use a common website, some aggregation may be possible. For example, although the website for sharing clinical trial data that Bayer, Boehringer Ingelheim, Eli Lilly, GlaxoSmithKline, Novartis, Roche, Sanofi, and ViiV Healthcare have agreed to use (www.ClinicalStudyDataRequest.com) does not allow data downloading, researchers working on the website are permitted to aggregate data from the different study sponsors.

The discussion thus far has assumed that a competitor would submit for marketing approval precisely the same molecule as that of the originator. However, certain jurisdictions, including the United States, allow applicants to submit modified molecules for approval through a pathway whereby they rely on approval of the originator's product and submit new data relating to the modification. In the United States, this is known as the 505(b)(2) pathway (Minsk et al., 2010). In the United States, data exclusivity regimes adopted with generic molecules in mind appear to apply to the 505(b)(2) case, so this route cannot be used until the data exclusivity of the originator's product expires.[*] However, such exclusivity may be absent in other countries. (see also the discussion of data protection and exclusivity laws in Appendix C). Moreover, in the case of pathways similar to 505(b)(2) in other countries, these countries may actually require detailed clinical trial data, in which case public release of even redacted clinical study reports could result in a risk of competitive harm, although how significant this risk might be is unclear.

---

[*] 21 U.S.C. § 355(b)(2).

data analysis, or even intentionally. Invalid secondary analyses may lead to inappropriate conclusions about the safety and effectiveness of therapies, which may in turn harm patients. Lastly, investigators who conduct clinical trials want some assurance that they will receive appropriate professional credit for their work and publications resulting from additional analyses of the data they collected.

The committee is aware that the likelihood or severity of any of these risks will be specific to the circumstances of a given trial. For trials involving sensitive or stigmatizing conditions, for example, the risk to privacy is great; for trials of innovative first-in-class agents, the risk to commercial interests is large. For other trials, these risks may be relatively small. Consequently, the committee does not recommend one access model for all trials and types of clinical trial data but instead presents the rationale for using various controls on access to clinical trial data and recommends operational strategies for their use. Current practices for mitigating the risks of data sharing include the de-identification of data; making data available for inspection and analysis but not for downloading; registration and the use of data use agreements (DUAs); and review of data requests, including review by an independent third party. Box 5-3 lists which specific controls are designed to address the various specific risks; further elaboration is provided below.

De-identification

De-identification is commonly used to protect the privacy of participants in a clinical trial (see also Appendix B). Various jurisdictions may differ on the degree to which the risk of re-identification must be reduced for the data to be considered sufficiently de-identified to justify more widespread sharing, particularly in the absence of specific informed consent of the data subjects.[2] In the United States, the Health Insurance Portability and Accountability Act (HIPAA) provides two methodologies for rendering health information "de-identified," but it does not set a specific numerical threshold for unacceptable re-identification risk. Similarly, the European Union's (EU's) Data Protection Directive and similar directives

---

[2] In general, privacy or data protection laws regulate or reserve the most stringent regulations for identifiable personal data—data that either directly or indirectly identify the data subjects. In the United States, for example, the Health Insurance Portability and Accountability Act (HIPAA) does not regulate health data that are "de-identified," which is defined as "health information that does not identify an individual and with respect to which there is no reasonable basis to believe the information can be used to identify an individual" (45 CFR 164.514). The European Union's Data Protection Directive 95/46, Recital 26, states that "the principles of data protection shall not apply to data rendered anonymous in such a way that the data subject is no longer identifiable."

BOX 5-3
Approaches to Mitigating the Risks of Sharing Individual
Participant Data and Clinical Study Reports (CSRs)

Participant Privacy
- De-identification and application of other privacy-enhancing technologies and algorithms
- Required registration
- DUA clause prohibiting the re-identification or misuse of data
- Security protections

Unfair Commercial Use
- DUA clauses
- Watermarking CSRs
- Making CSRs nondownloadable
- Review of data requests/restrictions on who gets access

Invalid Secondary Analyses
- Review of data requests/restrictions on access based on qualifications and/or merit of research proposal
- DUA clause requiring public posting of analysis plan
- DUA clause allowing sponsor/clinical trialist to review analyses before publication

Credit for Clinical Trialists/Sponsors
- DUA clause to credit data generator in any publication

---

around the world do not provide explicit guidelines for how data should be protected through de-identification or anonymization.[3] In Sweden, any possibility, however theoretical, that data can be re-identified is sufficient to render the data identifiable.[4] Thus, jurisdictions vary considerably in their standards for de-identification.

Frequently, the risk of re-identification depends on the context in which data are released. For example, are mitigating controls in place (e.g., release only in controlled environments or to recipients with strong

---

[3] The U.K. Information Commissioner's Office has published a code of practice providing examples of de-identification methods and issues to consider when assessing the level of identifiability of data, but it does not provide a full methodology or specific standards to follow (El Emam and Malin, 2014).

[4] E-mail communication, M. Barnes, B. Bierer, and R. Li, Multi-Regional Clinical Trials (MRCT) Center, to A. Claiborne, Institute of Medicine, regarding comments to the Institute of Medicine questions on data sharing, April 1, 2014.

data management policies and practices) that would reduce the likelihood of re-identification? What is the potential for harm or an invasion of privacy of the data subjects (e.g., due to sensitivity of the data) if re-identification were to occur? What are the possible motives and capacity of the recipient to re-identify the data? Providing some assurances to the public with respect to the risk of re-identification may require more than removing or masking direct or potential (quasi) identifiers.[5] At a minimum, recipients of data from data sharing initiatives should commit to not intentionally re-identifying the data subjects, for example, through a DUA (see the section below). In addition, all holders of even de-identified or anonymized data should adopt reasonable security safeguards to help prevent inadvertent, unauthorized access.

De-identifying data does not eliminate all risk of re-identification, and reducing that risk to zero, as by coarsening the data or combining cells in the data set that contain few individuals, often destroys or significantly impairs the utility of the data for subsequent research.

Protecting privacy is a particular challenge in the era of "big data," where the variety of data, the size of data sets, and the scope of data analysis are unprecedented. Inferences can be drawn about an individual even if there are no data about the individual that are traditionally considered identifying. Even if overt identifiers are removed from a data set, it may be possible to re-identify individuals by bringing auxiliary information from other sources to bear on the data set (Dwork, 2014). Moreover, it is possible to detect the presence of genomic DNA from a specific individual within an admixture of genomic DNA from many individuals (Homer et al., 2008). As one privacy scholar wrote, big data analytics "make certain facts newly inferable that anonymity promised to keep beyond reach" (Barocas and Nissenbaum, 2014, p. 56). Similarly, The President's Council of Advisors on Science and Technology (PCAST) declared that anonymization is now not "sufficiently robust to be a dependable basis for privacy protection where big data is [sic] concerned" (PCAST, 2014).

Successful re-identification attacks on properly de-identified or anonymized health or clinical data are rare, but they happen.[6,7] Reducing the risk of re-identification of data subjects is a valuable tool for ensuring that the benefits of data sharing outweigh the risks, but it should not be the

---

[5] Ibid.

[6] The well-publicized re-identification of the medical records of the governor of Massachusetts depended on using the governor's birthdate and zip code. These data would need to be removed from a de-identified data set under the HIPAA safe harbor requirements (DHS, 2005).

[7] E-mail communication, M. Barnes, B. Bierer, and R. Li, Multi-Regional Clinical Trials (MRCT) Center, to A. Claiborne, Institute of Medicine, regarding comments to the Institute of Medicine questions on data sharing, April 1, 2014.

only tool leveraged to protect the privacy of research participants. Entities storing clinical trial data for sharing should take advantage of innovations in data privacy and security protections and deploy additional safeguards to bolster protections against residual re-identification risk—for example, by deploying advanced cryptographic techniques when running analyses on encrypted data (Zeldovich, 2014) or relying on distributed data sets for analysis in lieu of centralized collection of data (which creates a single target for attack) (The White House Office of Science and Technology Policy and MIT, 2014). In addition, holders of clinical trial data may need to address differential privacy, such as through techniques that introduce random noise into a data set (Dwork, 2014; The White House Office of Science and Technology Policy and MIT, 2014). Stakeholders in responsible sharing of clinical trial data need to keep up to date with emerging privacy protection techniques being developed by computer scientists.

Making Data Available for Use But Not Downloadable

Several data sharing programs are granting some access to clinical trial data to secondary users but not allowing them to download the data to their own computers. The EMA is allowing users to view data online after simple registration; to download data, secondary users must agree to additional conditions. The consortium of drug companies ClinicalStudyDataRequest.com does not allow secondary users to download individual participant data to their computers; analyses must be carried out using standard software programs on the website in a secure workspace (ClinicalStudyDataRequest.com, 2014a). This approach helps protect sponsors from secondary users' carrying out analyses beyond those proposed in the data request, compromising participant privacy, or using data for their own regulatory submission. Secondary users can combine data from different clinical trials that are accessible on the website, for example, to carry out meta-analyses. However, secondary users may be concerned that this process may make their work more cumbersome or take longer.

Registration and Use of Data Use Agreements

Registration and use of DUAs (also called terms of use) can protect against many of the risks of data sharing and enhance the scientific value of additional analyses of shared data. DUAs are agreements executed between the party sharing the data and the data recipient that bind the recipient to certain conditions related to the data. The U.S. Secretary's Advisory Committee on Human Research Protections (SACHRP) has called for the use of DUAs, with penalties for violations, "under which the recipient would pledge to use the data only for the purposes specified; not to disclose the data to others (except insofar as needed to assure research integrity and except under specific publication conditions); and not to try at any point to re-identify subjects" (SACHRP, 2013). Common provisions in DUAs that may reduce risks to various parties currently include

- prohibitions on any attempt at re-identification or contact of individual trial participants,
- prohibitions on further sharing of the data unless permitted or required,
- prohibitions on the use of shared data to support a competitor sponsor's application for licensing of a product or new indication or for "unfair commercial use" (see Box 5-2),
- requirements to acknowledge in any publication or dissemination the trial whose data were shared so that the original trialists will gain appropriate professional credit for the value of their work for secondary analyses, and
- assignment of intellectual property rights for discoveries from the shared data.

Other provisions frequently included in DUAs are intended to enhance the scientific value of secondary analyses. They include

- requirements that secondary users seek to publish their analyses in peer-reviewed publications and make their statistical analysis plan available to other researchers;
- requirements to send copies of submitted manuscripts and publications to the trial investigators or study sponsor, with no right of revision or approval; and
- restrictions on using the data for purposes other than those originally proposed in the application to access the data.

Finally, to ensure that safety signals concerning medical products are used to protect the public health, DUAs may include requirements to notify industry sponsors and appropriate regulatory authorities of any findings that raise significant safety concerns.

The committee does not endorse all the above provisions in DUAs but believes that sponsors, funders, and intermediaries that hold and release clinical trial data should consider these provisions as potential options for increasing the benefits and reducing the risks of sharing clinical trial data. From a legal perspective, it is not clear whether and how these DUAs can be enforced if violated by secondary users, and the committee could not find any relevant case law. Nevertheless, the committee believes the terms in DUAs have a significant normative, symbolic, and deterrent value, setting standards for responsible behavior, even if their legal enforceability has not been tested in the courts.

Conclusion: DUAs are a useful strategy and best practice for increasing the benefits and mitigating the risks of sharing clinical trial data.

Review of Data Requests

Thus far, industry sponsors that have established data sharing arrangements have employed an additional level of control on data access beyond registration and use of DUAs—review of data requests, as employed, for example, by GlaxoSmithKline (GSK) and other sponsors via ClinicalStudyDataRequest.com (see Box 5-4). Proponents contend that review of data requests helps protect against invalid secondary uses of the data, which may occur for a number of reasons, including unfamiliarity with the data set and its limitations, invalid statistical methods, the

---

BOX 5-4
ClinicalStudyDataRequest.com

ClinicalStudyDataRequest.com is a multisponsor Web system, launched in January 2014 for requesting clinical trial data, which is based on a system initially launched in May 2013 by GlaxoSmithKline (GSK). Thus far, in addition to GSK, Bayer, Boehringer Ingelheim, Eli Lilly, Novartis, Roche, Sanofi, Takeda, UCB, and ViiV Healthcare have agreed to release data through the website.

The Web request system provides de-identified individual participant data from medicines that had received regulatory approval (in any country) or whose development had been terminated. As with the earlier system, ClinicalStudyDataRequest.com requires investigators to submit a research proposal to an independent review panel before a request for data is granted. The review panel (1) assesses whether the research proposal has a valid "scientific rationale and relevance to medical science or patient care" and (2) considers requesters' qualifications (e.g., statistical expertise) and potential conflicts of interest (Nisen and Rockhold, 2013). Once the review panel has accepted a data request and investigators have signed a data sharing agreement, access to individual participant data, analyzable data sets, and supporting or metadata documents—including the protocol, statistical analysis plan, clinical study report, blank annotated case record form, and data specifications—is granted through a password-protected secure Internet connection. Data are not downloadable. Finally, investigators that analyze shared data are required to post their analysis plan publicly and, after the study is completed, to post summary results and seek publication in a peer-reviewed journal (Hughes et al., 2014).

inherent inaccuracy of safety signals obtained without prespecification of adverse effects, or analyses aimed at reaching a preconceived conclusion. These data request submissions are reviewed either by the sponsor (e.g., Merck and as endorsed in Biotechnology Industry Organization [BIO] principles for data sharing), by an independent panel that applies criteria set by the sponsor on a case-by-case basis (e.g., the companies signed on to ClinicalStudyDataRequest.com), or by an independent intermediary organization to which the sponsor has transferred authority and jurisdiction for reviewing data requests (e.g., Johnson & Johnson's transfer of authority to Yale University Open Data Access [YODA]). The criteria used in reviewing requests may or may not be stated explicitly, and the review committee may or may not be publicly named (see Appendix D for a detailed description of the data sharing policies of the 12 largest pharmaceutical companies). Criteria for reviewing requests have focused on review of requesters' qualifications and the scientific merit and validity of the proposed research. One sponsor's independent review committee has published its experience during its first year (Strom et al., 2014).

Controlling Access Based on Qualifications

Sponsors that have implemented data sharing polices suggested to the committee that controlling access on the basis of qualifications may help reduce the risk of invalid secondary analyses. For example, requiring someone on the team to have expertise in biostatistics may reduce the likelihood that multiple analyses will be carried out without appropriate statistical correction. For example, Bayer, Eli Lilly, GSK, Merck, and Roche all require that data requesters have a biostatistician on their research team before granting requests. However, it is difficult to judge an individual's qualifications to carry out a proper statistical analysis. Some who are qualified to do so may not have a formal degree in statistics, while others who have a degree in statistics may lack the training or experience to carry out a rigorous biostatistical analysis of clinical trial data. Thus, a categorical requirement for formal biostatistics training may exclude some data user teams with appropriate expertise.

To address the problem of unwarranted malpractice claims driven by invalid secondary analyses, some have proposed restricting lawyers' access to clinical trial data (see Box 5-5). As noted earlier, the EMA reports that lawyers were among those most frequently requesting clinical trial data from the EMA—far more frequently than academic researchers.[8]

---

[8] Personal communication, Virtual WebEx Open Session, L. Brown and G. Fleming, to Committee on Strategies for Responsible Sharing of Clinical Trial Data, Institute of Medicine, regarding clinical trial data sharing: product liability, April 9, 2014.

BOX 5-5
Use of Shared Data for Malpractice Litigation

The benefits and risks of litigators' use of shared clinical trial data are hotly debated.

Plaintiffs' attorneys contend that malpractice suits have revealed serious problems with medical products that caused widespread harm to patients (e.g., COX-2 inhibitors, gabapentin).[a] From their perspective, lawsuits help protect patients from unsafe drugs and devices. Access to clinical trial data would help plaintiffs' attorneys identify new risks of therapies and obtain further evidence through the discovery process. Noting that in U.S. federal courts, the Daubert rule excludes invalid scientific evidence from being admitted into trial, these attorneys believe that concerns about "rogue science" are misplaced. In their view, moreover, contingency fees provide powerful incentives to bring only lawsuits that are based on sound scientific evidence.[a]

Defense attorneys have a sharply different perspective on the sharing of clinical trial data. Post hoc analyses can significantly overstate the risks of a therapy by including multiple subgroup analyses, varying the endpoints of an analysis, or selecting studies for inclusion in a meta-analysis in a biased manner. In their view, the Daubert rule does not reliably exclude statistically invalid subgroup analyses that identify a group of patients as more likely than not to be harmed by a therapy.[a] Moreover, the Daubert rule is applied differentially by judges and may not be used in a state court where a lawsuit is brought. From the perspective of defense attorneys, lawyers should not be categorically excluded from access to clinical trial data; like other secondary users, they should be able to obtain access to the data under controlled access by submitting a sound data analysis plan.[a] From this perspective, moreover, plaintiffs' lawyers do not need direct access to clinical trial data; they can obtain the data through the discovery process. In addition, plaintiffs' attorneys can draw on published reports by researchers who have conducted secondary analyses of the data.

Restricting litigators from direct access to clinical trial data poses difficult implementation challenges. The Yale University Open Data Access (YODA) policy states that YODA will deny access to data sought for purposes of litigation, but it does not address how those who do not self-identify as litigators might be identified. Prohibiting the downloading or copying of data may deter litigators from using only one result from multiple subgroup analyses without acknowledging the statistical limitations of such use. As discussed earlier, however, such prohibitions may also deter useful data analysis and aggregation by researchers. Similarly, provisions in data use agreements that the data not be used for litigation are difficult to enforce. Nonetheless, there may still be a normative, symbolic, or deterrent value in such restrictions.

---

[a] Personal communication, Virtual WebEx Open Session, L. Brown and G. Fleming, to Committee on Strategies for Responsible Sharing of Clinical Trial Data, Institute of Medicine, regarding clinical trial data sharing: product liability, April 9, 2014.

However, trying to restrict lawyers' access to clinical trial data may be impractical. Lawyers can arrange with academic researchers to obtain clinical trial data in order to seek evidence that sponsors knew about and failed to respond to serious adverse events. Furthermore, a lawyer may be part of a data requesting team that has an appropriate research question and analysis plan (Eichler, 2013).

> **Conclusion:** *Controlling access to data based on the requester's qualifications is not effective for mitigating risks and may present barriers to some qualified teams of requesters.*

Controlling Access Based on Data Access Requests

Several models for sharing clinical trial data entail reviewing the scientific rationale or purpose of data requests and the ability of the proposed research and data analysis plan to achieve the scientific objectives. The rationale for such review is to screen out data requests that lack a valid purpose or research or data analysis plan and therefore will not produce valid scientific knowledge that benefits the public. For example, requiring secondary users to prespecify a research question and submit a data analysis plan will reduce the risk of multiple comparisons leading to spurious conclusions because these requirements make it possible to identify secondary users who report a different analysis from what they originally proposed. However, at least one independent review panel does not see its role as performing scientific peer review, leaving that task to peer review of publications (Strom et al., 2014).

Review of a prespecified research question may also exclude secondary users whose analysis could benefit the public even though they lack a prespecified data analysis plan. For instance, an investigator may request a data set to generate new hypotheses for additional basic and clinical research but have no prespecified data analysis plan. As another example, a teacher of a biostatistics or evidence-based medicine course may wish to use a data set as a classroom exercise, to give students hands-on experience with analyzing clinical trial data.

Concerns about invalid secondary analyses are controversial. On the one hand, proponents of open science, who advocate public access to clinical trial data, argue that a free marketplace of ideas and vigorous debate are in the long run the best path to better understanding of clinical trial data (Goldacre, 2013a,b, 2014; Goldacre et al., 2014). From this perspective, sponsors and the original trial investigators may introduce serious bias into trials by withholding unfavorable data, manipulating variables, or carrying out inappropriate statistical analyses (Doshi et al., 2013). With some industry-sponsored trials, there is no peer review of the protocol or amendments. The resulting bias in the evidence base for clinical decisions harms patients. In this view, it is unfair to subject secondary analyses to more scrutiny than that received by the original trial. From this perspective, some invalid secondary analyses are an unavoidable side effect of sharing clinical trial data and gaining the benefits of correcting invalid original clinical trial reports and analyzing unpublished data. Moreover, proponents of open access argue that concerns about inaccurate secondary analyses are speculative (Doshi et al., 2013, p. 4), unlike documented cases of serious distortion in the evidence base for clinical care caused by biased published manuscripts and by unpublished data and trials (Doshi et al., 2013; Joober et al., 2012).

On the other hand, proponents of some controls over data access argue that biased primary analyses of clinical trial data and failure to publish unfavorable results will be addressed effectively by providing data to other investigators under controlled access. In their view, the reasonable controls currently being used by some drug manufacturers have not impeded the vast majority of requests for access to clinical trial data (Strom et al., 2014). Proponents of controls over access contend that with uncontrolled access to the CSRs and individual participant data, a secondary user of the data could carry out multiple analyses in an invalid manner. At least one team of clinical trialists has claimed that repeated challenges and accusations based on erroneous data and improper analyses can consume large amounts of time and effort; this team wrote that it wished to warn of the "dangers of open access to data when the peer review and editorial processes fail to do due diligence" (Wallentin et al., 2014).

Because a fundamental goal of responsible sharing of clinical trial data is to produce additional analyses that are scientifically valid, the committee believes some control over access to clinical trial data based on the research proposal may be beneficial, provided that the controls are not unduly burdensome for secondary users.

Conclusion: Controlling access on the basis of the purpose and/or scientific validity of the research proposal may be an effective strategy for mitigating risk, although overly restrictive controls are undesirable because they would inhibit valid secondary analyses and innovative scientific proposals.

Independent Review Panels

Use of review panels to control access to clinical trial data by reviewing and approving data requests raises important questions regarding implementation: Who decides whether data requestors gain access to the data, and what criteria are used to make the decision? One option is for the trial sponsor or investigator to make decisions about access. However, this arrangement may raise concern about conflicts of interest and bias and cause mistrust. Another option is for a "trusted intermediary" or "honest broker" to make the decisions. The intermediary may negotiate the conditions for data sharing (with the data provider retaining control over the data and their release) or take full responsibility for deciding who gets access and delivering the data to recipients (Mello et al., 2013). Trusted intermediaries may also accept and facilitate data analysis queries from secondary investigators if a model of "bringing the question to the data," as discussed in Chapter 6, is adopted. Moreover, an independent oversight panel could have the authority to use its discretion to alter the timing of data release; examples of how an urgent public health need might justify earlier release of the analytic data set supporting a pivotal publication were offered in Chapter 4. If the review of data requests is carried out by such a group that is independent of the sponsor and investigators in the original trial, high-profile concerns raised in the past about sponsors placing undue barriers and delays in the path of data requests can be avoided (Doshi et al., 2012; Godlee, 2009).

Conclusion: *It is best practice to designate an independent review panel, rather than the sponsor or investigator of a clinical trial, to be responsible for reviewing and approving requests for clinical trial data.*

The use of independent review panels also raises a number of practical issues that need to be resolved, including selection of the panel members, administration, funding, and compensation for the panel's services (ADNI, 2013; MCRT at Harvard, 2013; Nisen and Rockhold, 2013; PhRMA and EFPIA, 2013; YODA Project, 2013). Several large drug manufacturers have established programs for sharing clinical trial data using an independent review panel to determine access to the data. As stated above, GSK and nine additional industry sponsors have hired an independent panel of four members to review research requests (ClinicalStudyDataRequest. com, 2014b). Johnson & Johnson and Bristol-Myers Squibb have taken a slightly different approach and contracted with YODA and the Duke Clinical Research Institute, respectively. Currently, large pharmaceutical companies are paying for the cost of these services. However, investigators funded by public and nonprofit organizations generally lack the resources to establish their own independent review panels. Thus, public and nonprofit funders would need to provide support and funding to establish these panels for their investigators to use.

Composition of Independent Review Panels

In general, independent review panels are currently composed of persons with expertise in clinical research, clinical trials, biostatistics, and clinical medicine who have no conflicts of interest in deciding whether a data requester receives access. Some panels also have members with expertise in law and ethics, which is helpful if the panel is charged with reviewing whether consent forms from legacy trials allow data sharing.

Currently, many review panels established by pharmaceutical companies do not include representation of clinical trial participants, their communities, disease advocacy groups, or the public. But as discussed in Chapter 3, engaging these stakeholders and giving them a meaningful voice can help sponsors and investigators better understand their concerns and can suggest constructive ways of addressing those concerns and improving the sharing of clinical trial data generally.

There are several examples of how representatives of communities and patient and disease advocacy groups can contribute fresh perspectives and constructive ideas to research institutions and research projects. Furthermore, some research funders have required that patient and community representatives play formal roles in research organizations and projects. The 2005 National Research Council report *Ethical Considerations for Research on Housing-Related Health Hazards Involving Children* points out how community-based participatory research could enhance the scientific usefulness of such studies, reduce the risks of the research, and build trust among the communities being studied (NRC, 2005). The Centers for Disease Control and Prevention (CDC) has suggested that community-based participatory research may help increase the net benefits of research in cancer prevention and intervention by reducing disparities in cancer outcomes and by "addressing many of the challenges of traditional practice and research" (CDC and ATSDR, 1997; Simonds et al., 2013). The NIH-sponsored HIV Prevention Trials Network requires sites to have community advisory boards. Studies suggest that such community advisory boards may help investigators understand community concerns about proposed research and improve the informed consent process and consent forms (Morin et al., 2008). The California Institute for Regenerative Medicine, which provides public funding for stem cell research, has disease advocates serve on both the governing body and scientific panels that review grant applications (IOM, 2012). The 2014 NIH working group responding to the Institute of Medicine (IOM) report on the Clinical and Translational Science Awards (IOM, 2013) recommended having community or disease advocacy groups in all stages of planning for the awards and in oversight and administration (NCATS, 2014). In the health care delivery context, patients have been called on to play a key role. Taken together, these examples offer proof of the principle that stakeholders from disease advocacy groups and communities where research is carried out can enhance the mission of organizations funding and conducting clinical research.

> **Conclusion:** *Representatives of communities and patient and disease advocacy groups can contribute fresh perspective and constructive ideas to the bodies responsible for decisions about access to clinical trial data.*

Transparency in Data Processes and Procedures

Steps can be taken to enhance the trustworthiness of data sharing programs in several ways. First, the criteria for data sharing and the process for determining access should be publicly available. This transparency allows others to review the criteria and process, compare criteria and policies from different sponsors, and identify best practices. For instance, best practices regarding DUAs are likely to emerge as experience with different terms is shared. Public reporting of the number of requests for data and the number refused and for what reasons, as is done in the sharing program established by GSK, would further enhance trustworthiness (Strom et al., 2014); for example, the report on the program's first year of work reveals that the vast majority of data requests is granted. Going beyond these summary data, YODA will publicly post all data requests; the requester's research proposal and analysis plan; and, if access is denied, the reasons for refusal. This information will allow others to review the reasons for refusal and discuss whether they are appropriate.

> **Conclusion:** *It is best practice that policy and procedures regarding access to clinical trial data be transparent, including*
> - *public reporting of the policies and procedures for sharing clinical trial data (including criteria for determining access and conditions of use), as well as the names of individuals making decisions about access and serving on the governing body of the unit determining access; and*
> - *public reporting of a summary of the disposition of data sharing requests, including the number of requests and approvals and the reasons for disapprovals.*

CREATING A LEARNING SYSTEM

The experiences of early adopters of the sharing of clinical trial data will undoubtedly offer lessons and best practices from which others can learn. In fact, programs for sharing clinical trial data have already evolved in response to experience and feedback from stakeholders. For example,

YODA now has revised policies regarding the sharing of clinical trial data based on its experience with data sharing for Medtronic and on public comments it solicited on its draft policies to share data for Johnson & Johnson (YODA Project, 2013). In another noteworthy example, the EMA conducted a series of meetings and solicited public comments on draft regulations and revised its policies accordingly (EMA, 2014b). Policies on sharing clinical trial data can be expected to continue to evolve in the future. Sponsors will try different approaches, and comparing the outcomes of these approaches will provide useful information on what does and does not work in various contexts. Moreover, approaches to data sharing are likely to change as new approaches to clinical trials are introduced. Finally, new issues and challenges are likely to emerge as more experience is gained with data sharing.

RECOMMENDATION

The committee drew together the deliberations detailed in this chapter with the following overarching recommendation:

Recommendation 3: Holders of clinical trial data should mitigate the risks and enhance the benefits of sharing sensitive clinical trial data by implementing operational strategies that include employing data use agreements, designating an independent review panel, including members of the lay public in governance, and making access to clinical trial data transparent. Specifically, they should take the following actions:

- Employ data use agreements that include provisions aimed at protecting clinical trial participants, advancing the goal of producing scientifically valid secondary analyses, giving credit to the investigators who collected the clinical trial data, protecting the intellectual property interests of sponsors, and ultimately improving patient care.
- Employ other appropriate techniques for protecting privacy, in addition to de-identification and data security.
- Designate an independent review panel—in lieu of the sponsor or investigator of a clinical trial—if requests for access to clinical trial data will be reviewed for approval.
- Include lay representatives (e.g., patients, members of the public, and/or representatives of disease advocacy groups) on the independent review panel that reviews and approves data access requests.

- Make access to clinical trial data transparent by publicly reporting
  - the organizational structure, policies, procedures (e.g., criteria for determining access and conditions of use), and membership of the independent review panel that makes decisions about access to clinical trial data; and
  - a summary of the decisions regarding requests for data access, including the number of requests and approvals and the reasons for disapprovals.
- Learn from experience by collecting data on the outcomes of data sharing policies, procedures, and technical approaches (including the benefits, risks, and costs), and share information and lessons learned with clinical trial sponsors, the public, and other organizations sharing clinical trial data.

REFERENCES

ADNI (Alzheimer's Disease Neuroimaging Initiative). 2013. *ADNI overview.* http://www. adni-info.org/Scientists/ADNIOverview.aspx (accessed October 17, 2014).

Barocas, S., and H. Nissenbaum. 2014. Big data's end run around anonymity and consent. In *Privacy, big data, and the public good: Frameworks for engagement,* edited by J. Lane, V. Stodden, S. Bender, and H. Nissenbaum. New York: Cambridge University Press. Pp. 44-75.

Butte, A. 2014. *Clinical trials data sharing and the ImmPort experience.* Paper presented at IOM Committee on Strategies for Responsible Sharing of Clinical Trial Data: Meeting Two, February 3-4, Washington, DC.

CDC (Centers for Disease Control and Prevention) and ATSDR (Agency for Toxic Substances and Disease Registry). 1997. *Committee on community engagement: Principles of community engagement.* http://www.cdc.gov/phppo/pce (accessed October 17, 2014).

ClinicalStudyDataRequest.com. 2014a. *How it works: Access to data.* https://clinicalstudy datarequest.com/How-it-works-Access.aspx (accessed November 24, 2014).

ClinicalStudyDataRequest.com. 2014b. *Members of the independent review panel.* https://clinical studydatarequest.com/Members-of-the-Independent-Review-Panel.aspx (accessed November 24, 2014).

DHS (U.S. Department of Homeland Security). 2005. *Statement of Latanya Sweeney, PhD, associate professor of computer science, technology and policy, director, data privacy laboratory, Carnegie Mellon University, before the privacy and integrity advisory committee of the Department of Homeland Security ("DHS"), "privacy technologies for homeland security."* http://www.dhs.gov/xlibrary/assets/privacy/privacy_advcom_06-2005_testimony_ sweeney.pdf (accessed December 8, 2014).

Doshi, P., T. Jefferson, and C. Del Mar. 2012. The imperative to share clinical study reports: Recommendations from the Tamiflu experience. *PLoS Medicine* 9(4):e1001201.

Doshi, P., K. Dickersin, D. Healy, S. S. Vedula, and T. Jefferson. 2013. Restoring invisible and abandoned trials: A call for people to publish the findings. *British Medical Journal* 346:f2865.

Dwork, C. 2014. Differential privacy: A cryptographic approach to private data analysis. In *Privacy, big data, and the public good,* edited by J. Lane, V. Stodden, S. Bender, and H. Nissenbaum. New York: Cambridge University Press. Pp. 296-322.

Eichler, H. G. 2013. *Selecting data sharing activities*. Paper presented at IOM Committee on Strategies for Responsible Sharing of Clinical Trial Data: Meeting One, October 22-23, Washington, DC.

El Emam, K., and B. Malin. 2014. *Concepts and methods for de-identifying clinical trials data*. Paper commissioned by the Committee on Strategies for Responsible Sharing of Clinical Trial Data (see Appendix B).

EMA (European Medicines Agency). 2013. *Publication and access to clinical-trial data*. http://www.ema.europa.eu/docs/en_GB/document_library/Other/2013/06/WC500144730.pdf (accessed October 15, 2014).

EMA. 2014a. *European Medicines Agency policy on publication of clinical data for medicinal products for human use*. http://www.ema.europa.eu/docs/en_GB/document_library/Other/2014/10/WC500174796.pdf (accessed November 17, 2014).

EMA. 2014b. *Finalisation of the EMA policy on publication of and access to clinical trial data—targeted consultation with key stakeholders in May 2014*. http://www.ema.europa.eu/docs/en_GB/document_library/Report/2014/09/WC500174226.pdf (accessed October 17, 2014).

Godlee, F. 2009. We want raw data, now. *British Medical Journal* 339:b5405.

Goldacre, B. 2013a. Are clinical trial data shared sufficiently today? No. *British Medical Journal (Clinical Research Edition)* 347:f1880.

Goldacre, B. 2013b. My comments to IOM on IPD sharing. In *bengoldacre: passing thoughts*. http://bengoldacre.tumblr.com/post/64880190003/my-comments-to-iom-on-ipd-sharing (accessed December 16, 2014).

Goldacre, B. 2014. Commentary on Berlin et al. *Clinical Trials* 11(1):15-18.

Goldacre, B., F. Godlee, C. Heneghan, D. Tovey, R. Lehman, I. Chalmers, V. Barbour, and T. Brown. 2014. Open letter: European Medicines Agency should remove barriers to access clinical trial data. *British Medical Journal* 348:g3768.

Homer, N., S. Szelinger, M. Redman, D. Duggan, W. Tembe, J. Muehling, J. V. Pearson, D. A. Stephan, S. F. Nelson, and D. W. Craig. 2008. Resolving individuals contributing trace amounts of DNA to highly complex mixtures using high-density SNP genotyping microarrays. *PLoS Genetics* 4(8):e1000167.

Hughes, S., K. Wells, P. McSorley, and A. Freeman. 2014. Preparing individual patient data from clinical trials for sharing: The GlaxoSmithKline approach. *Pharmaceutical Statistics* 13(3):179-183.

Immune Tolerance Network. 2014. *Public studies on ITN TrialShare*. https://www.itntrialshare.org/public/catalog.html (accessed November 24, 2014).

IOM (Institute of Medicine). 2012. *The California Institute for Regenerative Medicine: Science, governance, and the pursuit of cures*. Washington, DC: The National Academies Press.

IOM. 2013. *The CTSA program at NIH: Opportunities for advancing clinical and translational research*. Edited by A. I. Leshner, S. F. Terry, A. M. Schultz, and C. T. Liverman. Washington, DC: The National Academies Press.

Joober, R., N. Schmitz, L. Annable, and P. Boksa. 2012. Publication bias: What are the challenges and can they be overcome? *Journal of Psychiatry & Neuroscience* 37(3):149-152.

Krumholz, H. M., and E. D. Peterson. 2014. Open access to clinical trials data. *Journal of the American Medical Association* 312(10):1002-1003.

Mello, M. M., J. K. Francer, M. Wilenzick, P. Teden, B. E. Bierer, and M. Barnes. 2013. Preparing for responsible sharing of clinical trial data. *New England Journal of Medicine* 369(17):1651-1658.

Minsk, A., L. Nguyen, and D. R. Cohen. 2010. The 505(b)(2) new drug application process: The essential primer. *FDLI Monograph Series* 1(6).

Morin, S. F., S. Morfit, A. Maiorana, A. Aramrattana, P. Goicochea, J. M. Mutsambi, J. L. Robbins, and T. A. Richards. 2008. Building community partnerships: Case studies of community advisory boards at research sites in Peru, Zimbabwe, and Thailand. *Clinical Trials* 5(2):147-156.

MRCT (Multi-Regional Clinical Trials) Center at Harvard. 2013. *Proceedings: Multi-Regional Clinical Trials Center (MRCT) at Harvard 2nd annual meeting.* Paper read at Multi-Regional Clinical Trials Center (MRCT) at Harvard 2nd Annual Meeting, December 4, 2013, Cambridge, MA.

NCATS (National Center for Advancing Translational Sciences). 2014. *NCATS Advisory Council Working Group on the IOM report: The CTSA program at NIH.* Bethesda, MD: NCATS.

NIH (U.S. National Institutes of Health). 2014. *NIH issues finalized policy on genomic data sharing.* http://www.nih.gov/news/health/aug2014/od-27.htm (accessed October 14, 2014).

Nisen, P., and F. Rockhold. 2013. Access to patient-level data from GlaxoSmithKline clinical trials. *New England Journal of Medicine* 369(5):475-478.

NRC (National Research Council). 2005. *Ethical considerations for research on housing-related health hazards involving children.* Washington, DC: The National Academies Press.

PCAST (President's Council of Advisors on Science and Technology). 2014. *Big data and privacy: A technological perspective.* http://www.whitehouse.gov/sites/default/files/microsites/ostp/PCAST/pcast_big_data_and_privacy_-_may_2014.pdf (accessed November 17, 2014).

PhRMA (Pharmaceutical Research and Manufacturers of America) and EFPIA (European Federation of Pharmaceutical Industries and Associations). 2013. *Principles for responsible clinical trial data sharing: Our commitment to patients and researchers.* http://www.phrma.org/sites/default/files/pdf/PhRMAPrinciplesForResponsibleClinicalTrialDataSharing.pdf (accessed October 16, 2014).

Rabesandratana, T. 2013. Europe. Drug watchdog ponders how to open clinical trial data vault. *Science* 339(6126):1369-1370.

SACHRP (Secretary's Advisory Committee on Human Research Protections). 2013. *SACHRP comment regarding the June 4, 2013 FDA request for comment relating to the availability of masked and de-identified non-summary safety and efficacy data.* http://www.hhs.gov/ohrp/sachrp/commsec/attachmentasecretarialletter21.pdf (accessed October 24, 2014).

Simonds, V. W., N. Wallerstein, B. Duran, and M. Villegas. 2013. Community-based participatory research: Its role in future cancer research and public health practice. *Preventing Chronic Disease* 10:E78.

Strom, B. L., M. Buyse, J. Hughes, and B. M. Knoppers. 2014. Data sharing, year 1—access to data from industry-sponsored clinical trials. *New England Journal of Medicine* 371: 2052-2054.

Wallentin, L., R. C. Becker, C. P. Cannon, C. Held, A. Himmelmann, S. Husted, S. K. James, H. S. Katus, K. W. Mahaffey, K. S. Pieper, R. F. Storey, P. G. Steg, and R. A. Harrington. 2014. Review of the accumulated PLATO documentation supports reliable and consistent superiority of ticagrelor over clopidogrel in patients with acute coronary syndrome. Commentary on: DiNicolantonio JJ, Tomek A, Inactivations, deletions, non-adjudications, and downgrades of clinical endpoints on ticagrelor: Serious concerns over the reliability of the PLATO trial, International Journal of Cardiology, 2013. *International Journal of Cardiology* 170(3):E59-E62.

The White House Office of Science and Technology Policy and MIT (Massachusetts Institute of Technology). 2014. *Big data privacy workshop: Advancing the state of the art in technology and practice, workshop summary report.* Cambridge, MA: MIT.

Wilbanks, J. 2014. *Open access to clinical data.* Paper presented at IOM Committee on Strategies for Responsible Sharing of Clinical Trial Data: Meeting Two, February 3-4, Washington, DC.

YODA (Yale University Open Data Access) Project. 2013. *Yale University Open Data Access (YODA) Project policy for the public availability of RHBMP-2 clinical trial data*. New Haven, CT: Yale University Center for Outcomes Research and Evaluation.

YODA Project. 2014. *Yale University Open Data Access (YODA) Project procedures to guide external investigator access to clinical trial data*. New Haven, CT: Yale University Center for Outcomes Research and Evaluation.

Zeldovich, N. 2014. *Using cryptography in databases and Web applications*. http://web.mit.edu/bigdata-priv/pdf/Nickolai-Zeldovich.pdf (accessed December 8, 2014).

6

The Future of Data Sharing in
a Changing Landscape

In Chapters 3 through 5, the committee recommends strategies and practical approaches for the responsible sharing of clinical trial data, addressing the who, what, when, and how of data sharing in the current environment. This chapter envisions the future that would emerge if stakeholders committed to responsible data sharing, modified their work processes to facilitate it, and possessed the resources and tools necessary to do so. This chapter also looks at the remaining infrastructure, technological, workforce, and sustainability challenges to achieving this future and provides the committee's recommendation for next steps in a path forward.

LOOKING FORWARD

The committee intends this report to be the beginning and not the end of discussions about how to develop a responsible global ecosystem for the responsible sharing of clinical trial data. More public discussions about how best to address the challenges of data sharing will be needed, ideally informed by the ongoing experience of data sharing initiatives. To help guide such discussion, the committee articulates its vision for the future:

- There are more platforms for sharing clinical trial data, with different data access models and sufficient total capacity to meet demand. Stakeholders are able to identify the platform that is most appropriate for their needs. The various initiatives are interoperable (e.g., data obtained from different platforms can easily be searched and combined to allow further analyses).

- A culture of sharing clinical trial data with effective incentives for sharing flourishes.
- Best practices for sharing clinical trial data are identified and modified in response to ongoing experience and feedback. The sharing of clinical trial data forms a "learning" ecosystem in which data on data sharing outcomes are routinely collected and continually used to improve how data sharing is conducted.
- There is adequate financial support for sharing clinical trial data, and costs are fairly allocated among stakeholders.
- Protections are in place to minimize the risks of data sharing (for example, threats to valid secondary analyses, participant privacy, intellectual property, and professional recognition) and to reduce disincentives for sharing.

Existing models described in previous chapters provide an initial foundation for building a global ecosystem for sharing clinical trial data. However, challenges need to be addressed if this future is to be realized. The following sections describe these infrastructure, technical, workforce, and sustainability challenges in greater detail, as well as the committee's views on a structure for further collaboration that will accomplish important next steps into the future. The final section presents the committee's recommendation for addressing these challenges and effecting this collaboration.

INFRASTRUCTURE CHALLENGES

If sponsors and investigators are to implement the recommendations in Chapters 3, 4, and 5, repositories with the capacity to hold and manage the vast amounts of incoming data will have to be created. Investigators are not in a position to hold and manage data from trials for an extended period of time; therefore, without a place to easily store the data after trials have been completed, investigators will have difficulty complying with the committee's recommendations for data sharing.

In addition to capacity, a data sharing infrastructure will need to be capable of managing data access according to the strategies laid out in Recommendation 3 in Chapter 5. As big data approaches become more widespread, newer technological solutions to data access may offer effective ways of achieving the benefits of sharing clinical trial data while mitigating its risks. These newer solutions are predicated on an approach to data query that differs from the traditional one with which most clinical trialists are familiar. In the traditional approach, data are brought to the query. That is, if a data requester wants to run a query, the requester obtains a copy of the data, installs the data on his/her own computer, and runs the query on the downloaded data. Because the data requester now holds a copy of the data, the original data holder has effectively lost control over access to the data.

The converse approach is bringing the query to the data: the data requester submits the query to the machine where the data reside, the query is run on that remote machine, and the results are returned back to the requester. Queries can, of course, be complex computations and analyses, not just simple search and retrieval queries. In this model, data holders retain control of the data, and the requester never has a copy of or control over the data.

This basic idea of bringing the query to the data can be implemented through many different configurations of databases and query servers. Three example configurations are described below to illustrate their representative benefits and challenges; many variations on each are possible. The committee makes no recommendation on data query architectures for data sharing because detailed consideration of this topic is beyond its charge and expertise.

Local Data Stores

In the simplest model, every data holder hosts its own data on its own server. External data requesters are allowed to establish user accounts on that server, perhaps with one of the access control models discussed in Chapter 5. The requester then can view and analyze the data but cannot download a copy of the data to his/her own machine.

Variants of this model currently exist for sharing clinical trial data (e.g., Yale University Open Data Access [YODA], in which a third party, Yale University, acts as the data holder for Johnson & Johnson). However, this model is infeasible for widespread data sharing because it is prohibitively expensive and inefficient for multiple data holders to handle access control, data provision, and user account services. Moreover, data requesters wishing to query multiple databases—for example, to carry out a meta-analysis—must establish multiple user accounts and navigate multiple access policies and procedures. Even after obtaining access to multiple data sets, the requester could not merge them.

One Single Centralized Data Store

The opposite of having each data holder maintain its own server is to collect all clinical trial data worldwide into one central database. This model benefits from economies of scale, and data requesters need submit their queries to only one database. However, a single global database of clinical trial results is unlikely to be adopted, given multiple global stakeholders, interests, and sensitivities as discussed in Chapter 3.

Federated Query Model

The federated query model combines the approach of bringing the query to the data with federated databases. Databases are federated when independent geographically dispersed databases are networked in such a way that they can respond to queries as if all the data were in a single virtual database. Thus, when data requesters submit a query to a federated query service, that query is routed to all databases participating in the federation. The provider of the query service may or may not be the "trusted intermediary" that adjudicates access control requests as discussed above. Federated query services can be purchased as a standalone technical service. Data holders maintain full control over their data, and neither the data requester nor the query service provider ever has direct access to the data. Federated query systems can protect against invasions of privacy, as discussed in Chapter 5. The U.S. Food and Drug Administration's (FDA's) Mini-Sentinel program is using a federated model to combine data sets for comparative effectiveness and outcomes research (Mini-Sentinel, 2014).

If all databases of clinical trial results were housed in a single global federated system that adopted a uniform technical approach to implementing access control, or even in a few federated systems, significant economies of scale and technical ease of data access would result. However, a large federated system could coexist with multiple trusted intermediaries purchasing query services from multiple providers.

A federated query approach can support access control models in which data requesters are able to query multiple databases simultaneously while data holders maintain control of their own data at all times. Yet while the technology and methods to implement a global federated data access system theoretically exist today, substantial challenges arise in practice. Different platforms making up the federated system need to be interoperable. Common data models and data exchange protocols that meet the needs of scientific analysts need to be defined and adopted. User authentication and authorization processes must be defined across different cultures, languages, and legal jurisdictions. Furthermore, secondary users may raise concerns that their data analyses will take more time and be more cumbersome than if they had all the data on their computers.

Conclusion: Currently there are insufficient platforms to store and manage clinical trial data, under a variety of access models, if all sponsors and investigators commit to data sharing.

TECHNICAL CHALLENGES

Just because data are accessible does not mean they are usable. Data are usable only if an investigator can search and retrieve them, can make sense of them, and can analyze them within a single trial or combine them across multiple trials. Given the large volume of data anticipated from the sharing of clinical trial data, the data must be in a computable form amenable to automated methods of search, analysis, and visualization.

To ensure such computability, data cannot be shared only as document files (e.g., PDF, Word). Rather, data must be in electronic databases that clearly specify the meaning of the data so that the database can respond correctly to queries. If data are spread over more than one database, the meaning of the data must be compatible across databases; otherwise, queries cannot be executed at all, or are executable but elicit incorrect answers. In general, such compatibility requires the adoption of common data models that all results databases would either use or be compatible with.

The meaning of the data in a database is specified through two basic mechanisms. The first is the *data model* or *database schema*, which, like column titles in a data table, describes the contents of each data field and defines the kinds of queries to which the database can respond. For example, for a database with a table column titled "Body Weight," all the cells under that column contain measures of weight, and this database can respond to queries about weight. A trial results database will have a data model that has the equivalent of many tables and table columns.[1] To be most useful for purposes of scientific reuse of data, this data model must include tables and columns for elements of the trial protocol that investigators will want to query for when they search for relevant trials, such as intervention names, primary outcomes, and study population characteristics (Sim and Niland, 2012). This *protocol data model* should be robust enough to respond to the complexity of typical scientific queries— for example, "Find me trials of metformin without exercise and diet for prevention of diabetes mellitus. Then give me access to their analyzable data sets." Although ClinicalTrials.gov contains study protocol information, its database currently is not robust enough to respond to such

---

[1] Relational databases follow a table structure, but there are other types of databases that are not based on tables. Relational databases are discussed here for illustrative purposes, recognizing that results databases may be of different types.

detailed queries (Tasneem et al., 2012). With the high level of investment required to enable sharing of clinical trial results, it is imperative that a sufficiently robust common protocol model be defined and adopted to ensure that descriptions of trials can be computationally searched, analyzed, and visualized across multiple databases. Leading protocol data models include CDISC (CDISC, 2014), the PICO ontology from the Cochrane Collaboration (Data.cochrane.org, 2014), and the Ontology of Clinical Research (Sim et al., 2013).

In addition to a common protocol data model, data standardization is required at the level of the study variables across trials (also termed the "data dictionary"). For example, if one trial collects body weight in kilograms, while another collects it as a categorical variable (e.g., 0-50 lb, 51-100 lb, etc.), while yet another collects only body mass index, scientific integration is greatly hampered if not impossible. If sharing of clinical trial data is to be useful for meta-analysis and large-scale data mining, trial protocols should ideally use common data elements for eligibility criteria and baseline and outcome variables. These data elements also should be indexed to standard clinical vocabularies (e.g., SNOMED) as appropriate. There are many common data element initiatives worldwide, from funding agencies (e.g., PROMIS and PhenX from the U.S. National Institutes of Health [NIH]), professional societies (e.g., the American Heart Association and American College of Cardiology Foundation), research collaboratives (e.g., PCORnet), industry collaboratives (e.g., CDISC), and nonprofit organizations (e.g., COMET). The adoption of common data elements has to date been slow to occur, in part because trialists are not aware of these initiatives (HIMSS, 2009) and in part because of a lack of incentives and clear value for doing so. Scientific value will accrue from data sharing only if investigators can easily access results data and can query, align, compute on, and visualize what will no doubt be a large amount of complex, heterogeneous data.

> **Conclusion:** *Current data sharing platforms are not consistently discoverable, searchable, and interoperable. Special attention is needed to the development and adoption of common protocol data models and common data elements to ensure the capacity for meaningful computation across disparate trials and databases.*

WORKFORCE CHALLENGES

An adequate workforce trained in the operational and technical aspects of data sharing is essential to meet the goals of responsible sharing of clinical trial data. As outlined in the 2012 report of the Advisory Committee to the NIH Director, there is a growing gap between the supply of trained quantitative research scientists at all levels (e.g., M.D., Ph.D., M.S., and B.S.) and the growing demand, stimulated in part by the recent explosion of big data in basic, translational, and clinical research (NIH, 2012a). In addition, the data on NIH-funded researchers indicate that the clinical trial and more generally the clinical research workforce is aging, and a new generation needs to be trained.

NIH's training mission has traditionally been focused on training doctoral-level researchers, with limited ability to train at the support staff level or to provide non-Ph.D.-level graduate training, such as that for a master's degree in clinical research or clinical trials (IOM, 2012, 2013b,c; NCATS, 2013; NIH, 2012b; Zerhouni, 2005). The need for the latter research support workforce is coupled with another key goal of the Clinical Translational Science Award (CTSA) program—training the scientific workforce needed for the translational sciences (NCATS, 2013). NIH's recent funding of CTSAs at more than 60 U.S. institutions offers an opportunity for training at various levels, as well as for short courses to address specific technical needs (NIH, 2014). Thus, the CTSA program could require CTSA institutions to provide support and training for designing clinical trials with an eye toward data sharing and its implementation. CTSA institutions could provide technical support and an infrastructure for sharing clinical trial data and also develop and disseminate best practices for data sharing among the CTSA consortium and partner institutions. As the academic homes for advancing innovative clinical and translational research, the leaders of National Center for Advancing Translational Sciences (NCATS) and CTSA institutions have a unique opportunity to create a professional culture conducive to sharing clinical trial data.

Conclusion: *Training for the sharing of clinical trial data needs to be part of the overall mission of funders of research training programs.*

Other stakeholders can and should contribute to workforce development as well. Large pharmaceutical, device, and biotechnology companies, as well as smaller industry sponsors when feasible, can contribute valuable hands-on, state-of-the-art training in data sharing. Foundations that sponsor medical research and training also can enlarge the scope of their programs to include data sharing. And international bodies that fund training of the clinical trial workforce can make training researchers in data sharing a core component of their initiatives. Making more clinical trial data available for analyses will yield few gains if too few data scientists are adequately trained to turn these data into knowledge.

Conclusion: *A workforce with the skills and knowledge to manage the operational and technical aspects of data sharing needs to be developed.*

SUSTAINABILITY CHALLENGES

To assess the benefits and burdens of sharing clinical trial data, it is essential to have sound estimates of the costs of different data sharing models. The only cost information in a peer-reviewed publication that the committee could identify is contained in a paper (Wilhelm et al., 2014) that breaks down the costs of data sharing in the Alzheimer's Disease Neuroimaging Initiative (ADNI), a longitudinal study, into four components:

1. Infrastructure and administration costs include the data repository, storage and curation of data, review of informed consent forms, and management of material transfer agreements.
2. Standardization costs include efforts to organize data and make them understandable to others.
3. Human resources costs encompass building and maintaining the infrastructure, providing data access, and responding to queries from potential users. The committee notes that responding to queries from potential secondary users is a challenge because staff that worked on a clinical trial are assigned to new projects after the trial's completion or leave the sponsor, data coordinating center, or institution that carried out the study. Responding to such queries is an important aspect of responsible sharing of clinical trial data: If there is no one to answer questions about the data from secondary users, the scientific usefulness of the shared data will be compromised. The committee also notes that the use of an Independent Review Board to determine access to clinical trial data may add further costs.
4. There are opportunity costs associated with not carrying out new research or new analyses of existing data.

The authors of this paper report that ADNI investigators estimated that data sharing would account for 10-15 percent of the total costs of the program and require about 15 percent of investigators' time (Wilhelm et al., 2014). The authors note problems with determining the costs of data sharing: "Meanwhile, there are few benchmarks by which to ascertain the costs of data sharing and as yet no prospectively derived metrics by which to reliably estimate the categorical costs."

Although this paper is helpful, the committee notes that it has several limitations. The authors examined only one study, a longitudinal neuroimaging study that collected large amounts of complex imaging data. Raw data from longitudinal neuroimaging studies may be much more extensive than complete analyzable data sets from clinical trials and thus more expensive to prepare, curate, and share. Costs were estimated by the study investigators without direct measurement, verification, or audit. The cost estimates did not include the costs of preparing the clinical study report (CSR) for a clinical trial that would not be submitted to regulatory agencies or manually redacting the CSRs from legacy trials for participant identifiers or commercially confidential information (Scott, 2013; Shoulson, 2014). The committee notes also that the figures in this paper may overestimate future data sharing costs if data collection templates and procedures are revised with data sharing in mind, as discussed further below.

Wilhelm and colleagues (2014, p. 1202) comment on inequities in the current business model for data sharing:

> The cost categories described are borne by those researchers who originally collected the data, with little if any cost to data users. Therefore, cost recovery in data sharing is needed and justifiable, especially because the current funding milieu provides limited support for data sharing.

The committee heard testimony about the current distribution of the costs of data sharing. Representatives of pharmaceutical companies that are carrying out or planning the sharing of clinical trial data testified that they are now paying all the costs of sharing data from trials they sponsor. In their view, other stakeholders should also contribute, and public sponsors should provide financial support for sharing data from trials they fund (Kuntz, 2013; Scott, 2013). In addition, the committee heard testimony from a biotechnology firm that for small companies with no revenue stream the cost of sharing clinical trial data would be prohibitive and a serious disincentive to investors (Moch, 2014). However, the committee also heard the counterargument from investors that if data sharing is carried out with appropriate controls to minimize invalid analyses (e.g., through review of data requests and analysis plans by independent review boards; see Chapter 5), investors will have greater confidence in promising trials and invest accordingly (Leff, 2014). The committee notes that small funders account for a significant proportion of new therapeutic discoveries. According to the Small Business Administration, 42 percent of new drug approvals in 2012 were granted to emerging sponsors (FDA, 2013). The committee notes further that there are precedents for reducing fees for small companies; the FDA, for example, charges small companies reduced application fees for new products. Public funders of clinical research such as NIH, whose budget has been declining in real dollars, may be reluctant to fund the sharing of clinical trial data if doing so would further reduce the funds available for new research grants. Finally, from a global perspective, the committee notes that the costs of data sharing may be prohibitive for clinical trialists in low-resource countries.

From the above findings, the committee concludes that the current business model for sharing clinical trial data is not sustainable. Furthermore, the current model for funding the sharing of clinical trial data does not distribute the costs equitably among the various stakeholders that participate in and benefit from such data sharing.

The committee is mindful that it was not constituted to address the issue of the cost of sharing clinical trial data and how to distribute those costs. In keeping with its charge to "outline strategies and suggest practical approaches to facilitate responsible data sharing," however, the committee presents the following conceptual framework regarding the costs of responsible sharing of clinical trial data.

First, responsible sharing of clinical trial data benefits the public and multiple stakeholders. Data sharing is a public good, as is the original research, leading to additional scientific knowledge regarding the effectiveness and safety of therapies, diagnostic tests, and the delivery of health care. In addition to patients and their physicians, other stakeholders benefit from this additional knowledge. These stakeholders include payers for health care (public insurance and health care payers at the state and local levels, private insurers, and employers that cover health insurance costs) that determine reimbursement based on evidence regarding the benefits and risks of therapies, as well as organizations that establish clinical practice guidelines (professional organizations and government agencies) (IOM, 2011).

Second, as a matter of fairness, those who benefit from responsible sharing of clinical trial data, including the users of shared data, should bear some of the costs of sharing. There is policy precedent for charging user fees to obtain access to data collected by others. The Health Information Technology for Economic and Clinical Health (HITECH) Act explicitly states that organizations that share data are entitled to reasonable cost recovery (infrastructure costs plus the marginal cost of delivering the data) (Evans, 2014). Any user fees will have to include provision for researchers from resource-poor areas, where the burden of disease and potential for benefit may be disproportionately great. Additional sources of funding for responsible sharing of clinical trial data may be identified; for example, private philanthropies may be interested in funding the development of infrastructure and the conduct of pilot projects for responsible sharing of clinical trial data or subsidizing data access in resource-poor countries.

Third, policies on equitably sharing the costs of responsible sharing of clinical trial data among stakeholders should be based on accurate information on the costs of data sharing for various kinds of clinical trials. Such cost data do not currently exist and would best be collected by impartial accounting and economics experts. Furthermore, there are no estimates of the potential savings that may result from sharing clinical trial data—which may include lower costs for secondary research conducted using shared data sets—for future clinical trials as a result of information gleaned from previous trials, or for health care because of lower use of ineffective or less effective therapies and reduced complications resulting from better safety data.

Fourth, the costs of responsible sharing of clinical trial data will decrease in the future if data collection and management are designed to facilitate data sharing. As an example, the Open Science Framework developed by the Center for Open Science makes transparent virtually all the metadata and data required for sharing on an ongoing, real-time basis as the research is being conducted (Open Science Framework, 2014). A shareable data set, with audit trails, is created in real time. Thus, the same technological platform used for both real-time data management and the conduct of research can be used for long-term data storage. After a trial has been completed, the study data, metadata, and relevant study documents can be made accessible almost immediately with minimal additional effort. In addition, as discussed above, another innovation with the potential to reduce the cost of data sharing is disease-specific standardized data elements and outcomes, as are currently being developed through the CDISC initiative, PCORnet, and other collaborative research enterprises. The lesson to be learned is that technological and procedural innovations that improve the quality of clinical trials can also reduce the costs of data sharing relative to current study procedures and data systems.

> **Conclusion:** *Currently, the costs of data sharing are borne by a small subset of sponsors, funders, and clinical trialists; for data sharing to be sustainable, its costs will need to be equitably distributed across both data generators and users.*

> **Conclusion:** *A market/landscape analysis of the costs of sharing clinical trial data and an economic analysis of sustainable and equitable funding options would provide an evidence base to facilitate the development of sustainable and equitable models for responsible data sharing.*

STRUCTURE FOR COLLABORATIVE NEXT STEPS

Sharing clinical trial data is a global health priority that is gathering momentum. The commissioning of the present study was intended to further the dialogue and begin to build a stronger foundation for a robust data sharing culture. But such data sharing is still nascent, and the challenges to achieving the vision outlined in this chapter are formidable. The committee has proposed guiding principles that need to be balanced in responsible sharing of clinical trial data and made recommendations addressing a number of the challenges to data sharing. To attempt to suggest how all specific issues should be resolved would, however, be presumptuous, imprudent, and beyond the committee's expertise and charge.

Several models for sharing clinical trial data exist today, and more can be expected in the future. Sponsors will try different approaches, and the outcomes of these approaches will provide useful information on what does and does not work in various contexts. New issues and challenges are likely to emerge as more experience is gained with sharing clinical trial data and as clinical trials themselves change. Thus, the sharing of clinical trial data will evolve in ways that cannot be predicted today.

Approaches to data sharing are likely to change and improve if stakeholders learn from experience and new approaches to clinical trials are introduced. Chapter 5 describes how pioneers in sharing clinical trial data, such as YODA and the European Medicines Agency (EMA), have revised their policies and procedures in response to feedback from stakeholders and early experience with data sharing. The committee proposes in that chapter (under Recommendation 3) that organizations sharing clinical trial data "learn from experience by collecting data on the outcomes of data sharing policies, procedures, and technical approaches (including the benefits, risks, and costs), and share information and lessons learned with clinical trial sponsors, the public, and other organizations sharing clinical trial data."

In this chapter, the committee has further developed the idea of improving the sharing of clinical trial data by drawing on experience in other areas of biomedical research and health care. The sharing of data from biobanks and genomic sequencing projects offers several insights. The U.K. Biobank has advocated "adaptive governance" for biobanks, characterized by willingness to adapt to unforeseen or emerging issues, flexibility, and nimbleness (Laurie and Sethi, 2013; O'Doherty et al., 2011a). Scholars who have consulted for biobanks regarding their governance also have advocated for adaptive governance (Kaye, 2014; O'Doherty et al., 2011b). Another aspect of adaptive governance in the context of responsible sharing of clinical trial data is using discretion to modify timelines for data sharing in exceptional circumstances, as discussed in Chapter 5.

Quality improvement in health care and industry builds on data-driven improvements. A "learning health care system" improves the quality of health care and reduces costs (IOM, 2013a). In the continuous quality improvement model, an opportunity for improvement is identified through outcome metrics, a broad-based team suggests how to improve the activity or process, and the impact of the intervention is tracked through ongoing monitoring of the metric, leading to a cycle of further improvements. "Learning" organizations have additional characteristics that facilitate improvement, including effective leadership, a culture that prizes improvement, and an emphasis on taking advantage of digital and Internet-based technology (IOM, 2013a). These organizational characteristics complement those advocated by proponents of adaptive governance.

In addition to individual funders and trusted intermediaries, the committee has considered the ecosystem of responsible sharing of clinical trial data as a whole. Although individual sponsors and trusted intermediaries can do a great deal within their own organizations to make the sharing of clinical trial data more responsible, effective, and efficient, other challenges can be addressed only in collaboration with other institutions.

First, different funders and intermediaries can share outcome data for different data sharing models with each other and the public (Strom et al., 2014). Sharing these outcomes will give individual organizations incentives to improve, develop common metrics, share lessons learned, and consider how to address common challenges.

Second, some challenges can be met only from a broader perspective than the standpoint of an individual funder or intermediary. Earlier in this report, the committee discussed how common data elements, interoperability, federated models for sharing data, a data set identification system, and sustainable and equitable business models would make the sharing of clinical trial data more useful and likely reduce costs as well. None of these elements can be developed by a single sponsor or trusted intermediary.

Third, the ecosystem for sharing clinical trial data consists of many types of organizations. In Chapter 3, the committee recommends that disease advocacy organizations, regulatory and research oversight agencies, Institutional Review Boards or Research Ethics Committees, research institutions and universities, medical journals, and membership and professional societies take certain steps to promote responsible sharing of clinical trial data. Many challenges will best be addressed through collaborative efforts involving different types of institutions. Chapter 3 presents the committee's analysis of the need for academic institutions and funders of clinical trials to provide incentives for investigators to share clinical trial data. One important need is to develop a way of tracking secondary analyses by other investigators that use a clinical trial data set so the original clinical trial and its investigators can receive appropriate professional recognition. Connecting a shared data set to subsequent publications of other investigators is a problem that other fields of science also are addressing (NRC, 2012). Still another problem requiring collaborative effort is how academic institutions should give appropriate professional recognition to a researcher who produces clinical trial data sets that other investigators use for secondary research. Universities might benefit from discussing with each other and with pretenure faculty and secondary users of data how to document and assess the scholarly contribution due to data that are shared.

RECOMMENDATION

This report articulates guiding principles and high-level recommendations to guide responsible sharing of clinical trial data. Several early adopters have established proof of principle that the sharing of clinical trial data can be accomplished. For responsible sharing of clinical trial data to become pervasive, sustained, and rooted as a professional norm, however, much additional work will need to be done. Many interrelated issues need to be resolved, and as changes occur in how clinical trials are designed and carried out, new issues and challenges undoubtedly will arise. Discussion among stakeholders and the exchange of ideas and empirical evaluations of different data sharing models will help best practices, incentives, and areas of agreement to emerge. To some extent, such discussion is already occurring. However, establishing forums for the discussion of issues and experiences among a broad range of stakeholders with varied interests can catalyze implementation. Because responsible sharing of clinical trial data is so multifaceted, people working on one aspect of data sharing need to be aware of how their work interacts with work on other aspects. The committee recommends that a combination of public, nonprofit, and industry funders, similar to the sponsors of this project, take the lead in convening these stakeholders. However, to ensure broad representation of stakeholder interests, including those of participants and investigators, it would be desirable for members of the convening body not to have a direct stake in clinical trials as sponsors, funders, or investigators. Ideally, the convener should be regarded as impartial and trusted by the multiple stakeholders who have countervailing interests in the sharing of clinical trial data. In the United Kingdom, for example, the Nuffield Council on Bioethics, the Academy of Medical Sciences, and the Medical Research Council each have issued several consensus reports on science and research policy (EAGDA, 2014); similar impartial, trusted bodies in other countries (such as the Rathenau Instituut in the Netherlands and the Canadian Academy of Health Sciences) could also play this role. Collaborations between convening organizations in different countries could help assure a global perspective. After a few initial meetings, it is likely that stakeholders most committed to responsible sharing of clinical trial data would agree on whether some ongoing forum or forums were desirable and if so, how they might be convened.

Recommendation 4: The sponsors of this study should take the lead, together with or via a trusted impartial organization(s), to convene a multistakeholder body with global reach and broad representation to address, in an ongoing process, the key infrastructure, technological, sustainability, and workforce challenges associated with the sharing of clinical trial data.

REFERENCES

CDISC (Clinical Data Interchange Standards Consortium). 2014. *CDISC vision and mission.* http://www.cdisc.org/CDISC-Vision-and-Mission (accessed October 17, 2014).

Data.cochrane.org. 2014. *PICO ontology.* http://data.cochrane.org/ontologies/pico (accessed October 17, 2014).

EAGDA (Expert Advisory Group on Data Access). 2014. *Establishing incentives and changing cultures to support data access.* http://www.wellcome.ac.uk/stellent/groups/corporatesite/@msh_peda/documents/web_document/wtp056495.pdf (accessed December 19, 2014).

Evans, B. J. 2014. Sustainable access to data for postmarketing medical product safety surveillance under the amended HIPAA Privacy Rule. *Health Matrix Clevel* 24:11-47.

FDA (U.S. Food and Drug Administration). 2013. *Section 1128 of the Food and Drug Administration Safety and Innovation Act (FDASIA): Small business report to Congress.* http://www.fda.gov/downloads/RegulatoryInformation/Legislation/Federal FoodDrugandCosmeticActFDCAct/SignificantAmendmentstotheFDCAct/FDASIA/UCM360058.pdf (accessed November 5, 2014).

HIMSS (Healthcare Information and Management Systems Society). 2009. *Defining and testing EMR usability: Principles and proposed methods of EMR usability evaluation and rating.* http://www.himss.org/files/HIMSSorg/content/files/himss_definingandtesting emrusability.pdf (accessed October 17, 2014).

IOM (Institute of Medicine). 2011. *Clinical practice guidelines we can trust.* Washington, DC: The National Academies Press.

IOM. 2012. *Envisioning a transformed clinical trials enterprise in the United States: Establishing an agenda for 2020: Workshop summary.* Washington, DC: The National Academies Press.

IOM. 2013a. *Best care at lower cost: The path to continuously learning health care in America.* Washington, DC: The National Academies Press.

IOM. 2013b. *The CTSA program at NIH: Opportunities for advancing clinical and translational research.* Edited by A. I. Leshner, S. F. Terry, A. M. Schultz, and C. T. Liverman. Washington, DC: The National Academies Press.

IOM. 2013c. *Sharing clinical research data: Workshop summary.* Washington, DC: The National Academies Press.

Kaye, J. 2014. *Adaptive governance.* Paper presented at IOM Committee on Strategies for Responsible Sharing of Clinical Trial Data: Meeting Four, May 5-7, Washington, DC.

Kuntz, R. 2013. *Yale University Open Data Access Project: A model for dissemination and independent analysis of clinical trial program data.* Paper presented at IOM Committee on Strategies for Responsible Sharing of Clinical Trial Data: Meeting One, October 22-23, Washington, DC.

Laurie, G., and N. Sethi. 2013. Towards principles-based approaches to governance of health-related research using personal data. *European Journal of Risk Regulation* 4(1):43-57.

Leff, J. 2014. *Strategies and practical approaches for responsible sharing of clinical trial data: Perspectives of trial sponsors and investors.* Paper presented at IOM Committee on Strategies for Responsible Sharing of Clinical Trial Data: Meeting Four, May 5-7, Washington, DC.

Mini-Sentinel. 2014. *Welcome to Mini-Sentinel*. http://mini-sentinel.org (accessed October 17, 2014).

Moch, K. I. 2014. *Clinical trial data sharing from the pre-revenue biotech perspective: Addressing the impact of limited resources on the implementation of data sharing technologies*. Paper presented at IOM Committee on Strategies for Responsible Sharing of Clinical Trial Data: Meeting Two, February 3-4, Washington, DC.

NCATS (National Center for Advancing Translational Sciences). 2013. *Scholar and research programs*. http://www.ncats.nih.gov/research/cts/ctsa/training/programs/scholar-trainee.html (accessed September 30, 2014).

NIH (U.S. National Institutes of Health). 2012a. *Data and informatics working group: Draft report to the advisory committee to the director*. Bethesda, MD: NIH.

NIH. 2012b. *Request for information (RFI): Enhancing community-engaged research through the Clinical and Translational Science Awards (CTSA) program*. http://grants.nih.gov/grants/guide/notice-files/NOT-TR-13-001.html (accessed September 30, 2014).

NIH. 2014. *Clinical and Translational Science Awards*. http://www.ncats.nih.gov/research/cts/ctsa/ctsa.html (accessed October 24, 2014).

NRC (National Research Council). 2012. *For attribution—developing data attribution and citation practices and standards: Summary of an international workshop*. Washington, DC: The National Academies Press.

O'Doherty, K. C., M. M. Burgess, K. Edwards, R. P. Gallagher, A. K. Hawkins, J. Kaye, V. McCaffrey, and D. E. Winickoff. 2011a. From consent to institutions: Designing adaptive governance for genomic biobanks. *Social Science & Medicine* 73(3):367-374.

O'Doherty, K. C., M. M. Burgess, K. Edwards, R. P. Gallagher, A. K. Hawkins, J. Kaye, V. McCaffrey, and D. E. Winickoff. 2011b. From consent to institutions: Designing adaptive governance for genomic biobanks. *Social Science & Medicine* 73(3):367-374.

Open Science Framework. 2014. *Project management with collaborators, project sharing with the public*. https://osf.io (accessed October 24, 2014).

Scott, J. 2013. *Access to anonymised patient level data from GSK clinical trials*. Paper presented at IOM Committee on Strategies for Responsible Sharing of Clinical Trial Data: Meeting One, October 22-23, Washington, DC.

Shoulson, I. 2014. *Cultural and financial incentives for data sharing: Recognition and promotion*. Paper presented at IOM Committee on Strategies for Responsible Sharing of Clinical Trial Data: Meeting Two, February 3-4, Washington, DC.

Sim, I., and J. C. Niland. 2012. Study protocol representation. In *Clinical research informatics*, edited by R. L. Richesson and J. E. Andrews. New York: Springer. Pp. 155-174.

Sim, I., S. W. Tu, S. Carini, H. P. Lehmann, B. H. Pollock, M. Peleg, and K. M. Wittkowski. 2013. The Ontology of Clinical Research (OCRe): An informatics foundation for the science of clinical research. *Journal of Biomedical Informatics* 52:78-91.

Strom, B. L., M. Buyse, J. Hughes, and B. M. Knoppers. 2014. Data sharing, year 1—access to data from industry-sponsored clinical trials. *New England Journal of Medicine* 371: 2052-2054.

Tasneem, A., L. Aberle, H. Ananth, S. Chakraborty, K. Chiswell, B. J. McCourt, and R. Pietrobon. 2012. The database for Aggregate Analysis of ClinicalTrials.gov (AACT) and subsequent regrouping by clinical specialty. *PLoS ONE* 7(3):e33677.

Wilhelm, E. E., E. Oster, and I. Shoulson. 2014. Approaches and costs for sharing clinical research data. *Journal of the American Medical Association* 311(12):1201-1202.

Zerhouni, E. A. 2005. Translational and clinical science—time for a new vision. *New England Journal of Medicine* 353(15):1621-1623.

Appendix A

Study Approach

STUDY PROCESS

During the course of its deliberations, the committee gathered information through a variety of mechanisms: (1) three 1.5-day workshops held in person in Washington, DC, in October 2013, February 2014, and May 2014 and one virtual workshop held in April 2014, all of which were open to the public; (2) release in January 2014 of a document presenting a framework for discussion, which invited public feedback on a set of issues relevant to this report and is described in greater detail in the section below; (3) reviews of the scientific literature and commissioning of two papers on special topics, including de-identification of clinical trial data (see Appendix B) and drug regulation in selected developing countries;[1] and (4) personal communication between committee members and staff and individuals who have been directly involved in or have special knowledge of the issues under consideration.

FRAMEWORK FOR DISCUSSION AND PUBLIC FEEDBACK

As directed by the committee's charge, a document presenting a framework for discussion ("the Framework") was publicly released in January 2014. The Framework articulated the committee's preliminary

---

[1] The commissioned paper, "The Interaction Between Open Trial Data and Drug Regulation in Selected Developing Countries," was used by the committee in support of its analysis in this report. This paper is available on this report's website (www.iom.edu/datasharing).

observations on guiding principles that underpin the responsible sharing of clinical trial data, a nomenclature for data sharing, and a description of a selected set of data sharing activities. The Framework did not contain conclusions or recommendations but rather served to elicit feedback from a variety of stakeholders to inform the second phase of this study and the conclusions and recommendations contained in this final report. The committee invited comments on a set of specific topics for public feedback on difficult issues that were likely to be complex and on which the public and stakeholders were likely to have differing perspectives.

In addition to the public release of the Framework, several medical journals wrote editorials on the committee's work and encouraged their readership to send comments. In response to these efforts, the committee received 85 written comments from a variety of individuals and organizations, including academic researchers from across the globe, industry (pharmaceutical, device, and biologic) representatives (from both individual companies and trade associations), clinicians and health care organizations, patient/disease advocacy representatives, and others. Staff collected and compiled all comments for the committee's review, calling particular attention to cross-cutting themes and unique perspectives.

CLINICAL TRIALS LITERATURE REVIEW

Search Parameters:
- Date range: 2000-present
- International, English only

Databases:
- OVID Medline
- OVID Embase
- Scopus
- Web of Science
- Grey literature reports (NIH, FDA, EMA [European Medicines Agency], WHO)

Email Alerts:
- LexisNexis—major newspapers (*New York Times*, *Wall Street Journal*, *Washington Post*)
- Alerts received on a weekly schedule

Search Strategy:

("Clinical Trials" or "Clinical Trials as Topic" or "Clinical trial (topic)")

AND

("Data sharing" or "Information dissemination"[2] or "Data-sharing" or "Data transparency")

AND (with the following key words searched individually)

- "Resource constraints" or "Resource limitations"
- "Implementation"
- "Incentives" or "Disincentives" and "Academic"/or "Outcome research" or
- "Changing norms"
- "Protection of human subjects" "/or" "/"
- "Patient privacy" or "Patient confidentiality" or Privacy
- "Intellectual property"
- Legal or Jurisprudence or "Legal issues" or "Legal aspects" or Law
- "Scientific standards" or "Rogue analyses"
- "Data quality" or "Quality control"
- "Informed consent"
- "Competition law" or "Antitrust"
- "Liability"
- "Data exclusivity"
- "Infrastructure"
- "Governance"
- "Resource poor setting"
- "Public health"
- "Risks"
- "Benefits"
- "Challenges"

---

[2] Note that "information dissemination" is the MeSH (Medical Subject Headings) term for data sharing.

COMMITTEE MEETING AGENDAS

Meeting One: October 22-23, 2013

The National Academies
2101 Constitution Avenue, NW
Washington, DC 20418

October 22, 2013 (Day 1)
CLOSED SESSION (9:30 AM-2:20 PM)

October 22, 2013 (Day 1)
OPEN SESSION (2:30 PM-4:45 PM)

OPEN Session Objectives
- Review statement of task with sponsors
- Receive testimony from invited speakers and the public on attributes of responsible data sharing activities

National Academy of Sciences Building, NAS 125
2101 Constitution Avenue, Washington, DC

2:30 PM	**Welcome and Introductory Remarks** *(begin open session)* *Bernard Lo, Committee Chair* *The Greenwall Foundation*
2:40 PM	**The Charge to the Committee: A Discussion with the Sponsors**

Objective: Receive remarks from invited sponsor representatives to discuss background, purpose, and context for the study, including needs the study could address. Provide opportunity for the committee and sponsors to clarify the study scope and task through question and answer and open discussion.

- *Kathy Hudson, U.S. National Institutes of Health*
- *Richard Moscicki, U.S. Food and Drug Administration*
- *Elizabeth (Betsy) Myers, Doris Duke Charitable Foundation*
- *John Orloff, Novartis*
- *Nicola Perrin, The Wellcome Trust*

4:30-4:45 PM	**Closing Remarks** *(end open session)* *Bernard Lo, Committee Chair*

October 22, 2013 (Day 1)
CLOSED SESSION (4:45 PM–5:45 PM)

October 23, 2013 (Day 2)
OPEN SESSION (8:00 AM–5:45 PM)

8:00 AM   **Welcome and Introductory Remarks** *(begin open session)*
Bernard Lo, Committee Chair

8:15–8:45 AM   **Clinical Trial Data and Challenges to Data Sharing**
Robert Califf, Duke University (by WebEx)
Discussion

8:45–9:15 AM   **Preparing for Responsible Sharing of Clinical Trial Data**
Michelle Mello, Harvard University
Discussion

SESSION 1: CLINICAL TRIAL DATA TYPES AND SHARING ACTIVITIES

Objectives: Characterize the spectrum of "data" generated in the conduct of clinical trials and review existing and proposed data sharing activities. Explore the benefits, risks, and burdens associated with sharing different types of data.

9:15–9:45 AM   **Clinical Trial Data:** What types of data (and associated materials) might be shared? Who holds these data? Under what circumstances are they now shared, and why are they shared? What analyses are possible using summary vs. analytic data sets vs. clinical study reports (CSRs) vs. participant-level data?

Panel discussion: Each panelist to briefly introduce himself/herself and provide 5 minutes of prepared comments, followed by a moderated discussion.

- *Pat Teden, Teden Consulting (by WebEx)*
- *Deborah Zarin, U.S. National Institutes of Health*
Moderator: David DeMets, University of Wisconsin–Madison

9:45–10:00 AM   **BREAK**

10:00 AM-12:00 PM **Selected Data Sharing Activities:** What are the drivers and goals of proposed and existing data sharing activities? What data are shared, with whom, and how? What are some of the barriers to and risks, burdens, and benefits of data sharing, and how do different data sharing activities address these issues?

Panel discussion: Each panelist to briefly introduce himself/herself and provide 8 minutes of prepared comments, followed by a moderated discussion.

- *Adam Asare, Immune Tolerance Network Trial Share*
- *Hans-Georg Eichler, European Medicines Agency*
- *Charles Hugh-Jones, Project Data Sphere*
- *Frank Rockhold, GlaxoSmithKline*
- *Joseph Ross, Yale University Open Data Access Project*
Moderator: Joanne Waldstreicher, Johnson & Johnson

12:00-1:00 PM **Lunch**

SESSION 2: PRINCIPLES FOR RESPONSIBLE SHARING OF CLINICAL TRIAL DATA

Objectives: Explore the perspectives of those conducting, sponsoring, or participating in clinical trials and those disseminating and using clinical trial data. Identify interests, values, and concerns to consider in the development of guiding principles for sharing clinical trial data.

Panel discussion: Each panelist to briefly introduce himself/herself and provide 5 minutes of prepared comments, followed by moderated discussion.

1:00-2:20 PM **Research Community Perspectives**
- *Kay Dickersin, Johns Hopkins Bloomberg School of Public Health*
- *Louis Fiore, VA Boston Healthcare System*
- *Ben Goldacre, London School of Hygiene and Tropical Medicine (WebEx)*
- *Rebecca Kush, CDISC*
- *Eric Perakslis, Center for Biomedical Informatics, Harvard Medical School*
- *Lesley Stewart, University of York*
- *Madhukar Trivedi, University of Texas, Southwestern*
Moderator: Jeffrey Drazen, New England Journal of Medicine

2:20-2:45 PM   **Research Participant Perspectives**
- *Deborah Collyar, Patient Advocates In Research*
- *Sharon Hesterlee, Parent Project Muscular Dystrophy*

Moderator: Deven McGraw, Manatt, Phelps & Phillips, LLP

2:45-3:00 PM   **BREAK**

3:00-3:50 PM   **Study Sponsor Perspectives**
- *Elaine Collier, National Center for Advancing Translational Sciences*
- *Nicole Hamblett, Cystic Fibrosis Therapeutics Development Network-Seattle Children's Hospital*
- *Richard Kuntz, Medtronic (by WebEx)*
- *Justin McCarthy, Pfizer*

Moderator: Arti Rai, Duke University School of Law

3:50-4:30 PM   **Scientific and Medical Journal Perspectives**
- *Catherine DeAngelis,* Journal of the American Medical Association *(former)*
- *Charlotte Haug,* Norwegian Journal of Medicine
- *Elizabeth Loder,* British Medical Journal

Moderator: Steven Goodman, Stanford University

4:30-5:30 PM   **Public Comment Period**

5:30-5:45 PM   **Closing Comments and Discussion** *(end open session)*
Bernard Lo, Committee Chair

MEETING TWO: FEBRUARY 3-4, 2014

**The National Academies
Keck Center, Room 208
500 Fifth Street, NW
Washington, DC 20001**

Workshop Objectives:
- Seek public comment on the discussion framework document released in January 2014.
- Discuss the elements and activities of data sharing outlined in the discussion framework document, and review the completeness of the set of selected models as a heuristic framework for the committee's analytic process to be undertaken as part of the study.

- Identify key benefits of sharing and risks of not sharing clinical trial data, and key challenges and risks of sharing clinical trial data.
- Discuss the landscape of laws, regulations, and policies under which data sharing occurs, focusing on competition and intellectual property laws and protection of clinical trial research participants.
- Discuss incentives for data sharing and challenges in the implementation and ongoing conduct of data sharing activities.
- Seek public comment on potential strategies and approaches to facilitate responsible data sharing.

February 3, 2014 (Day 1)
OPEN SESSION (1:00 PM-5:00 PM)

1:00 PM   **Welcome and Introductory Remarks** *(begin open session)*
               Bernard Lo, Committee Chair
               The Greenwall Foundation

1:05 PM   **Overview of the Framework for Discussion**
               Bernard Lo, Committee Chair

SESSION 1: CLINICAL TRIAL DATA ELEMENTS AND SHARING ACTIVITIES: PUBLIC FEEDBACK

Objectives: Identify the key purposes, benefits, risks, and challenges of each model described in the discussion framework. Where relevant, explore how each model's benefits and burdens are differentially experienced by research sponsors and investigators, study participants, regulatory agencies, patient groups, and the public. Consider whether other models of sharing might be included in the analytic framework.

Series of Panel Discussions

1:20-1:45 PM   **Model 1 – Open Access**
               - *Atul Butte, Stanford University School of Medicine*
               - *John Wilbanks, Sage Bionetworks*
               Moderator: Ida Sim, University of California, San Francisco, School of Medicine

1:45-2:10 PM **Model 2 – Controlled Access to Individual Company, Institution, or Researcher Data**
- *Joe Ross, Yale University School of Medicine*
- *Ira Shoulson, Georgetown University*
Moderator: Steve Goodman, Stanford University School of Medicine

2:10-2:35 PM **Model 3 – Controlled Access to Pooled or Multiple Data Sources**
- *Laurie Ryan, Alzheimer's Disease Neuroimaging Initiative*
- *Jessica Scott, GlaxoSmithKline*
Moderator: Steve Goodman, Stanford University School of Medicine

2:35-3:00 PM **Model 4 – Closed Partnership/Consortium**
- *Lynn D. Hudson, Critical Path Institute*
Moderator: Ida Sim, University of California, San Francisco, School of Medicine

3:00-3:25 PM **Moderated Discussion and Public Response:** Invited panelists have the opportunity to present benefits, risks, and challenges of other models from their perspective. What, if any, changes or additions to the descriptions of the models might be considered? Are there other models substantially different from those the committee has proposed that could be included?

Moderator: Steve Goodman, Stanford University School of Medicine

3:25-3:40 PM **BREAK**

3:40-4:45 PM **Guiding Principles for Clinical Trial Data Sharing:** Invited discussants to consider the suggested guiding principles for data sharing. Discuss how the principles can be operationalized to balance the benefits and risks of data sharing.

- *Barbara Bierer, Brigham and Women's Hospital*
- *Susan Bull, The Ethox Centre, University of Oxford*
- *Phil Fontanarosa, JAMA*
Moderator: Patricia A. King, Georgetown University Law Center

4:45-5:00 PM   **Brief Preliminary Public Comment Period**

5:00 PM   **Closing Remarks** *(end open session)*
                  Bernard Lo, Committee Chair

                  February 4, 2014 (Day 2)
                  OPEN SESSION (9:00 AM-5:30 PM)

9:00 AM   **Welcome and Introductory Remarks** *(begin open
                  session)*
                  Bernard Lo, Committee Chair

SESSION 2: LEGAL, REGULATORY, AND POLICY CONTEXT

Objectives: Discuss the landscape of laws, regulations, and policies under which data sharing occurs, focusing on protection of clinical trial research participants and competition and intellectual property laws.

Legal, Regulatory, and Policy Context: Protection of Research Participants

9:05-9:35 AM   **International Legal and Policy Context**
                  Mark Barnes, Ropes & Gray LLP and Harvard Multi-Regional Clinical Trials (MRCT) Network

9:35-10:20 AM   **Discussion Panel: Informed Consent:** Issues and barriers for retrospective data sharing (trials already conducted or under way). Current legal framework— United States (Common Rule and the U.S. Food and Drug Administration [FDA]) and international. Suggestions to facilitate sharing while guarding principles and requirements for informed consent for prospective data sharing (trials not yet conducted or initiated). Legal and policy framework needed to facilitate prospective data sharing. Principles and elements of the consent document and process. Operational and institutional issues, especially Institutional Review Board (IRB)/Ethics Committee Review.

                  • *David Forster, Western IRB*
                  • *Pearl O'Rourke, Harvard University*
                  Moderator: Elizabeth G. Nabel, Harvard Medical School, Brigham and Women's Hospital

10:20-10:30 AM   **Erika Von Mutius,** University of Munich

10:30-10:45 AM   **BREAK**

10:45-11:45 AM   **Discussion Panel: Privacy:** Current legal framework of
                   privacy protections—global legal/regulatory structure,
                   with an emphasis on European Union (EU) and
                   United States and high-level description of other non-
                   EU/U.S. jurisdictions. How can a global infrastructure
                   or common global approach to data sharing address
                   or take into account disparate data privacy protection
                   requirements and different cultural standards? Privacy
                   risks presented by data sharing (including to patients,
                   researchers, and institutions). Current de-identification
                   and re-identification technology and standards.
                   Defining "de-identified" and "anonymized" data;
                   purposes and uses of identifiable/nonanonymized
                   data—when/for what scientific or other purposes are
                   identifiable data required? Fair information practices
                   and approaches to privacy protection.

                   - *Mark Barnes, Ropes & Gray LLP*
                   - *Barbara Evans, University of Houston Law School*
                   - *Robert Gellman, Privacy and Information Policy
                     Consultant*
                   - *Bradley Malin, Vanderbilt University*
                   *Moderator: Deven McGraw, Manatt, Phelps & Phillips,
                   LLP*

11:45 AM-   **LUNCH**
12:30 PM

SESSION 3: INCENTIVES FOR SHARING AND
IMPLEMENTATION OF DATA SHARING ACTIVITIES

*Objectives: Discuss how recognition and promotion structures and processes
can provide incentives or disincentives to share data. Identify these incentives
and norms in academia, industry, government, and other sectors as relevant.
Explore potential strategies to lower disincentives or other barriers to data
sharing. Discuss potential negative or unintended consequences of sharing data
and explore potential strategies to mitigate these consequences or challenges.*

12:30-1:15 PM   **Discussion Panel: Scientific Standards and Data Integrity/Quality:** The impact of secondary analyses of data. What methods should be in place to ensure that potential consequences are balanced? Strategies to provide an understanding of how different analyses may lead to different conclusions. Approaches to address potential negative consequences and support the scientific integrity of the original and derivative works. Standards and expectations for secondary use. Provide examples where data sharing made a positive difference in understanding and where data sharing led to detrimental outcomes or analyses that did not meet scientific standards.

- *Peter Doshi, Johns Hopkins University*
- *John Ioannidis, Stanford University School of Medicine*
  Moderator: Jeffrey Drazen, New England Journal of Medicine

1:15-2:15 PM   **Legal, Regulatory, and Policy Context: Intellectual Property and Competition Law:** Speakers to address: Intellectual property law and patent issues, data exclusivity rules and regulatory landscape, definition of "commercially confidential information," and antitrust considerations for data sharing.

- *Jorge Contreras, American University, Washington College of Law*
- *Trevor Cook, WilmerHale*
- *Aliza Y. Glasner, Georgetown University*
- *Benjamin Roin, Petrie-Flom Center, Harvard Law School*
  Moderator: Arti Rai, Duke University School of Law

2:15-3:00 PM   **Discussion Panel: Cultural and Financial Incentives for Data Sharing—Recognition and Promotion:** Recognition and promotion norms in academia— including academic promotion/tenure structures; approaches to academic credit for clinical trialists— and their impact on incentives to share data. Industry staffing/promotion structures; cultural issues relating to data sharing.

- *Ann Bonham, Association of American Medical Colleges (AAMC)*
- *Michael Rosenblatt, Merck*
- *Ira Shoulson, Georgetown University*

Moderator: Joanne Waldstreicher, Johnson & Johnson

3:00-3:15 PM	**BREAK**

3:15-4:00 PM   **Discussion Panel: Resource Considerations and Implementation Barriers:** Benefits, risks, and challenges associated with having staff to answer inquiries and questions from secondary users of data. Handling of data queries/requests; allocation of responsibilities for housing data and maintaining needed records. Issues pertaining to sharing of data in settings of limited resources (e.g., developing or resource-poor countries or small companies/biotech).

- *Atul Butte, Stanford University School of Medicine*
- *Matt Gross, SAS*
- *Kenneth I. Moch, Chimerix*
- *Janet Wittes, Statistics Collaborative*

Moderator: Tim Coetzee, National MS Society

SESSION 4: OVERARCHING AND CROSS-CUTTING ISSUES

Objectives: Discuss and explore the practical implications of the proposed guiding principles in light of the panel discussions held during this public workshop. Discuss selected cross-cutting questions and issues posed by the committee in the discussion framework. Suggest strategies and practical approaches to facilitate responsible data sharing.

4:00-4:45 PM   **Discussion Panel: Cross-Cutting Proposed Guiding Principles and Discussion Framework Questions**

Panelists to discuss:
- Because most large clinical trials are global in nature, how can clinical trial data be shared in that global context? How can different national regulations for research participants' privacy protections; approval of drugs and devices; data exclusivity; and intellectual property laws, resources, and health priorities be taken into account?

- How might strategies and approaches regarding data sharing take into account clinical trials conducted in resource-poor settings; trials designed by citizen-scientists using data they contribute directly; and trials designed through participatory research?
- How might different types of clinical trial data, and different uses of shared data, be prioritized for sharing? What would be the rationale for placing a higher priority on certain types of data or analyses? What might be the advantages and disadvantages of distinguishing highest-priority sharing of clinical trial data from subsequent sharing activities?
- What might be the advantages and disadvantages to various stakeholders of sharing different types of data sets, at different points in time after the completion of a clinical trial?
- Should programs or approaches calling for or requiring new data sharing apply only to new trials undertaken from the date of a new program forward, or retroactively apply to clinical trials started before the data sharing program was initiated?
- What might be done to minimize the risks to patients and to public health from the dissemination of findings from invalid analyses of shared clinical trial data?
- What measures should be deployed to minimize the privacy and confidentiality risks to trial participants? For example, are current anonymization or de-identification methodologies sufficient?
- Under what circumstances are identifiable data needed to fulfill articulated purposes of a data sharing activity? Under what circumstances might re-identification of trial participants be beneficial (for the participants or the public)? Have there been there examples of instances of re-identification of trial participants (e.g., for safety reasons to warn a patient of a potential risk, or for questionable and potentially unethical reasons), and what were the impacts?
- What incentives and protections might be established to encourage clinical trial sponsors and clinical investigators to continue to conduct clinical trials in the future, without unduly restricting the sharing of certain types of data? How do we protect or provide incentives for researchers to share data?

- What is the appropriate responsibility of the primary investigator(s) or research institution(s) to support secondary users in their interpretation of shared data, and what infrastructure or resources are needed to enable such ongoing support? For those with experience in data sharing, what is the burden of providing such support to help others understand and use the provided information?
- What would be appropriate outcome measures to assess the usefulness of different models of clinical trial data sharing, and how can they be used to guide improvements in data sharing practices?

- *Susan Bull, The Ethox Centre, University of Oxford*
- *John Ioannidis, Stanford University School of Medicine*
- *Ira Shoulson, Georgetown University*
Moderator: Bernard Lo, Committee Chair

4:45 PM   **Public Comment Period**

5:15 PM   **Closing Comments** *(end open session)*
              Bernard Lo, Committee Chair

MEETING THREE: APRIL 9, 2014
Virtual WebEx

April 7, 2014 (Day 1)
CLOSED SESSION (10:30 AM-5:00 PM)

April 8, 2014 (Day 2)
CLOSED SESSION (10:30 AM-5:00 PM)

April 9, 2014 (Day 3)
CLOSED SESSION (11:00 AM-12:00 PM)

OPEN SESSION (12:00 PM-1:30 PM)

12:00-1:30 PM   **Clinical Trial Data Sharing: Product Liability**

Objective: Discuss the product liability litigation concerns of requiring drug and device manufacturers to make clinical trial data public.

Panel discussion:Each panelist will provide an 8- to 10-minute presentation, followed by moderated discussion with the committee.

- Loren Brown, DLA Piper
- George Fleming, Fleming, Nolan, and Jez L.L.C.
- William Sage, University of Texas, School of Law

Moderator: Arti Rai, Committee Member

CLOSED SESSION (1:30 PM-3:30 PM)

MEETING FOUR: MAY 5-7, 2014

Public Workshop
Keck Center, Room 100
The National Academies
500 Fifth Street, NW
Washington, DC 20001

May 5, 2014 (Day 1)
OPEN SESSION (9:30 AM-5:00 PM)

Overall Workshop Objectives:
- Discuss the benefits, risks, and challenges of data sharing with medical product developers outside of large pharmaceutical companies, including small biotechnology/venture capital, diagnostics and other devices, and disease- and condition-specific organizations.
- Discuss incentives and disincentives in the global clinical trial landscape, particularly within research institutions, including universities, organizations that carry out data sharing, funders, journals, and other organizations involved in clinical trials.
- Discuss guiding principles and characteristics for the optimal infrastructure and governance for sharing clinical trial data.

9:30 AM   **Welcome and Introductory Remarks**
                 Bernard Lo, Committee Chair
                 The Greenwall Foundation

9:40-10:00 AM   **Introductory Presentation: Vision for the Future of Clinical Trials: Implications for Data Sharing**
                 Bernard Munos, M.B.A. (confirmed), InnoThink Center for Research in Biomedical Innovation

SESSION 1: STRATEGIES AND PRACTICAL APPROACHES FOR RESPONSIBLE SHARING OF CLINICAL TRIAL DATA: PERSPECTIVES OF TRIAL SPONSORS AND INVESTORS

Objectives: Hear from investors and sponsors of clinical research (e.g., biotechnology, diagnostic, device, and patient-supported research trials), who will discuss the benefits, risks, and challenges of sharing clinical trial data from their perspective and how those may align with or differ from those associated with large drug trials. Identify strategies and practical approaches to overcome challenges and barriers to responsible data sharing identified by these sponsors.

10:00-11:15 AM   **Discussion Panel**

Small Biotechnology/Venture Capital
- *Jonathan Leff (confirmed), Partner and Chairman, Deerfield Institute*

Device/Diagnostic Companies
- *Rick Kuntz, M.D., M.S. (confirmed), Senior Vice President and Chief Scientific, Clinical and Regulatory Officer, Medtronic, Inc.*
- *Steven Gutman, M.D. (confirmed), Strategic Advisor, Myraqa*

Disease- and Condition-Specific Organizations
- *Robert N. McBurney, Ph.D. (confirmed), Chief Executive Officer, Accelerated Cure Project for MS*
Moderator: Sharon Terry, Committee Member

11:15 AM   **BREAK**

SESSION 2: STRATEGIES AND PRACTICAL APPROACHES FOR INCENTIVIZING RESPONSIBLE SHARING OF CLINICAL TRIAL DATA: PERSPECTIVES OF INVESTIGATORS AND LEADERS OF ACADEMIC MEDICAL CENTERS

Objectives: Understand current norms and attitudes toward clinical trial data sharing. Identify new and current incentives that might facilitate clinical trial data sharing and practical steps within the broad clinical trial enterprise (including major research fields, international and limited-resource settings, data coordinating centers). Discuss incentives and disincentives in the global clinical trial landscape and the academic research model and strategies for overcoming disincentives.

11:30 AM- 12:30 PM	**Discussion Panel: Clinical Trial Investigators and Leaders of Academic Medical Centers and Data Coordinating Centers**

- *Rory Collins, Ph.D., Professor of Medicine and Epidemiology, University of Oxford and Chief Executive, UK Biobank (via WebEx, May 6)*
- *Steve Cummings, M.D. (confirmed), Professor Emeritus, Department of Medicine (General Internal Medicine), UCSF, and Director, San Francisco Coordinating Center*
- *Clay Johnston, M.D., Ph.D. (confirmed by WebEx), Dean, School of Medicine, University of Texas at Austin, former Director of UCSF Clinical and Translational Science Institute*
- *Quarraisha Abdool Karim, Ph.D., M.S., Associate Professor, Columbia University and Associate Scientific Director, CAPRISA (Center for the AIDS Programme of Research in South Africa) (via WebEx, May 6)*
- *Paula K. Shireman, M.D. (confirmed), Vice Dean for Research, University of Texas Health Science Center San Antonio*
Moderator: Bernard Lo, Committee Chair

12:30 PM	**LUNCH**

SESSION 3: STRATEGIES AND PRACTICAL APPROACHES FOR RESPONSIBLE SHARING OF CLINICAL TRIAL DATA: GOVERNANCE AND INFRASTRUCTURE

Objectives: Identify guiding principles and characteristics for the optimal infrastructure and governance for responsible sharing of clinical trial data. Discuss optimal and practical governance models that account for the global nature of clinical trials, in which relevant laws, policies and practices vary by jurisdiction.

1:30-3:00 PM	**Discussion Panel: Operational Principles for the Governance for Sharing Clinical Trial Data**

- *Philip E. Bourne, Ph.D. (confirmed), Associate Director for Data Science (ADDS), National Institutes of Health*
- *Glenn Cohen, J.D. (confirmed), Professor of Law and Co-Director, Petrie-Flom Center for Health Law Policy, Biotechnology & Bioethics*

- *Jane Kaye, D.Phil., LL.B. (via WebEx, May 7), Director, Centre for Law, Health and Emerging Technologies, Oxford: (HeLEX) based in the Department of Public Health at the University of Oxford*
- *Bartha Knoppers, Ph.D., LL.M., LL.B. (confirmed), Director, Centre of Genomics and Policy, McGill University*

Moderator: Tim Coetzee, Committee Member

3:00-4:30 PM   **Discussion Panel: Characteristics for the Optimal Infrastructure of Data Sharing**

- *Philip E. Bourne, Ph.D. (confirmed), Associate Director, Data Science (ADDS), National Institutes of Health*
- *Rory Collins, Ph.D., Professor of Medicine and Epidemiology, University of Oxford and Chief Executive, UK Biobank (via WebEx, May 6)*
- *Harlan Krumholz, M.D. (confirmed), Director, Yale University Open Data Access (YODA) Project*
- *Frank Rockhold, Ph.D. (confirmed), GSK Sr. Vice President GCSP*
- *Paula K. Shireman, M.D. (confirmed), Vice Dean for Research, University of Texas Health Science Center San Antonio*

Moderator: Ida Sim, Committee Member

4:30-5:00 PM   **Public Comment Period**

5:00 PM   **ADJOURN**

May 6, 2014 (Day 2)
OPEN SESSION (9:30 AM-11:30 AM)

SESSION 4: CONTINUATION FROM MAY 5

9:30-10:15 AM   **Clinical Trial Investigator Perspectives**
Quarraisha Abdool Karim, Ph.D., M.S.
Associate Professor, Columbia University and Associate Scientific Director, CAPRISA (Center for the AIDS Programme of Research in South Africa) (confirmed)

10:15-10:30 AM   **BREAK**

10:30-11:30 AM   **Characteristics for the Optimal Infrastructure of Data Sharing and Incentivizing Data Sharing**
Rory Collins, Ph.D., Professor of Medicine and Epidemiology, University of Oxford and Chief Executive, UK Biobank (confirmed)

May 7, 2014 (Day 3)
OPEN SESSION (9:00 AM-9:45 AM)

9:00-9:45 AM   **Operational Principles for the Governance for Sharing Clinical Trial Data**
Jane Kaye, D.Phil., LL.B., Director, Centre for Law, Health and Emerging Technologies, Oxford: (HeLEX) based in the Department of Public Health at the University of Oxford (confirmed)

DATA SHARING PUBLIC COMMENTS AND CONTRIBUTIONS

Contributors

Name	Organization
Alves, Teresa	Health Action International Europe, International Society of Drug Bulletins, Medicines in Europe Forum, and Transatlantic Consumer Dialogue
Aquino, John	Bloomberg BNA
Azoulay, Daniel	AP-HP Hôpitaux Universitaires Henri Mondor
Barnes, Mark	Harvard MRCT (Multi-Regional Clinical Trials) Center
Beckett, William	Harvard Medical School
Berger, Philip	University of Toronto, St. Michael's Hospital
Bierut, Laura	Washington University School of Medicine in St. Louis
Brannin, Nancy L.	Clinician
Brewer, Alina	Preeclampsia Foundation

Name	Organization
Cantekin, Erdem	University of Pittsburgh School of Medicine
Charles, H. Cecil	Duke University
Cheah, Phaik	Faculty of Tropical Medicine, Mahidol University
Davies, Gerry	PreDiCT-TB Consortium
Detmer, Don	University of Virginia School of Medicine
Dixon, Dennis	Unknown
Espeland, Mark	Wake Forest School of Medicine
Federici, Tara	AdvaMed
Feigal, Ellen	California Institute for Regenerative Medicine
Ferguson, Stephen	Cook Group, Inc.
Francer, Jeffrey	PhRMA (Pharmaceutical Research and Manufacturers of America)
Gellman, Robert	Privacy and Information Policy Consultant
Goldacre, Ben	Author
Gutierrez, Querol	Universitat Autonoma de Barcelona
Hauze, Joyce	Xogene Services
Holbrook, Anne	McMaster
Holmes, J.	Unknown
Johnson, Lorraine	Consumers United for Evidence-Based Healthcare
Jureidini, Jon	University of Adelaide
Kalamegham, Rasika	American Association for Cancer Research
Kush, Rebecca	Clinical Data Interchange Standards Consortium
Lehman, Dale	Alaska Pacific University
Levett, Paul	George Washington University
Levit, Laura	ASCO (American Society of Clinical Oncology

Name	Organization
Li, Rebecca	Harvard MRCT
Lin, Edward	Emory University School of Medicine
Mayer, Mark	Chief Medical Officer Roundtable
McLean, Samuel	University of North Carolina School of Medicine
Miller, Pamella	*New England Journal of Medicine*
Murray, Jeff	University of Iowa
NA	The Cancer Imaging Archive (TCIA)
NA	Global Health Network
NA	Harvard MRCT
NA	Novo Nordisk
NA	The Radiological Society of North America (RSNA)
NA	Roche
O'Donnel, D.	Unknown
Offermann, Margaret	Federation of America Societies for Experimental Biology
O'Neill, Onera	The Wellcome Trust
Potter, Bill	U.S. National Institutes of Health
Radecki, Ryan	University of Texas Medical School
Rivas, Maria	AbbVie
Rosenblatt, Michael	Merck and Co., Inc.
Rouse, Dwight	NIH funded clinical trialist
Sanjuan, Judit Rius	Médecins Sans Frontières/Doctors Without Borders (MSF)
Scott, James	University of Utah, School of Medicine
Scott, Jessica	GSK (GlaxoSmithKline)
Shahzamani, Azin	Genentech, Inc.

Name	Organization
Shorish, Yasmeen	James Madison University
Shuttes, James	Unknown
Sprosen, Tim	Clinical Trial Service Unit & Epidemiological Studies Unit (CTSU), Nuffield Department of Population Health, University of Oxford
States, David	Brown Foundation Institute of Molecular Medicine & University of Texas Health Science Center at Houston
Taichman, Darren	ICMJE (International Committee of Medical Journal Editors)
Vinson, Eric	Northwest Portland Area Indian Health Board
Wang, Yajie	CSPCC: VA (Clinical Studies Program Coordination Center: U.S. Department of Veterans Affairs) VA Palo Alto Healthy Care Center
Weitzman, Stephen A.	The Wellcome Trust
Womack, Andrew W.	BIO (Biotechnology Industry Organization)

Specific Topics for Public Feedback

Global Implementation and Practical Consideration

- Because most large clinical trials are global in nature, how can clinical trial data be shared in that global context? How can different national regulations for research participants' privacy protections; approval of drugs and devices; data exclusivity; and intellectual property laws, resources, and health priorities be taken into account?
- How might strategies and approaches regarding data sharing take into account clinical trials conducted in resource-poor settings, trials designed by citizen-scientists using data they contribute directly, and trials designed through participatory research?

Timing and Prioritization

- How might different types of clinical trial data, and different uses of shared data, be prioritized for sharing? What would be the rationale for placing a higher priority on certain types of data or analyses? What might be the advantages and disadvantages of distinguishing highest-priority sharing of clinical trial data from other sharing activities?

- What might be the advantages and disadvantages to various stakeholders of sharing different types of data sets, at different points in time, after the completion of a clinical trial?
- Should programs or approaches calling for or requiring new data sharing apply only to new trials undertaken from the date of a new program forward, or retroactively apply to clinical trials started before the data sharing program was initiated?

Mitigating Risks

- What might be done to minimize the risks to patients and to public health from the dissemination of findings from invalid analyses of shared clinical trial data?
- What measures should be deployed to minimize the privacy and confidentiality risks to trial participants? For example, are current anonymization or de-identification methodologies sufficient?
- Under what circumstances are identifiable data needed to fulfill articulated purposes of a data sharing activity? Under what circumstances might re-identification of trial participants be beneficial (for the participants or the public)? Have there been there examples of instances of re-identification of trial participants (e.g., for safety reasons to warn a patient of a potential risk, or for questionable and potentially unethical reasons), and what were the impacts?

Enhancing Incentives

- What incentives and protections might be established to encourage clinical trial sponsors and clinical investigators to continue to conduct clinical trials in the future, without unduly restricting the sharing of certain types of data? How do we protect or provide incentives for researchers to share data?
- What is the appropriate responsibility of the primary investigator(s) or research institution(s) to support secondary users in their interpretation of shared data, and what infrastructure or resources are needed to enable such ongoing support? For those with experience in data sharing, what is the burden of providing such support to help others understand and use the provided information?

Measuring Impact

- What would be appropriate outcome measures to assess the usefulness of different models of clinical trial data sharing, and how can they be used to guide improvements in data sharing practices?

Appendix B

Concepts and Methods for De-identifying Clinical Trial Data[1]

INTRODUCTION

Context

Very detailed health information about participants is collected during clinical trials. A number of different stakeholders would typically have access to individual-level participant data (IPD), including the study sites, the sponsor of the study, statisticians, Institutional Review Boards (IRBs), and regulators. By IPD we mean individual-level data on trial participants, which is more than the information that is typically included, for example, in clinical study reports (CSRs).

There is increasing pressure to share IPD more broadly than occurs at present. There are many reasons for such sharing, such as transparency in the trial and wider disclosure of adverse events that may have transpired, or to facilitate the reuse of such data for secondary purposes, specifically in the context of health research (Gøtzsche, 2011; IOM, 2013; Vallance and Chalmers, 2013). Many funding agencies tasked with the oversight of research, as well as its funding, are requiring that data collected by the projects they support be made available to others (MRC, 2011; NIH, 2003; The Wellcome Trust, 2011). There are current efforts by regulators, such as the European Medicines Agency (EMA) (2014a,b), to examine how to

---

[1] This background report was commissioned by the Institute of Medicine Committee on Strategies for Responsible Sharing of Clinical Trial Data, written by Khaled El Emam, University of Ottawa, and Bradley Malin, Vanderbilt University.

make IPD from clinical trials shared more widely (IOM, 2013). In many cases, however, privacy concerns have been stated as a key obstacle to making these data available (Castellani, 2013; IOM, 2013).

One way in which privacy issues can be addressed is through the protection of the identities of the corresponding research participants. Such "de-identified" or "anonymized" health data (the former term being popular in North America, and the latter in Europe and other regions) are often considered to be sufficiently devoid of personal health information in many jurisdictions around the world. Many privacy laws therefore allow the data to be used and disclosed for any secondary purposes with participant consent. As long as the data are appropriately de-identified, many privacy concerns associated with data sharing can be readily addressed.

It should be recognized that de-identification is not, by any means, the only privacy concern that needs to be addressed when sharing clinical trial data. In fact, there must be a level of governance in place to ensure that the data will not be analyzed or used to discriminate against or stigmatize the participants or certain groups (e.g., religious or ethnic) associated with the study. This is because discrimination and stigmatization can occur even if the data are de-identified.

This paper describes a high-level risk-based methodology that can be followed to de-identify clinical trial IPD. To contextualize our review and analysis of de-identification, we also touch upon additional governance mechanisms, but we acknowledge that a complete treatment of governance is beyond the scope of this paper. Rather, the primary focus here is only on the privacy protective elements.

Data Recipients, Sponsors, and Adversaries

Clinical trial data may be disclosed by making them completely public or through a request mechanism. The data recipient may be a qualified investigator (QI) who must meet specific criteria. There may be other data recipients who are not QIs as well. If the data are made publicly available with no restrictions, however, then other types of users may access the data, such as journalists and nongovernmental organizations (NGOs). In our discussions we refer to the data recipient as the QI as a primary exemplar, although this is not intended to exclude other possible data recipients (it does make the presentation less verbose).

Data are being disclosed to the QI by the sponsor. We use the term "sponsor" generally to refer to all data custodians who are disclosing IPD, recognizing that the term may mean different entities depending on the context. It may not always be the case that the sponsor is a pharmaceutical company or a medical device company. For example, a regulator may decide to disclose the data to a QI, or a pharmaceutical company may provide the data to an academic institution, whereupon that institution becomes the entity that discloses the data.

The term "adversary" is often used in the disclosure control literature to refer to the role of the individual or entity that is trying to re-identify data subjects. Other terms used are "attacker" and "intruder." Discussions about the QI being a potential adversary are not intended to paint QIs as having malicious objectives. Rather, in the context of a risk assessment, one must consider a number of possible data recipients as being potential adversaries and manage the re-identification risk accordingly.

Data Sharing Models

A number of different ways to provide access to IPD have been proposed and used, each with different advantages and risks (Mello et al., 2013). First, there is the traditional public data release where anyone can get access to the data with no registration or conditions. Examples of such releases include the publicly available clinical trial data from the International Stroke Trial (IST) (Sandercock et al., 2011) and data posted to the Dryad online open access data repository (Dryad, undated; Haggie, 2013).

A second form of data sharing, which is more restrictive, occurs when there exists a formal request and approval process to obtain access to clinical trial data, such as the GlaxoSmithKline (GSK) trials repository (Harrison, 2012; Nisen and Rockhold, 2013); Project Data Sphere (whose focus is on oncology trial data) (Bhattacharjee, 2012; Hede, 2013); the Yale University Open Data Access (YODA) Project, which is initially making trial data from Medtronic available (CORE, 2014; Krumholz and Ross, 2011); and the Immunology Database and Analysis Portal (ImmPort, n.d.), which is restricted to researchers funded by the Division of Allergy, Immunology, and Transplantation of the National Institute of Allergy and Infectious Diseases (DAIT/NIAID), other approved life science researchers, National Institutes of Health employees, and other preauthorized government employees (ImmPort, n.d.). More recently, pharmaceutical companies have created the ClinicalStudyDataRequest.com website, which facilitates data requests to multiple companies under one portal. Following this restrictive model, a request can be processed by the study sponsor or by a delegate of the sponsor (e.g., an academic institution).

A hybrid of the above approaches is a quasi-public release, in which the data user must agree to some terms of use or sign a "click-through" contract. Click-through contracts are online terms of use that may place restrictions on what can be done with the data and how the data are handled. Regardless, anyone can still download such data. For example, public analytics competition data sets, such as the Heritage Health Prize (El Emam et al., 2012), and data-centric software application development competitions, such as the Cajun Code Fest (Center for Business and Information Technologies, 2013), fall into this category. In practice, however, click-through terms are not common for the sharing of clinical trial IPD.[2]

A form of data access that does not require any data sharing occurs when analysts request that the data controller perform an analysis on their behalf. Because this does not involve the sharing of IPD, it is a scenario that we do not consider further in this paper.

Data Sharing Mechanisms

Different mechanisms can be used to share IPD. Clinical trial IPD can be shared either as *microdata* or through an *online portal*. The term "microdata" is commonly used in the disclosure control literature to refer to individual-level raw data (Willenborg and de Waal, 1996, 2001). These microdata may be in the form of one or more flat files or relational databases.

When disclosed as microdata, the data are downloaded as a raw data file that can be analyzed by QIs on their own machines, using their own software if they wish to do so. The microdata can be downloaded through a website, sent to the QI on a disc, or transferred electronically. If access is through a website, the QI may have to register, sign a contract, or go through other steps before downloading the data.

When a portal is used, the QI can access the data only through a remote computer interface, such that the raw data reside on the sponsor's computers and all analysis performed is on the sponsor's computers. Data users do not download any microdata to their own local computers through this portal. Under this model, all actions can be audited.

A public online portal allows anyone to register and get access to the IPD. Otherwise, the access mechanism requires a formal request process.

De-identification is relevant in both of the aforementioned scenarios. When data are provided as microdata, the de-identification process ensures that each record is protected from the QI and his/her staff as the potential adversary. When data are shared through the portal, a QI or his/her staff may inadvertently recognize a data subject because that data subject is a neighbor, relative, coworker, or famous person (see Box B-1).

The different approaches for sharing clinical trial IPD are summarized in Figure B-1.

---

[2] Although the EMA has recently proposed using an online portal to share the CSRs using a simple terms-of-use setup, this was not intended to apply to IPD.

BOX B-1
Types of Re-identification Attacks

For public data, the sponsor needs to make a worst-case assumption and protect against an adversary who is targeting the data subjects with the highest risk of re-identification.

For a nonpublic data set, we consider three types of attacks:

- a deliberate re-identification by the data recipient (or his/her staff and subcontractors);
- an inadvertent re-identification by the data recipient (or his/her staff and subcontractors); and
- a data breach, where data are accidentally exposed to a broader audience.

These three cases are relevant when microdata are being disclosed. If the data are made available through a portal, we assume that the sponsor will ensure that stringent controls and appropriate auditing are in place, which manages risks from the first and third types of attack. In such a case, the second type of attack, where data may be inadvertently re-identified, becomes the primary risk that needs to be managed. An example is if the statistician working with the data inadvertently recognizes someone he or she knows.

Scope of Data to Be De-identified

It is important to make a distinction between biological, and particularly genomic, data and other types of data. Many clinical trials are creating biorepositories. These may have a pseudonym or other unique identifier for the participant, and a sample of data. The de-identification methods we describe in this paper are applicable to clinical, administrative, and survey data. Genomic data raise a different set of issues. These issues are addressed directly in a later section of this paper.

	Microdata	Online Portal
Public	LEAST CONTROL BY SPONSOR LIMIT CONSTRAINTS ON QI	
Formal Request		MOST CONTROL BY SPONSOR SIGNIFICANT CONSTRAINTS ON QI
	Risks	**Risks**
	• Deliberate re-identification • Inadvertent re-identification • Accidental release and re-identification	• Inadvertent re-identification

FIGURE B-1 Different approaches for sharing clinical trial data.
NOTE: QI = qualified investigator.

Clinical trial data can be shared at multiple levels of detail. For example, the data can be raw source data or analysis-ready data. We assume that the data are analysis-ready and that no data cleansing is required before de-identification.

Existing Standards for De-identification

Various regulations associated with data protection around the world permit the sharing of de-identified (or similarly termed) data. For instance, European Union (EU) Data Protection Directive 95/46/EC, which strictly prohibits secondary uses of person-specific data without individual consent, provides an exception to the ruling in Recital 26, which states that the "principles of protection shall not apply to data rendered anonymous in such a way that the data subject is no longer identifiable." However, what does it mean for data to be "identifiable"? How do we know when they are no longer identifiable? The Data Protection Directive, and similar directives around the world, do not provide explicit guidelines regarding how data should be protected. An exception to this rule is a code of practice document published by the U.K. Information Commissioner's Office (ICO) (2012). And although this document provides examples of de-identification methods and issues to consider when assessing the level of identifiability of data, it does not provide a full methodology or specific standards to follow.

There are, however, de-identification standards provided in the Privacy Rule of the U.S. Health Insurance Portability and Accountability Act of 1996 (HIPAA) and subsequent guidance published by the Office for Civil Rights (OCR) at the U.S. Department of Health and Human Services (HHS) (HHS, 2012). This rule is referred to by many regulatory frameworks around the world, and the principles are strongly related to those set forth in the United Kingdom's code of practice document mentioned above.

Two of the key existing standards for the de-identification of health microdata are described in the HIPAA Privacy Rule. It should be recognized that HIPAA applies only to "covered entities" (i.e., health plans, health care clearinghouses, and health care providers that transmit health information electronically) in the United States. It is likely that in many instances the sponsors of clinical trials will not fall into this class. However, these de-identification standards have been in place for approximately a decade, and there is therefore a considerable amount of real-world experience in their application. They can serve as a good launching point for examining best practices in this area. For the disclosure of clinical trial data, the HIPAA Privacy Rule de-identification standards offer a practically defensible foundation even if they are not a regulatory requirement.

According to section 164.514 of the HIPAA Privacy Rule, "health information that does not identify an individual and with respect to which there is no reasonable basis to believe that the information can be used to identify an individual is not individually identifiable health information." Section 164.514(b) of the Privacy Rule contains the implementation specifications that a covered entity, or affiliated business associate, must follow to meet the de-identification standard. In particular, the Privacy Rule outlines two routes by which health data can be designated as de-identified. These are illustrated in Figure B-2.

The first route is the "Safe Harbor" method. Safe Harbor requires the manipulation of 18 fields in the data set as described in Box B-2. The Privacy Rule requires that a number of these data elements be "removed." However, there may be acceptable alternatives to actual removal of values as long as the risk of reverse engineering the original values is very small. Compliance with the Safe Harbor standard also requires that the sponsor

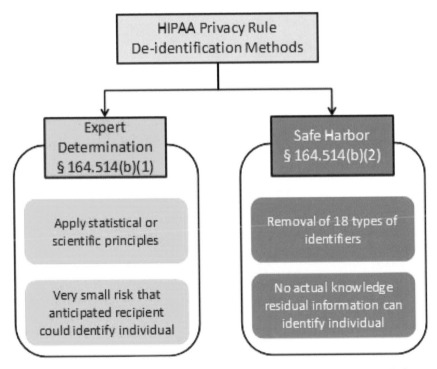

FIGURE B-2 The two de-identification standards in the HIPAA Privacy Rule. SOURCE: Reprinted from a document produced by OCR (HHS, 2012).

BOX B-2
The Safe Harbor De-identification Standard

1. Names;
2. All geographic subdivisions smaller than a state, including street address, city, county, precinct, zip code, and their equivalent geocodes, except for the initial three digits of a zip code if, according to the current publicly available data from the Bureau of the Census:
   a) The geographic unit formed by combining all zip codes with the same three initial digits contains more than 20,000 people; and
   b) The initial three digits of a zip code for all such geographic units containing 20,000 or fewer people is changed to 000.
3. All elements of dates (except year) for dates directly related to an individual, including birth date, admission date, discharge date, date of death; and all ages over 89 and all elements of dates (including year) indicative of such age, except that such ages and elements may be aggregated into a single category of age 90 or older;
4. Telephone numbers;
5. Fax numbers;
6. Electronic mail addresses;
7. Social Security Numbers;
8. Medical record numbers;
9. Health plan beneficiary numbers;
10. Account numbers;
11. Certificate/license numbers;
12. Vehicle identifiers and serial numbers, including license plate numbers;
13. Device identifiers and serial numbers;
14. Web universal resource locators (URLs);
15. Internet protocol (IP) address numbers;
16. Biometric identifiers, including finger and voice prints;
17. Full face photographic images and any comparable images; and
18. Any other unique identifying number, characteristic, or code.

---

not have any actual knowledge that a data subject can be re-identified. Assumptions of the Safe Harbor method are listed in Box B-3.

The application of Safe Harbor is straightforward, but there clearly are instances in which dates and more fine-grained geographic information are necessary. In practice the Safe Harbor standard would remove critical geospatial and temporal information from the data (see items 2 and 3 in Box B-2), potentially reducing the utility of the data. Many meaningful analyses of clinical trial data sets require the dates and event order to be clear. For example, in a Safe Harbor data set, it would not be possible to include the dates when adverse events occurred.

In recognition of the limitations of de-identification via Safe

---

BOX B-3
Assumptions of the HIPAA Safe Harbor Method

- There are only two quasi-identifiers that need to be manipulated in a data set: dates and zip codes.
- The adversary does not know who is in the data set (i.e., would not know which individuals participated in the clinical trial).
- All dates are quasi-identifiers.

Harbor, the HIPAA Privacy Rule provides for an alternative in the form of the Expert Determination method. This method has three general requirements:

- The de-identification must be based on *generally accepted statistical and scientific principles and methods for rendering information not individually identifiable*. This means that the sponsor needs to ensure that there is a body of work that justifies and evaluates the methods that are used for the de-identification and that these methods must be generally known (i.e., undocumented methods or proprietary methods that have never been published would be difficult to classify as "generally accepted").
- The risk of re-identification needs to be *very small*, such that the information could not be used, alone or in combination with other reasonably available information, by an anticipated recipient to identify an individual who is a subject of the information. However, the mechanism for measuring re-identification risk is not defined in the HIPAA Privacy Rule, and what would be considered *very small* risk also is not defined. Therefore, the de-identification methodology must include some manner of measuring re-identification risk in a defensible way and have a repeatable process to follow that allows for the definition of *very small* risk.
- Finally, the *methods and results of the analysis that justify such determination* must be documented. The basic principles of de-identification are expected to be consistent across all clinical trials, but the details will be different for each study, and these details also need to be documented.

These conditions are reasonable for a de-identification methodology and are consistent with the guidance that has been produced by other agencies and regulators (Canadian Institute for Health Information, 2010; ICO,

2012). They also serve as a set of conditions that must be met for the methods described here.

Unique and Derived Codes Under HIPAA

According to the 18th item in Safe Harbor (see Box B-2), "any unique identifying number, characteristic, or code" must be removed from the data set; otherwise it would be considered personal health information. However, in lieu of removing the value, it may be hashed or encrypted. This would be called a "pseudonym." For example, the unique identifier may be a participant's clinical trial number, and this is encrypted with a secret key to create a pseudonym. A similar scheme for creating pseudonyms would be used under the Expert Determination method.

However, in the HIPAA Privacy Rule at § 164.514(c), it is stated that any code that is *derived* from information about an individual is considered identifiable data. However, such pseudonyms are practically important for knowing which records belong to the same clinical trial participant and constructing the longitudinal record of a data subject. Not being able to create derived pseudonyms means that random pseudonyms must be created. To be able to use random pseudonyms, one must maintain a crosswalk between the individual identity and the random pseudonym. The crosswalk allows the sponsor to use the same pseudonym for each participant across data sets and to allow re-identification at a future date if the need arises. These crosswalks, which are effectively linking tables between the pseudonym and the information about the individual, arguably present an elevated privacy risk because clearly identifiable information must now be stored somehow. Furthermore, the original regulations did not impose any controls on this crosswalk table.

For research purposes, the Common Rule will also apply. Under the Common Rule, which guides IRBs, if the data recipient has no means of getting the key, for example, through an agreement with the sponsor prohibiting the sharing of keys under any circumstances or through organizational policies prohibiting such an exchange, then creating such derived pseudonyms is an acceptable approach (HHS, 2004, 2008b).

Therefore, there is an inconsistency between the Privacy Rule and the Common Rule in that the former does not permit derived pseudonyms, while the latter does. This is well documented (Rothstein, 2005, 2010). However, in the recent guidelines from OCR, this is clarified to state that "a covered entity may disclose codes derived from PHI (protected health information) as part of a de-identified data set if an expert determines that the data meets the de-identification requirements at §164.514(b)(1)" (HHS, 2012, p. 22). This means that a derived code, such as an encryption or hash function, can be used as a pseudonym as long as there is assurance that the means to reverse that pseudonym are tightly controlled. There is now clarity and consistency among rules in that if there is a defensible mechanism whereby reverse engineering a derived pseudonym has a very small probability of being successful this is permitted.

Is It Necessary to Destroy Original Data?

Under the Expert Determination method, the re-identification risk needs to be managed assuming that the adversary is "an anticipated recipient" of the data. This limits the range of adversaries that needs to be considered because, in our context, the anticipated recipient is the QI.

However, under the EU Data Protection Directive, the adversary may be the "data controller or any other person." The data controller is the sponsor or the QI receiving the de-identified data. There are a number of challenges with interpreting this at face value.

One practical issue is that the sponsor will, by definition, be able to re-identify the data because the sponsor will retain the original clinical trial data set. The Article 29 Working Party has proposed that, effectively, the sponsor needs to destroy or aggregate the original data to be able to claim that the data provided to the QI are truly de-identified (Article 29 Data Protection Working Party, 2014). This means that the data are not de-identified if there exists another data set that can re-identify it, even in the possession of another data controller. Therefore, because the identified data exist with the sponsor, the data provided to the QI cannot be considered de-identified. This is certainly not practical because the original data are required for legal reasons (e.g., clinical trial data need to be retained for an extended period of time whose duration depends on the jurisdiction). Such a requirement would discourage de-identification by sponsors and push them to share identifiable data, which arguably would increase the risk of re-identification for trial participants significantly.

In an earlier opinion the Article 29 Data Protection Working Party (2007) emphasized the importance of "likely reasonable" in the definition of identifiable information in the 95/46/EC Directive. In that case, if it is not likely reasonable that data recipients would be able to readily re-identify the anonymized data because they do not have access to the original data, those anonymized data would not be considered personal information. That would seem to be a more reasonable approach that is consistent with interpretations in other jurisdictions.

Is De-identification a Permitted Use?

Retroactively obtaining participant consent to de-identify data and use them for secondary analysis may introduce bias in the data set (El

Emam, 2013). If de-identification is a permitted use under the relevant regulations, then de-identification can proceed without seeking participant consent. Whether that is the case will depend on the prevailing jurisdiction.

Under HIPAA and extensions under the Health Information Technology for Economic and Clinical Health (HITECH) Act Omnibus Rule, de-identification is a permitted use by a covered entity. However, a business associate can de-identify a data set only if the business associate agreement explicitly allows for that. Silence on de-identification in a business associate agreement is interpreted as not permitting de-identification.

In other jurisdictions, such as Ontario, the legislation makes explicit that de-identification is a permitted use (Perun et al., 2005).

Terminology

Terminology in this area is not always clear, and different authors and institutions use the same terms to mean different things or different terms to mean the same thing (Knoppers and Saginur, 2005). Here, we provide the terminology and definitions used in this paper.

The International Organization for Standardization (ISO) Technical Specification on the pseudonymization of health data defines relevant terminology for our purposes. The term "anonymization" is defined as a "process that removes the association between the identifying data set and the data subject" (ISO, 2008). This is consistent with current definitions of "identity disclosure," which corresponds to assigning an identity to a data subject in a data set (OMB, 1994; Skinner, 1992). For example, an identity disclosure would transpire if the QI determined that the third record (ID = 3) in the example data set in Table B-1 belonged to Alice Brown. Thus, anonymization is the process of reducing the probability of identity disclosure to a very small value.

Arguably, the term "anonymization" would be the appropriate term to use here given its more global utilization. However, to remain consistent with the HIPAA Privacy Rule, we use the term "de-identification" in this paper.

Beyond identity disclosure, organizations (and privacy professionals) are, at times, concerned about "attribute disclosure" (OMB, 1994; Skinner, 1992). This occurs when a QI learns a sensitive attribute about a participant in the database with a sufficiently high probability, even if the Q1 does not know which specific record belongs to that patient (Machanavajjhala et al., 2007; Skinner, 1992). For example, in Table B-1, all males born in 1967 had a creatine kinease lab test. Assume that an adversary does not know which record belongs to Almond Zipf (who has record ID = 17; see Table B-2). However, because Almond is male and was born in 1967,

TABLE B-1 An Example of Data Used to Illustrate a Number of Concepts Referred to Throughout This Paper

	Quasi-identifiers		Other Variables	
ID	Sex	Year of Birth	Lab Test	Lab Result
1	Male	1959	Albumin, Serum	4.8
2	Male	1969	Creatine Kinase	86
3	Female	1955	Alkaline Phosphatase	66
4	Male	1959	Bilirubin	Negative
5	Female	1942	BUN/Creatinine Ratio	17
6	Female	1975	Calcium, Serum	9.2
7	Female	1966	Free Thyroxine Index	2.7
8	Female	1987	Globulin, Total	3.5
9	Male	1959	B-type Natriuretic Peptide	134.1
10	Male	1967	Creatine Kinase	80
11	Male	1968	Alanine Aminotransferase	24
12	Female	1955	Cancer Antigen 125	86
13	Male	1967	Creatine Kinase	327
14	Male	1967	Creatine Kinase	82
15	Female	1966	Creatinine	0.78
16	Female	1955	Triglycerides	147
17	Male	1967	Creatine Kinase	73
18	Female	1956	Monocytes	12
19	Female	1956	HDL Cholesterol	68
20	Male	1978	Neutrophils	83
21	Female	1966	Prothrombin Time	16.9
22	Male	1967	Creatine Kinase	68
23	Male	1971	White Blood Cell Count	13.0
24	Female	1954	Hemoglobin	14.8
25	Female	1977	Lipase, Serum	37
26	Male	1944	Cholesterol, Total	147
27	Male	1965	Hematocrit	45.3

NOTE: BUN = blood urea nitrogen; HDL = high-density lipoprotein

the QI will discover something new about him—that he had a test often administered to individuals showing symptoms of a heart attack. All known re-identification attacks are identity disclosures and not attribute disclosures (El Emam et al., 2011a).[3] Furthermore, privacy statutes and

---

[3] This statement does not apply to genomic data. See the summary of evidence on genomic data later in this paper for more detail.

TABLE B-2 Identities of Participants from the Hypothetical Data Set

ID	Name
1	John Smith
2	Alan Smith
3	Alice Brown
4	Hercules Green
5	Alicia Freds
6	Gill Stringer
7	Marie Kirkpatrick
8	Leslie Hall
9	Douglas Henry
10	Fred Thompson
11	Joe Doe
12	Lillian Barley
13	Deitmar Plank
14	Anderson Hoyt
15	Alexandra Knight
16	Helene Arnold
17	Almond Zipf
18	Britney Goldman
19	Lisa Marie
20	William Cooper
21	Kathy Last
22	Deitmar Plank
23	Anderson Hoyt
24	Alexandra Knight
25	Helene Arnold
26	Anderson Heft
27	Almond Zipf

regulations in multiple jurisdictions, including the HIPAA Privacy Rule, the Ontario Personal Health Information Protection Act (PHIPA), and the EU Data Protection Directive, consider identity disclosure only in their definitions of personal health information. Although participants may consider certain types of attribute disclosure to be a privacy violation, it is not considered so when the objective is anonymization of the data set.

Technical methods have been developed to modify the data to protect against attribute disclosure (Fung et al., 2010). However, these methods have rarely, if ever, been used in practice for the disclosure of health data. One possible reason for this is that they distort the data to such an extent that the data are no longer useful for analysis purposes. There are other, nontechnical approaches that are more appropriate for addressing the risks of attribute disclosure, and in the final section on governance we provide a description of how a sponsor can protect against attribute disclosure. Therefore, our focus in this paper is on identity disclosure.

HOW TO MEASURE THE RISK OF RE-IDENTIFICATION

We begin with some basic definitions that are critical for having a meaningful discussion about how re-identification works. Along the way, we address some of the controversies around de-identification that have appeared in the literature and the media.

Categories of Variables

It is useful to differentiate among the different types of variables in a clinical trial data set. The way the variables are handled during the de-identification process will depend on how they are categorized. We make a distinction among three types of variables (Samarati, 2001; Sweeney, 2002):

- **Directly identifying variables.** Direct identifiers have two important characteristics: (1) one or more direct identifiers can be used to uniquely identify an individual, either by themselves or in combination with other readily available information; and (2) they often are not useful for data analysis purposes. Examples of directly identifying variables include names, email addresses, and telephone numbers of participants. It is uncommon to perform data analysis on clinical trial participant names and telephone numbers.
- **Indirectly identifying variables (quasi-identifiers).** Quasi-identifiers are the variables about research participants in the data set that a QI can use, either individually or in combination, to re-identify a record. If an adversary does not have background knowledge of a variable, it cannot be a quasi-identifier. The means by which an adversary can obtain such background knowledge will determine which attacks on a data set are plausible. For example, the background knowledge may be available because the adversary knows a particular target individual in the disclosed clinical trial data set, an individual in the data set has a visible characteristic that is also described in the data set, or the background knowledge exists in a public or semipublic registry. Examples of quasi-identifiers include sex, date of birth or age, locations (such as

postal codes, census geography, and information about proximity to known or unique landmarks), language spoken at home, ethnic origin, aboriginal identity, total years of schooling, marital status, criminal history, total income, visible minority status, activity difficulties/reductions, profession, event dates (such as admission, discharge, procedure, death, specimen collection, visit/encounter), codes (such as diagnosis codes, procedure codes, and adverse event codes), country of birth, birth weight, and birth plurality.

- **Other variables.** These are the variables that are not really useful for determining an individual's identity. They may or may not be clinically relevant.

Individuals can be re-identified because of the directly identifying variables and the quasi-identifiers. Therefore, our focus is on these two types of variables.

Classifying Variables

An initial step in being able to reason about the identifiability of a clinical trial data set is to classify the variables into the above categories. We consider the process for doing so below.

Is It an Identifier?

There are three conditions for a field to be considered an identifier (of either type). These conditions were informed by HHS's de-identification guidelines (HHS, 2012).

Replicability

The field values must be sufficiently stable over time so that the values will occur consistently in relation to the data subject. For example, the results of a patient's blood glucose level tests are unlikely to be replicable over time because they will vary quite a bit. If a field value is not replicable, it will be challenging for an adversary to use that information to re-identify an individual.

Distinguishability

The variable must have sufficient variability to distinguish among individuals in a data set. For example, in a data set of only breast cancer patients, the diagnosis code (at least at a high level) will have little variation. On the other hand, if a variable has considerable variation among the data subjects, it can distinguish among individuals more precisely. That diagnosis field will be quite distinguishable in a general insurance claims database.

Knowability

An adversary must know the identifiers about the data subject in order to re-identify them. If a variable is not knowable by an adversary, it cannot be used to launch a re-identification attack on the data.

When we say that a variable is knowable, it also means that the adversary has an identity attached to that information. For example, if an adversary has a zip code and a date of birth, as well as an identity associated with that information (such as a name), then both the zip code and date of birth are knowable.

Knowability will depend on whether an adversary is an acquaintance of a data subject. If the adversary is an acquaintance, such as a neighbor, coworker, relative, or friend, it can be assumed that certain things will be known. Things known by an acquaintance will be, for example, the subject's demographics (e.g., date of birth, gender, ethnicity, race, language spoken at home, place of birth, and visible physical characteristics). An acquaintance may also know some socioeconomic information, such as approximate years of education, approximate income, number of children, and type of dwelling.

A nonacquaintance will know things about a data subject in a number of different ways, in decreasing order of likelihood:

- The information can be inferred from other knowable information or other variables that determined to be identifiers. For example, birth weight can often be inferred from weeks of gestation. If weeks of gestation are included in the database, birth weight can be determined with reasonable accuracy.
- The information is publicly available. For example, the information is in a public registry, or it appears in a newspaper article (say, an article about an accident or a famous person). Information can also become public if self-revealed by individuals. Examples are information posted on social networking sites and broadcast email announcements (e.g., births). It should be noted that only information that many people would self-reveal should be considered an identifier. If there is a single example or a small number of examples of people who are revealing everything about their lives (e.g., a quantified self-enthusiast who is also an exhibitionist), this does not mean that this kind of information is an identifier for the majority of the population.

- The information is in a semipublic registry. Access to these registries may require a nominal fee or application process.
- The information can be purchased from commercial data brokers. Use of commercial databases is not inexpensive, so an adversary would need to have a strong motive to use such background information.

Some of these data sources can be assessed objectively (e.g., whether there is relevant public information). In other cases, the decision will be subjective and may vary over time.

A Suggested Process for Determining Whether a Variable Is an Identifier

A simple way to determine whether a variable is an identifier is to ask an expert, internal or external to the sponsor, to do so. There are other, more formal processes that can be used as well.

There are two general approaches to classifying variables. In one approach, two analysts who know the data and the data subject population classify the variables independently; then some measure of agreement is computed. A commonly used measure of agreement is Cohen's Kappa (Cohen, 1960). If this value is above 0.8, there is arguably general consensus, and the two analysts will meet to resolve the classifications on which they had disagreements. The results of this exercise are then retained as documentation.

If the Kappa value is less than 0.8, there is arguably little consensus. In such a case, it is recommended that a group of individuals at the sponsor site review the field classifications and reach a classification consensus. This consensus then needs to be documented, along with the process used to reach it. This process provides the data custodian with a defensible classification of variables.

Is It a Direct or Indirect Identifier?

Once a variable has been determined to be an identifier, it is necessary to determine whether it is a direct or indirect (quasi-) identifier. If the field uniquely identifies an individual (e.g., a Social Security Number), it will be treated as a direct identifier. If it is not unique, the next question is whether it is likely to be used for data analysis. If so, it should be treated as a quasi-identifier. This is an important decision because the techniques often used to protect direct identifiers distort the data and their truthfulness significantly.

Is it possible to know which fields will be used for analysis at the time that de-identification is being applied? In many instances, an educated

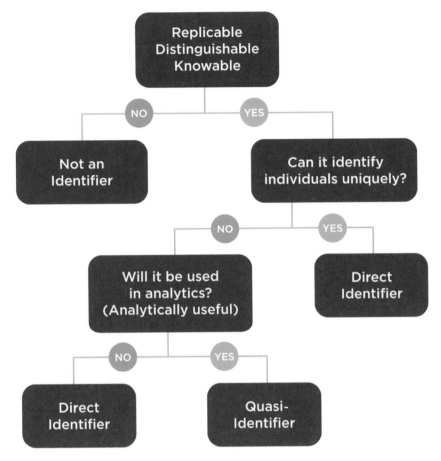

FIGURE B-3 Decision rule for classifying identifiers.
SOURCE: Reprinted with permission from El Emam and colleagues, 2014.

judgment can be made, for example, about potential outcome variables and confounders.

The overall decision rule for classifying variables is shown in Figure B-3.

How Is Re-identification Probability Measured?

Measurement of re-identification risk is a topic that has received extensive study over multiple decades. We examine it at a conceptual level to illustrate key concepts. This discussion builds on the classification of variables described above.

The Risk of Re-identification for Direct Identifiers

We define risk as the probability of re-identifying a trial participant. In practice, we consider the risk of re-identification for direct identifiers to be 1. If a direct identifier does exist in a clinical trial data set, then by definition it will be considered to have a very high risk of re-identification.

Strictly speaking, the probability is not always 1. For example, consider the direct identifier "Last Name." If a trial participant is named "Smith," it is likely that there are other people in the trial named "Smith," and this is even more likely in the community where that participant lives. However, assuming that the probability of re-identification is equal to 1 is a simplification that has little impact in practice, errs on the conservative side, and makes it possible to focus attention on the quasi-identifiers, which is where, in many instances, the most data utility lies.

Two methods can be applied to protect direct identifiers. The first is suppression, or removal of the variable. For example, when a clinical trial data set is disclosed, all of the names of the participants are stripped from the data set. The second method is to create a pseudonym (ISO, 2008). Pseudonymization is also sometimes called "coding" in the health research literature (Knoppers and Saginur, 2005).[4] There are different schemes and technical methods for pseudonymization, such as single and double coding, reversible or irreversible pseudonyms, and encryption and hashing techniques. If executed well, pseudonymization ensures that the probability of re-identification is very small. There is no need to measure this probability on the data after suppression or pseudonymization because in almost all cases that value is going to be very small.

Quasi-identifiers, however, cannot be protected using such procedures. This is because the resulting data, in almost all cases, will not be useful for analytic purposes. Therefore, a different set of approaches is required for measuring and de-identifying quasi-identifiers.

The Risk of Re-identification for Quasi-identifiers

Equivalence Classes

All the records that share the same values on a set of quasi-identifiers are called an "equivalence class." For example, consider the quasi-identifiers in Table B-1—sex and age. All the records in Table B-1 for males born in 1967 (i.e., records 10, 13, 14, 17, and 22) form an equivalence class.

---

[4] A case can made for just using the term "coding" rather than the term "pseudonymization" because it is easier to remember and pronounce. That is certainly a good reason to use the former term as long as the equivalence of the two terms is noted, because "pseudonymization" is the term used in an ISO technical specification.

Equivalence class sizes for a data concept, such as age, potentially change during de-identification. For example, there may be five records for males born in 1967. When the precision of age is reduced to a 5-year interval, there are eight records for males born between 1965 and 1969 (i.e., records 2, 10, 11, 13, 14, 17, 22, and 27). In general, there is a trade-off between the level of detail provided for a data concept and the size of the corresponding equivalence classes, with more detail being associated with smaller equivalence classes.

The most common way to measure the probability of re-identification for a record in a data set is for the probability to be equal to 1 divided by the size of its equivalence class. For example, record number 14 is in an equivalence class of size five, and therefore its probability of re-identification is 0.2. Record number 27 is in an equivalence class of size one and therefore its probability of re-identification is equal to 1 divided by 1. Records that are in equivalence classes of size one are called "uniques." In Table B-3, we have assigned the probability to each record in our example.

This probability applies under two conditions: (1) the adversary knows someone in the real world and is trying to find the record that matches that individual, and (2) the adversary has selected a record in the data set and is trying to find the identity of that person in the real world. Both of these types of attacks on health data have occurred in practice, and therefore both perspectives are important to consider. An example of the former perspective is when an adversary gathers information from a newspaper and attempts to find the data subject in the data set. An example of the latter attack is when the adversary selects a record in the data set and tries to match it with a record in the voter registration list.

A key observation here is that the probability of re-identification is not based solely on the uniques in the data set. For example, record number 18 is not a unique, but it still has quite a high probability of re-identification. Therefore, it is recommended that the risk of re-identification be considered, and managed, for both uniques and non-uniques.

Maximum Risk

One way to measure the probability of re-identification for the entire data set is through the maximum risk, which corresponds to the maximum probability of re-identification across all records. From Table B-3, it can be seen that there is a unique record, such that the maximum risk is 1 for this data set.

TABLE B-3 The Data Set in Table B-1 with the Probabilities of Re-identification per Record Added

ID	Quasi-identifiers		Probability of Re-identification
	Sex	Year of Birth	
1	Male	1959	0.33
2	Male	1969	1
3	Female	1955	0.33
4	Male	1959	0.33
5	Female	1942	1
6	Female	1975	1
7	Female	1966	0.33
8	Female	1987	1
9	Male	1959	0.33
10	Male	1967	0.2
11	Male	1968	1
12	Female	1955	0.33
13	Male	1967	0.2
14	Male	1967	0.2
15	Female	1966	0.33
16	Female	1955	0.33
17	Male	1967	0.2
18	Female	1956	0.5
19	Female	1956	0.5
20	Male	1978	1
21	Female	1966	0.33
22	Male	1967	0.2
23	Male	1971	1
24	Female	1954	1
25	Female	1977	1
26	Male	1944	1
27	Male	1965	1

Average Risk

The average risk corresponds to the average across all records in the data set. In the example of Table B-3, this amounts to 0.59. By definition, the average risk for a data set will be no greater than the maximum risk for the same data set.

Which Risk Metric to Use

As the data set is modified, the risk values may change. For example, consider Table B-4, in which year of birth has been generalized to decade of birth. The maximum risk is still 1, but the average risk has declined to 0.33. The average risk will be more sensitive than the maximum risk to modifications to the data.

TABLE B-4 The Data Set in Table B-1 After Year of Birth Has Been Generalized to Decade of Birth, with the Probabilities of Re-identification per Record Added

	Quasi-identifiers		Probability of Re-identification
ID	Sex	Decade of Birth	
1	Male	1950-1959	0.33
2	Male	1960-1969	0.125
3	Female	1950-1959	0.167
4	Male	1950-1959	0.33
5	Female	1940-1949	1
6	Female	1970-1979	0.33
7	Female	1960-1969	0.33
8	Female	1980-1989	1
9	Male	1950-1959	0.33
10	Male	1960-1969	0.125
11	Male	1960-1969	0.125
12	Female	1950-1959	0.167
13	Male	1960-1969	0.125
14	Male	1960-1969	0.125
15	Female	1960-1969	0.33
16	Female	1950-1959	0.167
17	Male	1960-1969	0.125
18	Female	1950-1959	0.167
19	Female	1950-1959	0.167
20	Male	1970-1979	1
21	Female	1960-1969	0.33
22	Male	1960-1969	0.125
23	Male	1970-1979	0.33
24	Female	1950-1959	0.167
25	Female	1970-1979	0.33
26	Male	1940-1949	1
27	Male	1960-1969	0.125

Because the average risk is no greater than the maximum risk, the latter is generally used when a data set is going to be disclosed publicly (El Emam, 2013). This is because a dedicated adversary who is launching a demonstration attack against a publicly available data set will target the record(s) in the disclosed clinical trial data set with the maximum probability of re-identification. Therefore, it is prudent to protect against such an adversary by measuring and managing maximum risk.

The average risk, by comparison, is more suitable for nonpublic data disclosures. For nonpublic data disclosures, some form of data sharing agreement with prohibitions on re-identification can be expected. In this case, it can be assumed that any data subject may be targeted by the adversary.

As a general rule, it is undesirable to have unique records in the data set after de-identification. In the example of Table B-1, there are unique records both in the original data set and after year of birth has been changed to decade of birth (see Table B-4). For example, record 26 is unique in Table B-4. Unique records have a high risk of re-identification. Also, as a general rule, it is undesirable to have records with a probability of re-identification equal to 0.5 in the data set.

With average risk, one can have data sets with an acceptably small average risk but with unique records or records in equivalence classes of size 2. To avoid that situation, one can use the concept of "strict average risk." Here, maximum risk is first evaluated to ensure that it is at or below 0.33. If that condition is met, average risk is computed. This two-step measure ensures that there are no uniques or doubles in the data set.

In the example data set in Table B-4, the strict average risk is 1. This is because the maximum risk is 1, so the first condition is not met. However, the data set in Table B-5 has a strict average risk of 0.33. Therefore, in practice, maximum risk or strict average risk would be used to measure re-identification risk.

Samples and Populations

The above examples are based on the premise that an adversary knows who is in the data set. Under those conditions, the manner in which the risk metrics have been demonstrated is correct. We call this a "closed" data set. There are situations in which this premise holds true. For instance, one such case occurs when the data set covers everyone in the population. A second case is when the data collection method itself discloses who is in the data set. Here are several examples in which the data collection method makes a data set closed:

- If everyone attending a clinic is screened into a trial, an adversary who knows someone who attends the clinic will know that that individual is in the trial database.
- A study of illicit drug use among youth requires parental consent, which means that parents will know if their child is in the study database.
- The trial participants self-reveal that they are taking part in a particular trial, for example, on social networks or on online forums.

If it is not possible to know who is in the data set, the trial data set can be considered to be a sample from some population. We call this an "open" data set. Because the data set is a sample, there is some uncertainty about

TABLE B-5 The Generalized Data Set with No Uniques or Doubles

| ID | Quasi-identifiers | | Probability of Re-identification |
	Sex	Decade of Birth	
1	Male	1950-1959	0.33
2	Male	1960-1969	0.125
3	Female	1950-1959	0.167
4	Male	1950-1959	0.33
6	Female	1970-1979	0.33
7	Female	1960-1969	0.33
9	Male	1950-1959	0.33
10	Male	1960-1969	0.125
11	Male	1960-1969	0.125
12	Female	1950-1959	0.167
13	Male	1960-1969	0.125
14	Male	1960-1969	0.125
15	Female	1960-1969	0.33
16	Female	1950-1959	0.167
17	Male	1960-1969	0.125
18	Female	1950-1959	0.167
19	Female	1950-1959	0.167
21	Female	1960-1969	0.33
22	Male	1960-1969	0.125
23	Male	1970-1979	0.33
24	Female	1950-1959	0.167
25	Female	1970-1979	0.33
27	Male	1960-1969	0.125

whether a person is in the data set or not. This uncertainty can reduce the probability of re-identification.

When the trial data set is treated as a sample, the maximum and average risk need to be estimated from the sample data. The reason is that in a sample context, the risk calculations depend on the equivalence class size in the population as well. Therefore, the population equivalence class sizes need to be estimated for the same records. Estimates are needed because in most the cases, the sponsor will not have access to the population data.

There is a large body of work on these estimators in the disclosure control literature (e.g., Dankar et al., 2012; Skinner and Shlomo, 2008). A particularly challenging estimation problem is deciding whether a unique record in the sample is also a unique in the population. If a record is unique in the sample, it may be because the sampling fraction is so small that all records in the sample are uniques. Yet a record may be unique in the sample because it is also unique in the population.

Under these conditions, appropriate estimators need to be used to compute the maximum and average risk correctly. In general, when the data set is treated as a sample, the probability of re-identification will be no greater than the probability associated with situations in which the data set is not treated as a sample (i.e., the adversary knows who is in the data set).

Re-identification Risk of Participants with Rare Diseases

It is generally believed that clinical trials conducted on rare diseases will always have a high risk of re-identification. It is true that the risk of re-identification will, in general, be higher than that for nonrare diseases. However, it is not necessarily too high. If the data set is open with a small sampling fraction and one is using (strict) average risk, the risk of re-identification may be acceptably small. The exact risk value will need to be calculated on the actual data set to make that determination.

Taking Context into Account

Determining whether a data set is disclosed to the public or a more restricted group of recipients illustrates how context is critical. In the case of the recipient, for instance, it informs us which metric is more appropriate. However, this is only one aspect of the context surrounding a data set, and a more complete picture can be applied to make more accurate assessments of re-identification risk.

For a public data release, we assume that the adversary will launch a demonstration attack, and therefore it is necessary to manage maximum risk. There are no other controls that can be put in place. For a nonpublic data set, we consider three types of attacks that cover the universe of attacks: deliberate, inadvertent, and breach (El Emam, 2013; El Emam and Arbuckle, 2013).

A **deliberate attack** transpires when the adversary deliberately attempts to re-identify individuals in the data set. This may be a deliberate decision by the leadership of the data recipient (e.g., the QI decides to re-identify individuals in order to link to another data set) or by a rogue employee associated with the data recipient. The probability that this type of attack will be successful can be computed as follows:

$$Pr(\text{re-id, attempt}) = Pr(\text{re-id} \mid \text{attempt}) \times Pr(\text{attempt}) \tag{1}$$

where the term $Pr(\text{attempt})$ captures the probability that a deliberate attempt to re-identify the data will be made by the data recipient. The actual value for $Pr(\text{attempt})$ will depend on the security and privacy controls that the data recipient has in place and the contractual controls that are being imposed as part of the data sharing agreement. The second term, $Pr(\text{re-id} \mid \text{attempt})$, corresponds to the probability that the attack will be successful in the event that the recipient has chosen to commit the attack. This conditional can be measured from the actual data.

An **inadvertent attack** transpires when a data analyst working with the QI (or the QI himself/herself) inadvertently re-identifies someone in the data set. For instance, this could occur when the recipient is already aware of the identity of someone in the data set, such as a friend; relative, or, more generally, an acquaintance. The probability of successful re-identification in this situation can be computed as follows:

$$Pr(\text{re-id, acquaintance}) = Pr(\text{re-id} \mid \text{acquaintance}) \times$$
$$Pr(\text{acquaintance}) \tag{2}$$

There are defensible ways to compute $Pr(\text{acquaintance})$ (El Emam, 2013), which evaluates the probability of an analyst's knowing someone in the data set. For example, if the trial is of a breast cancer treatment, then $Pr(\text{acquaintance})$ is the probability of the analyst's knowing someone who has breast cancer. The value for $Pr(\text{re-id} \mid \text{acquaintance})$ needs to be computed from the data. Box B-4 considers the question of whether it is always necessary to be concerned about the risk of inadvertent re-identification.

A **breach** will occur if there is a data breach at the QI's facility. The probability of this type of attack being successful is

$$Pr(\text{re-id, breach}) = Pr(\text{re-id} \mid \text{breach}) \times Pr(\text{breach}) \tag{3}$$

BOX B-4
Is It Always Necessary to Be Concerned About
the Risk of Inadvertent Re-identification?

In the context of data release through an online portal, an argument can be made that the sponsor imposes significant security and privacy controls and re- quires the qualified investigator (QI) to sign a contract that contains the relevant prohibitions (e.g., a prohibition on re-identification attacks). This means that the probability of re-identification under these two conditions is likely to be very small (but that should still be confirmed).

For inadvertent re-identification, what is the likelihood that an analyst will know someone in the data set? If the clinical trial was conducted in Japan and the data analyst at the QI is in New York, is there a chance that the QI will know a Japanese participant? The reasonable answer is no, in that inadvertent re-identification will be highly unlikely when the plausibility of a relationship between the participant and the analyst is negligible. Specifically, this means that Pr(acquaintance) will be negligibly small. Does that lead us to the conclusion that the data should not be de-identified at all? The answer is no because the Japanese participants will still expect that the data about them are de-identified to some extent. The public per- ception of the possibility of disclosing data that have a high risk of re-identification needs to be considered.

---

where the term Pr(breach) captures the probability that a breach will occur. What should Pr(breach) be? Publicly available data about the prob- ability of a breach can be used to determine this value; the value of the conditional in this case, Pr(re-id | breach), will be computed from these data. Data for 2010 show that 19 percent of health care organizations suf- fered a data breach within the previous year (HIMSS Analytics, 2010); data for 2012 show that this number rose to 27 percent (HIMSS Analytics, 2012). These organizations were all following the HIPAA Security Rule. Note that these figures are averages and may be adjusted to account for variation.

For a nonpublic data release, then, there are three types of attacks for which the re-identification risk needs to be measured and managed. The risk metrics are summarized in Table B-6. The overall probability of re-identification will then be the largest value among the three equations.

Setting Thresholds: What Is Acceptable Risk?

There are quite a few precedents for what can be considered an acceptable amount of risk. These precedents have been in use for many decades, are consistent internationally, and have persisted over time as

TABLE B-6 Data Risk Metrics

Data Risk	Metric to Use
Pr(re-id | attempt)	Strict average risk
Pr(re-id | acquaintance)	Strict average risk
Pr(re-id | breach)	Strict average risk or maximum risk, depending on the assumptions

well (El Emam, 2013). It should be noted, however, that the precedents set to date have been for assessments of maximum risk.

In commentary about the de-identification standard in the HIPAA Privacy Rule, HHS notes in the *Federal Register* (HHS, 2000) that

> the two main sources of disclosure risk for de-identified records about individuals are the existence of records with very unique characteristics (e.g., unusual occupation or very high salary or age) and the existence of external sources of records with matching data elements which can be used to link with the de-identified information and identify individuals (e.g., voter registration records or driver's license records) ... an expert disclosure analysis would also consider the probability that an individual who is the target of an attempt at re-identification is represented on both files, the probability that the matching variables are recorded identically on the two types of records, the probability that the target individual is unique in the population for the matching variables, and the degree of confidence that a match would correctly identify a unique person.

It is clear that HHS considers unique records to have a high risk of re-identification, but such statements also suggest that non-unique records have an acceptably low risk of re-identification.

Yet uniqueness is not a universal threshold. Historically, data custodians (particularly government agencies focused on reporting statistics) have used the "minimum cell size" rule as a threshold for deciding whether to de-identify data (Alexander and Jabine, 1978; Cancer Care Ontario, 2005; Health Quality Council, 2004a,b; HHS, 2000; Manitoba Center for Health Policy, 2002; Office of the Information and Privacy Commissioner of British Columbia, 1998; Office of the Information and Privacy Commissioner of Ontario, 1994; OMB, 1994; Ontario Ministry of Health and Long-Term Care, 1984; Statistics Canada, 2007). This rule was originally applied to counting data in tables (e.g., number of males aged 30-35 living in a certain geographic region). The most common minimum cell size in practice is 5, which implies that the maximum probability of re-identifying a record is $1/5$, or 0.2. Some custodians, such as certain public health offices, use a smaller minimum count, such as 3 (CDC and HRSA, 2004; de Waal and Willenborg, 1996; NRC, 1993; Office of the Privacy Commissioner of Quebec, 1997; U.S. Department of Education,

2003). Others, by contrast, use a larger minimum, such as 11 (in the United States) (Baier et al., 2012; CMS, 2008, 2011; Erdem and Prada, 2011; HHS, 2008a) and 20 (in Canada) (El Emam et al., 2011b, 2012). Based on our review of the literature and the practices of various statistical agencies, the largest minimum cell size is 25 (El Emam et al., 2011b). It should be recognized, however, that there is no agreed-upon threshold, even for what many people would agree is highly sensitive data. For example, minimal counts of 3 and 5 were recommended for HIV/AIDS data (CDC and HRSA, 2004) and abortion data (Statistics Canada, 2007), respectively. Public data releases have used different cell sizes in different jurisdictions. The variability is due, in part, to different tolerances for risk, the sensitivity of data, whether a data sharing agreement is in place, and the nature of the data recipient.

A minimum cell size criterion amounts to a maximum risk value. Yet in some cases, this is too stringent a standard or may not be an appropriate reflection of the type of attack. In such a case, one can use the average risk, as discussed in the previous section. This makes the review of cell size thresholds suitable for both types of risk metrics.

It is possible to construct a decision framework based on these precedents with five "bins" representing five possible thresholds, as shown in Figure B-4. At one extreme is data that would be considered identifiable when the cell size is smaller than 3. Next to that are data that are de-identified with a minimal cell size of 3. Given that this is the least de-identified data set, one could choose to disclose such data sets only to trusted entities where the risks are minimal (for example, where a data sharing agreement is in place and the data recipient has good security and privacy practices). At the other end of the spectrum is the minimal cell size of 20. This high level of de-identification is appropriate when the data are publicly released, with no restrictions on or tracking of what is done with the data and who has accessed them.

If the extreme situations cannot be justified in a particular disclosure, an alternative process is needed for choosing one of the intermediate values. In Figure B-4, this is a choice between a value of 5 and a value of 20.

The above framework does not preclude the use of other values (for example, a sponsor may choose to use a threshold value of 25 observations per cell). However, this framework does ground the choices based on precedents of actual data sets.

What Is the Likelihood of Re-identifying Clinical Trial Data Sets?

There has been concern in the health care and privacy communities that the risk of re-identification in data is quite high and that de-identification is not possible (Ohm, 2010). This argument is often sup-

<3 (>0.33)	3 (0.33)	5 (0.2)	11 (0.09)	20 (0.02)
identifiable data	highly trusted data disclosure			highly untrusted data disclosure

FIGURE B-4 Commonly used risk thresholds based on the review/references in the text.

ported by examples of a number of publicly known re-identification attacks. A systematic review of publicly known re-identification attacks found, however, that when appropriate re-identification standards are used, the risk of re-identification is indeed very small (El Emam et al., 2011a).[5] It was only when no de-identification at all was performed on the data or the de-identification applied was not consistent with or based on best practices that data sets were re-identified with a high success rate. Therefore, the evidence that exists today suggests that using current standards and best practices does provide reasonably strong protections against re-identification.

HOW TO MANAGE RE-IDENTIFICATION RISK

Managing re-identification risk means (1) selecting an appropriate risk metric, (2) selecting an appropriate threshold, and (3) measuring the risk in the actual clinical trial data set that will be disclosed. The choice of a metric is a function of whether the clinical trial data set will be released publicly. For public data sets, it is prudent to use maximum risk in measuring risk and setting thresholds. For nonpublic data sets, a strong case can be made for using average risk (El Emam, 2013; El Emam and Arbuckle, 2013).

How to Choose an Acceptable Threshold

Selecting an acceptable threshold within the range described earlier requires an examination of the context of the data themselves. The re-identification risk threshold is determined based on factors characterizing the QI and the data themselves (El Emam, 2010). These factors have been suggested and have been in use informally by data custodians for at least

---

[5] Note that this conclusion does not apply to genomic data sets. A discussion of genomic data sets is provided in the last section of this paper.

the last decade and a half (Jabine, 1993a,b). They cover three dimensions (El Emam et al., 2010), as illustrated in Figure B-5:

- **Mitigating controls.** This is the set of security and privacy practices that the QI has in place. A recent review identifies a collection of practices used by large data custodians and recommended by funding agencies and IRBs for managing sensitive health information (El Emam et al., 2009).
- **Invasion of privacy.** This entails evaluation of the extent to which a particular disclosure would be an invasion of privacy to the participants (a checklist is available in El Emam et al. [2009]). There are three considerations: (1) the sensitivity of the data (the greater the sensitivity of the data, the greater the invasion of privacy), (2) the potential injury to patients from an inappropriate disclosure (the greater the potential for injury, the greater the invasion of privacy), and (3) the appropriateness of consent for disclosing the data (the less appropriate the consent, the greater the invasion of privacy) (see Box B-5).
- **Motives and capacity.** This dimension compasses the motives and the capacity of the QI to re-identify the data, considering such issues as conflicts of interest, the potential for financial gain from re-identification, and whether the data recipient has the skills and financial capacity to re-identify the data (a checklist is available in El Emam et al. [2009]).

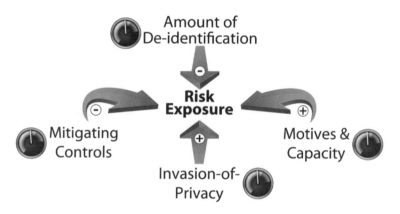

FIGURE B-5 Factors to consider when deciding on an acceptable level of re-identification risk.
SOURCE: Reprinted with permission from El Emam and colleagues, 2014.

BOX B-5
Consent and De-identification

As noted earlier, there is no legislative or regulatory requirement to obtain consent from participants to share their de-identified data. There are additional ongoing efforts to ensure that consent forms do not create barriers to data sharing (Health Research Authority, 2013).

Consideration of consent in this context, then, is only to account for situations in which consent has been provided by trial participants or notice has been given to participants. In such cases, the sharing of clinical trial data is not considered as invasive to privacy as opposed to cases in which consent is not sought. Multiple levels of notice and consent can exist for disclosure of de-identified data. These are as follows, in increasing order of invasion of privacy:

- Participants may have consented for the disclosure of personal health data from the trial for the purpose of secondary analysis. This may be a specific or broad consent for secondary analysis. That the sponsor is trying to de-identify the data reflects extra caution and privacy-protective behavior on the part of the sponsor.
- Participants may have consented to the disclosure of only de-identified data for secondary analysis. This may be specific or broad secondary analysis.
- The sponsor does not have express consent for sharing the data but is consulting with representatives of the trial participants (e.g., patient advocacy groups) and the trial sites to address any sensitivities and to determine the best way to notify participants that their data will be shared.
- The sponsor does not have express consent and is not planning any consultations or notice.

From a risk management perspective, the first option above is the least invasive of participant privacy, while the last is the most invasive. The practical consequence is that the acceptable threshold (or the definition of "very small risk") will be lower under the most invasive scenario.

In general, many of these elements can be managed through contracts (e.g., a prohibition on re-identification, restrictions on linking the data with other data sets, and disallowing the sharing of the data with other third parties). For example, if the mitigating controls are low, which means that the QI has poor security and privacy practices, the re-identification threshold should be set at a lower level. This will result in more de-identification being applied. However, if the QI has very good security and privacy practices in place, the threshold can be set higher. Checklists for evaluating these dimensions, as well as a scoring scheme, are available (El Emam, 2013).

If the sponsor is disclosing the data through an online portal, the sponsor has control of many, but not all, of the mitigating controls. This provides additional assurances to the sponsor that a certain subset of controls will be implemented to the sponsor's satisfaction.

Once a threshold has been determined, the actual probability of re-identification is measured in the data set. If the probability is higher than the threshold, transformations of the data need to be performed. Otherwise, the data can be declared to have a very small risk of re-identification.

The implication here is that the amount of data transformation needed will be a function of these other contextual factors. For example, if the QI has good security and privacy practices in place, the threshold chosen will be higher, which means that the data will be subjected to less de-identification.

The security and privacy practices of the QI can be manipulated through contracts. The contract signed by the QI can impose a certain list of practices that must be in place, which are the basis for determining the threshold. Therefore, they must be in place by the QI to justify the level of transformation performed on the data.

This approach is consistent with the limited data set (LDS) method for sharing data under HIPAA. However, this method does not ensure that the risk of re-identification is very small, and therefore the data will still be considered personal health information.

For public data releases, there are no contracts and no expectation that any mitigating controls will be in place. In that case, the lowest probability thresholds (or highest cell size thresholds) are used.

Methods for Transforming the Data

There are a number ways to transform a data set to reduce the probability of re-identification to a value below the threshold. Many algorithms for this purpose have been proposed by the computer science and statistics communities. They vary in quality and performance. Ideally, algorithms adopted for clinical trial data sets should minimize the modifications to the data while ensuring that the measured probability is below the threshold.

Four general classes of techniques have worked well in practice:

- **Generalization.** This is when the value of a field is modified to a more general value. For example, a date of birth can be generalized to a month and year of birth.
- **Suppression.** This is when specific values in the clinical trial data set are removed from the data set (i.e., induced missingness). For example, a value in a record that makes it an outlier may be suppressed.

- **Randomization.** This denotes adding noise to a field. The noise can come from a uniform or other type of distribution. For example, a date may be shifted a week forward or backward.
- **Subsampling.** This is used to disclose a random subset of the data rather than the full data set to the QI.

In practice, a combination of these techniques is applied for any given data disclosure. Furthermore, these techniques can be customized to specific field types. For example, generalization and suppression can be applied differently to dates and zip codes to maximize the data quality for each (El Emam and Arbuckle, 2013).

The application of these techniques can reduce the risk of re-identification. For example, consider the average risk in Table B-3, which is 0.59. There is a reduction in average risk to 0.33 when the year of birth is generalized to decades in Table B-4. By suppressing some records, it was possible to further reduce the average risk to 0.22 in Table B-5. Each transformation progressively reduces the risk.

The Use of Identifier Lists

Thus far we have covered a sufficient number of topics that we can start performing a critical appraisal of some commonly used de-identification methods and the extent to which they can ensure that the risk of re-identification is very small. We focus on the use of identifier lists. The reason is that this approach is quite common and is being adopted to de-identify clinical trial data.

The HIPAA Privacy Rule's Safe Harbor Standard

We first consider the variable list in the HIPAA Privacy Rule Safe Harbor method.

The Safe Harbor list contains a number of direct identifiers and two quasi-identifiers (i.e., dates and zip codes), as summarized earlier in Box B-2. It should be evident that in applying a fixed list of variables, there is no assurance that all of the quasi-identifiers have been accounted for in the risk measurement and the transformation of the data set. For example, other quasi-identifiers, such as race, ethnicity, and occupation, may be in the data set, but they will be ignored. Even if the probability of re-identification under Safe Harbor is small (Benitez and Malin, 2010), this low probability may not carry over with more quasi-identifiers than the two in the original list.

The empirical analysis that was conducted before the Safe Harbor standard was issued assumed that the data set is a random sample from the U.S. population. This assumption may have variable validity in real data sets. However, there will be cases when it is definitely not true. For example, consider a data set that consists of only the records in Table B-1. Now, assume that an adversary can find out who is in the data set. This can happen if the data set covers a well-defined population. If the trial site is known, it can be reasonably assumed that the participants in the trial who received treatment at that site live in the same geographic region. If the adversary knows that Bob was born in 1965, lives in the town in which the site is situated, and was in the trial, the adversary knows that Bob is in the data set, and therefore the 27th record must be Bob. This re-identification occurs even though this table meets the requirements of the Safe Harbor standard. Members of a data set may be known if their inclusion in the trial is revealing (e.g., a trial in a workplace where participants have to wear a visible device, parents who must consent to have their teenage children participate in a study, or adolescents who must miss a few days of school to participate in a study). Therefore, this standard can be protective only if the adversary cannot know who is in the data set. This will be the case if the data set is a random sample from the population.

If these assumptions are met, the applicability of Safe Harbor to a clinical trial data set will be defensible, but only if there are no international participants. If a clinical trial data set includes participants from sites outside the United States, the analysis that justifies using this standard will not be applicable. For example, there is a difference of two orders of magnitude between the median number of individuals living in U.S. zip codes and in Canadian postal codes. Therefore, translating the zip code truncation logic in Safe Harbor to Canadian postal codes would not be based on defensible evidence.

Safe Harbor also has some weaknesses that are specific to the two quasi-identifiers that are included.

In some instances, there may be dates in a clinical trial data set that are not really quasi-identifiers because they do not pass the test highlighted earlier. For example, consider an implantable medical device that fires, and each time it does so there is a time and date stamp in the data stream. The date of a device's firing is unlikely to be a quasi-identifier because it is not knowable, but it is a date.

Safe Harbor states that all three-digit zip codes with fewer than 20,000 inhabitants from the 2010 census must be replaced with "000"; otherwise the three-digit zip code may be included in the data set. The locations of three-digit zip codes with fewer than 20,000 inhabitants are shown in Figure B-6. However, in some states there is only one zip code with fewer than 20,000 inhabitants. For example, if a data set is disclosed with "000" for the residential three-digit zip code for participants in a site in New

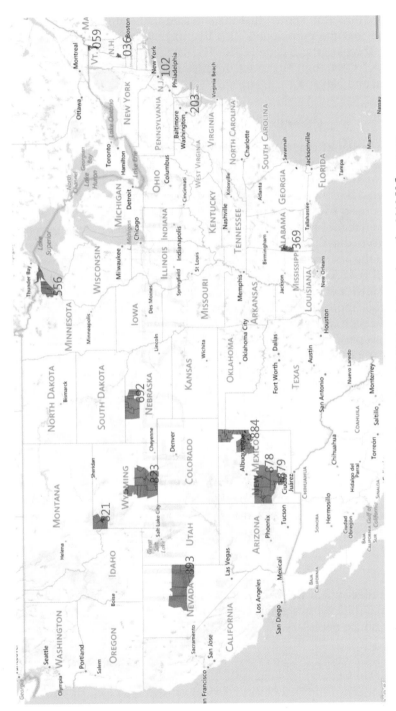

FIGURE B-6 Inhabited three-digit zip codes with fewer than 20,000 inhabitants from the 2010 U.S. census.

Hampshire (and it is known that the site is in that state), it is reasonable to assume that the participants also live in that state and to infer that their true three-digit zip code is 036. The same conclusion can be drawn about "000" three-digit zip codes in states such as Alabama, Minnesota, Nebraska, and Nevada.

Other Examples of Identifier Lists

More recent attempts at developing a fixed list of quasi-identifiers to de-identify clinical trial data have indicated that including any combination of two quasi-identifiers (from the prespecified list) is acceptable (Hrynaszkiewicz et al., 2010). Data sets with more than two quasi-identifiers need to go through a more thorough evaluation, such as the risk management approach described earlier. However, this approach suffers from the same limitations as the Safe Harbor standard with respect to the assumption of two quasi-identifiers always having acceptably small risk. An additional limitation is that the authors of the list in Hrynaszkiewicz et al. (2010) present no empirical evaluation demonstrating that this approach consistently produces data sets with a low risk of re-identification, whereas at least the Safe Harbor list is based on empirical analysis performed by the Census Bureau.

More important, a number of de-identification standards proposed by sponsors have followed similar approaches for sharing clinical trial data from participants globally (see the standards at ClinicalStudyDataRequest.com). Ideally, methods that can provide stronger assurances should be used to de-identify such data.

Putting It All Together

Now that we have gone through the various key elements of the de-identification process, we can put them together into a comprehensive data flow. This flow is illustrated in Figure B-7. The steps in this process are as follows.

Step 1: Determine direct identifiers in the data set.

Determine which fields in the data set are direct identifiers. If the clinical trial data set has already been stripped of direct identifiers, this step may not be necessary.

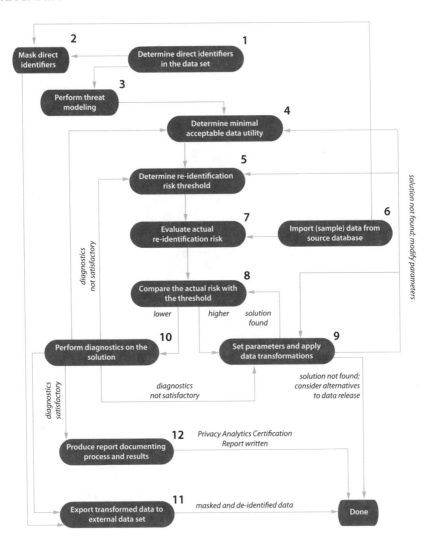

FIGURE B-7 The overall de-identification process.
SOURCE: Reprinted with permission from El Emam and colleagues, 2014.

Step 2: Mask (transform) direct identifiers.

Once the direct identifiers have been determined, masking techniques must be applied to those direct identifiers. Masking techniques include the following: (1) removal of the direct identifiers, (2) replacement of the direct identifiers with random values, or (3) replacement of the direct identifiers with pseudonyms. Once masking has been completed there is virtually no risk of re-identification from direct identifiers. If the database has already been stripped of direct identifiers, this step may not be necessary.

Step 3: Perform threat modeling.

Threat modeling consists of two activities: (1) identification of the plausible adversaries and what information they may be able to access, and (2) determination of the quasi-identifiers in the data set.

Step 4: Determine minimal acceptable data utility.

It is important to determine in advance the minimal relevant data based on the quasi-identifiers. This is essentially an examination of what fields are considered most appropriate given the purpose of the use or disclosure. This step concludes with the imposition of practical limits on how some data may be de-identified and the analyses that may need to be performed later on.

Step 5: Determine the re-identification risk threshold.

This step entails determining what constitutes acceptable risk. As an outcome of the process used to define the threshold, the mitigating controls that need to be imposed on the QI, if any, become evident.

Step 6: Import (sample) data from the source database.

Importing data from the source database may be a simple or complex exercise, depending on the data model of the source data set. This step is included explicitly in the process because it can consume significant resources and must be accounted for in any planning for de-identification.

Step 7: Evaluate the actual re-identification risk.

The actual risk is computed from the data set using the appropriate metric (maximum or strict average). To compute risk, a number of parameters need to be set, such as the sampling fraction.

Step 8: Compare the actual risk with the threshold.

This step entails comparing the actual risk with the threshold determined in Step 5.

Step 9: Set parameters and apply data transformations.

If the measured risk is higher than the threshold, anonymization methods, such as generalization, suppression, randomization, and subsampling, are applied to the data. Sometimes a solution cannot be found within the specified parameters, and it is necessary to go back and reset the parameters. It may also be necessary to modify the threshold and adjust some of the assumptions behind the original risk assessment. Alternatively, some of the assumptions about acceptable data utility may need to be renegotiated with the data users.

Step 10: Perform diagnostics on the solution.

If the measured risk is lower than the threshold, diagnostics should be performed on the solution. Diagnostics may be objective or subjective. An objective diagnostic will evaluate the sensitivity of the solution to violations of assumptions that were made. For example, an assumption may be that an adversary might know the diagnosis code of a patient, or if there is uncertainty about the sampling fraction of the data set, a sensitivity to that value can be performed. A subjective diagnostic will determine whether the utility of the data is sufficiently high for the intended purposes of the use or disclosure.

If the diagnostics are satisfactory, the de-identified data are exported, and a report documenting the de-identification is produced. On the other hand, if the diagnostics are not satisfactory, the re-identification parameters may need to be modified; the risk threshold adjusted; and the original assumptions about minimal, acceptable utility renegotiated with the data user.

Step 11: Export transformed data to external data set.

Exporting the de-identified data to the destination database may be a simple or complex exercise, depending on the data model of the destination database. This step is included explicitly in the process because it can consume significant resources and must be accounted for in any planning for de-identification.

ASSESSING THE IMPACT OF
DE-IDENTIFICATION ON DATA QUALITY

As noted above, Safe Harbor and similar methods that significantly restrict the precision of the fields that can be disclosed can result in a nontrivial reduction in the quality of de-identified data. Therefore, in this section, we focus on data quality when statistical methods are used to de-identify data.

The evidence on the impact of de-identification on data utility is mixed. Some studies show little impact (Kennickell and Lane, 2006), while others show significant impact (Purdam and Elliot, 2007). There is also evidence that data utility will depend on the type of analysis performed (Cox and Kim, 2006; Lechner and Pohlmeier, 2004). In general, if de-identification is accomplished using precise risk measurement and strong optimization algorithms to transform the data, data quality should remain high.

Ensuring that the analysis results produced after de-identification are similar to the results that would be obtained on the original data sets is critical. It would be problematic if a QI attempted to replicate the results from a published trial and were unable to do so because of extensive distortion caused by the de-identification that was applied. Therefore, the amount of distortion must be minimized.

However, de-identification always introduces some distortion, and there is a trade-off between data quality and the amount of de-identification performed to protect privacy. This trade-off can be represented as a curve between data utility and privacy protection, as illustrated in Figure B-8.

Consider, then, that there is a minimal amount of data utility that would be tolerable to ensure that the results of the original trial can be replicated to a large extent. On the other hand, there is a re-identification probability threshold that cannot be exceeded. As shown in Figure B-8, this will leave a small range of possible solutions. To ensure that the de-identification solution is truly within this narrow operating range, it is necessary to perform a pilot evaluation on one or more representative clinical trial data sets and compare the before and after analysis results using exactly the same analytic techniques.

Obtaining similar results for a de-identified clinical trial data set that is intended for public release will be more challenging than disclosing the data set to a QI with strong mitigating controls. The reason is that the amount of de-identification will vary, being more in the former case. This may limit a sponsor's ability to disclose data publicly, or there may have to be a strong replicability caveat on the public data set. For a nonpublic data set when a QI is known, the sponsor may impose a minimal set of mitigating controls through a contract or by providing the data through

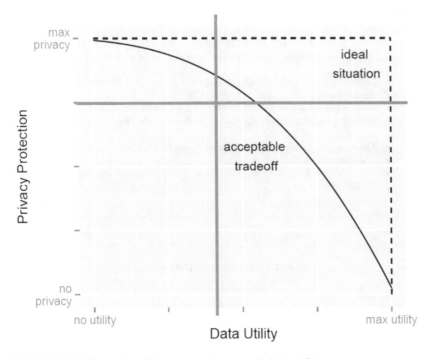

FIGURE B-8 The trade-off between privacy and data utility.

an online portal to ensure that the de-identification applied to the data set is not excessive.

GOVERNANCE

Governance is necessary for the sponsor to manage the risks when disclosing clinical trial data, and it requires that a set of additional practices be in place. What would be characterized as high-maturity sponsors will have a robust governance process in place.

Governance Practices

Some governance practices are somewhat obvious, such as the need to track all data releases; trigger alerts for data use expirations; and ensure that the documentation for the de-identification for each data release has, in fact, been completed. Other practices are necessary to ensure that participant privacy is adequately protected in practice. Elements of governance practices are listed in Box B-6.

BOX B-6
Elements of Governance Practices

- Developing and maintaining global anonymization documentation
- Process and tools for tracking all data releases
- Process and tools for triggering alerts for data use expirations
- Ensuring that documentation for the de-identification for each data release is complete and indexed
- On occasion, commissioning controlled re-identification attacks
- Implementing a QI audit process
- Ensuring that there is ethics review that covers protections against attribute disclosure

---

Controlled Re-identification

The U.K. ICO has recommended that organizations that disclose data also perform controlled re-identification attacks on their disclosed data sets (ICO, 2012). Doing so will allow them to obtain independent evidence on how well their de-identification practices are working and determine whether there are any potential weaknesses that they need to start addressing.

Controlled re-identification attacks are commissioned by the sponsor. With limited funding, these attacks often use publicly available information to attack databases. If additional funding is available, those who conduct these attacks can purchase and use commercial databases to re-identify data subjects.

Appropriate Contracts

Additional governance elements become particularly important when a sponsor discloses data to a QI under a contract. This contract will document the mitigating controls as part of the conditions for receiving the data. The sponsor should then have an audit regime in place to ensure that QIs have indeed put these practices in place. The sponsor may select high-risk QIs for audit, select randomly, or combine the two. Another approach is to ask QIs to conduct third-party audits and report the results back to the sponsor on a regular basis for as long as they are using the data set. The purpose of the audit is to ensure that the mitigating controls are indeed in place.

Enterprise De-identification Process

At an enterprise level, sponsors need to have an enterprise de-identification process that will be applied across all clinical trial data sets. This process includes the appropriate thresholds and controls for data releases, as well as templates for data sharing agreements and terms of use of data. The global process ensures consistency across all data releases. This process must then be enacted for each clinical trial data set, and this may involve some customization to address specific characteristics of a given data set.

The cost of such a process will depend on the size of the sponsor and the heterogeneity of its clinical trials and therapeutic areas. However, in the long term such an approach can be expected to have a lower total cost because there will be more opportunities for reuse and learning.

In practice, many sponsors have standard case report forms (CRFs) for a subset of the data they collect in their clinical trials. For example, there may be standard CRFs for demographics or for standardized measures and patient-reported outcomes. The global process can classify the variables in these standard CRFs as direct and quasi-identifiers and articulate the techniques that should be used to transform those variables. This will reduce the anonymization effort per clinical trial by a nontrivial amount.

Protecting Against Attribute Disclosure

At the beginning of this paper, we briefly mentioned attribute disclosure, but did not address how to protect against it. Such protections can be implemented as part of governance. However, in general, modifying the data to protect against attribute disclosure means reducing the plausible inferences that can be drawn from the data. This can be detrimental to the objective of learning as much as possible from the data and building generalizable statistical models from the data. Furthermore, to protect against attribute disclosure, one must anticipate all inferences and make data modifications to impede them, which may not be possible.

Some inferences may be desirable because they may enhance understanding of the treatment benefits or safety of a new drug or device, and some inferences will be stigmatizing to the data subjects. One will not want to make modifications to the data that block the former type of inferences.

For nonpublic data releases, it is recommended that there be an ethics review of the analysis protocols. As part of the ethics review process, the ethics committee or council will examine the potential for stigmatizing attribute disclosure. This is a subjective decision and will have to take into account current social norms and participant expectations (see also the discussion in El Emam and Arbuckle [2013]). The ethics review may be performed on the secondary analysis protocol by the QI's institutional IRB, or by a separate committee reporting to the sponsor or even within the sponsor. Such an approach will maximize data integrity but also provide assurance that attribute disclosure is addressed. An internal sponsor ethics review council will include a privacy professional, an ethicist, a lay person representing the participants, a person with knowledge of the clinical trials business at the sponsor, and a brand or public relations person.

For public data releases, there is no analysis protocol or a priori approval process, and therefore it will be challenging to provide assurances about attribute disclosure.

De-identifying Genomic Data

There have been various proposals to apply the types of generalization and randomization strategies discussed in this paper to genomic data, and *omics data more generally (e.g., RNA expression or proteomic records) (Li et al., 2012; Lin et al., 2002, 2004; Malin, 2005). However, evidence suggests that such methods may not be suitable for the anonymization of biomarkers that constitute a large number of dimensions. The main reasons are that they can cause significant distortion of long sequences, and the assumptions that need to be made to de-identify sequences of patient events (e.g., visits and claims) will not apply to *omic data. At the same time, there are nuances that are worth considering. For context, we address concerns around genomic data specifically, while noting that similar allusions can be made to other types of data.

First, it is important to recognize that many of the attacks that have been carried out on genomic data require additional information (Malin et al., 2011). In certain cases, for instance, the re-identification of genomic data is accomplished through the demographics of the corresponding research participant; the associated clinical information (Loukides et al., 2010b); or contextual cues associated with the collection and dissemination of the data, such as the set of health care providers visited by the participant (Malin and Sweeney, 2004). For example, a recently reported re-identification attack on participants in the Personal Genome Project (PGP) was based almost entirely on information derived from publicly accessible profiles—notably birth date (or month and year), gender, and geographic indicators of residence (e.g., zip code) (Sweeney et al., 2013). Other individuals in the PGP were re-identified based on the fact that they uploaded compressed files that incorporated their personal names as file names when uncompressed. This attack used the same type of variables that can be protected using the techniques described in this paper. Moreover, it has been shown that many of the protection strategies discussed in this paper can be tailored to support genome-phenome association discovery (e.g., through anonymization of standardized clinical codes [Heatherly et al., 2013; Loukides et al., 2010a]).

This fact is true for attacks that factor genomic data into the attack as well. For instance, it was recently shown that an adversary could use publicly available databases that report on Y-chromosome–surname correlations to ascertain the surname of a genome sequence lacking an individual's name (Haggie, 2013). However, for this attack to be successful, it required additional information about the corresponding individual. Specifically, the attacker also needed to know the approximate area of residence (e.g., U.S. state) and approximate age of the individual. Although such information may be permitted within a Safe Harbor de-identification framework, a statistical assessment of the potential identifiability of such information would indicate that such ancillary information might constitute an unacceptably high rate of re-identification risk. At the same time, it should be recognized that, even when such information was made available, the attack reported in Haggie (2013) was successful 12 percent of the time and unsuccessful 5 percent of the time. In other words, there is variability in the chance that such attacks will be successful.

More direct attacks are, however, plausible. There is evidence that a sequence of 30 to 80 independent single nucleotide polymorphisms (SNPs) could uniquely identify a single person (Lin et al., 2004). Unlike the surname inference attack mentioned above, a direct attack would require that the adversary already have identified genotype data for a target individual. Yet linking an individual using his or her genome would permit the adversary to learn any additional information in the new resource, such as the individual's health status. Additionally, a recent demonstration with data from openSNP and Facebook suggests that in certain instances, the genomic status of an individual can be inferred from the genome sequences of close family members (Humbert et al., 2013).

Beyond direct matching of sequences, there is also a risk of privacy compromise in "pooled" data, where only summary statistics are reported. For instance, it has been shown that it is possible to determine whether an individual is in a pool of cases or controls for a study by assessing the likelihood that the individual's sequence is "closer" to one group or the other (Homer et al., 2008; Jacobs et al., 2009; Wang et al., 2009). Despite such vulnerability, it has also been shown that the likelihood of success for this attack becomes lower as the number of people in each group increases. In fact, for studies with a reasonable number of participants (more than 1,000), it is safe to reveal the summary statistics of all common (not rare) genomic regions (Sankararaman et al., 2009).

However, one of the challenges with genomic data is that it is possible to learn phenotypic information directly. When such information can be ascertained with certainty, it can then be used in a re-identification attack. For example, predictions (varying in accuracy) of height, facial morphology, age, body mass index, approximate skin pigmentation, eye color, and diagnosis of cystic fibrosis or Huntington's chorea from genetic information have been reported (Kayser and de Knijff, 2011; Kohn, 1991; Lowrance and Collins, 2007; Malin and Sweeney, 2000; Ou et al., 2012; Silventoinen et al., 2003; Wjst, 2010; Zubakov et al., 2010), although it should be noted that there have been no full demonstrations of attacks using such inferences. Also, because of the errors in some of these predictions (excluding Mendelian disorders that are directly dependent on a mutation in a certain portion of the genome), it is not clear that they would be sufficiently reliable for re-identification attacks.

Although traditional generalization and randomization strategies may not provide a sufficient balance between utility and privacy for high-dimensional *omics data, a solution to the problem may be possible with the assistance of modern cryptography. In particular, secure multiparty computation (SMC) corresponds to a set of techniques (and protocols) that allow quite sophisticated mathematical and statistical operations to be performed on encrypted data. In the process, individual records would never be disclosed to the user of such a resource. This type of protection would not prevent inference through summary-level statistics, but it would prevent direct attacks on individuals' records. SMC solutions have been demonstrated that have been tailored to support frequency queries (Kantarcioglu et al., 2008), genomic sequence alignment (Chen et al., 2012), kinship (and other comparison) tests (Baldi et al., 2011; He et al., 2014), and personalized medical risk scores (Ayday et al., 2013a,b). Nonetheless, the application of these methods to genetic data is still in the early stages of research, and it may be a few more years before some large-scale practical results are seen.

REFERENCES

Alexander, L., and T. Jabine. 1978. Access to social security microdata files for research and statistical purposes. *Social Security Bulletin* 41(8):3-17.

Article 29 Data Protection Working Party. 2007. *Opinion 4/2007 on the concept of personal data.* WP136. http://ec.europa.eu/justice/policies/privacy/docs/wpdocs/2007/wp136_en.pdf (accessed December 19, 2014).

Article 29 Data Protection Working Party. 2014. *Opinion 05/2014 on anonymization techniques.* WP216. http://ec.europa.eu/justice/data-protection/article-29/documentation/opinion-recommendation/files/2014/wp216_en.pdf (accessed December 19, 2014).

Ayday, E., J. L. Raisaro, and J.-P. Hubaux. 2013a. Privacy-enhancing technologies for medical tests using genomic data. *20th Annual Network and Distributed System Security Symposium (NDSS)*, San Diego, CA, February 2013.

Ayday, E., J. L. Raisaro, J.-P. Hubaux, and J. Rougemont. 2013b. Protecting and evaluating genomic privacy in medical tests and personalized medicine. *Proceedings of the 12th ACM Workshop on Workshop on Privacy in the Electronic Society* 95-106.

Baier, P., S. Hinkins, and F. Scheuren. 2012. *The electronic health records incentive program eligible professionals public use file.* http://www.cms.gov/Regulations-and-Guidance/Legislation/EHRIncentivePrograms/DataAndReports.html (accessed December 19, 2014).

Baldi, P., R. Baronio, E. De Cristofaro, P. Gasti, and G. Tsudik. 2011. Countering GATTACA: Efficient and secure testing of fully-sequenced human genomes. *Proceedings of the 18th ACM Conference on Computer and Communications Security* 691-702.

Benitez, K., and B. Malin. 2010. Evaluating re-identification risks with respect to the HIPAA Privacy Rule. *Journal of the American Medical Informatics Association* 17(2):169-177.

Bhattacharjee, Y. 2012. Pharma firms push for sharing of cancer trial data. *Science* 38(6103):29.

Canadian Institute for Health Information. 2010. *"Best practice" guidelines for managing the disclosure of de-identified health information.* http://www.ijpc-se.org/documents/hhs10.pdf (accessed December 19, 2014).

Cancer Care Ontario. 2005. *Cancer Care Ontario data use and disclosure policy.* Toronto, ON: Cancer Care Ontario.

Castellani, J. 2013. Are clinical trial data shared sufficiently today?: Yes. *British Medical Journal* 347(1):f1881.

CDC (Centers for Disease Control and Prevention) and HRSA (Health Resources and Services Administration). 2004. *Integrated guidelines for developing epidemiologic profiles: HIV Prevention and Ryan White CARE Act community planning.* Atlanta, GA: CDC. http://www.cdph.ca.gov/programs/aids/Documents/GLines-IntegratedEpiProfiles.pdf (accessed December 19, 2014).

Center for Business and Information Technologies. 2013. *Cajun Code Fest.* http://cajuncodefest.org (accessed November 9, 2012).

Chen, Y., B. Peng, X. Wang, and H. Tang. 2012. Large-scale privacy-preserving mapping of human genomic sequences on hybrid clouds. *Proceeding of the 19th Network and Distributed System Security Symposium,* San Diego, CA, February 2012.

CMS (Centers for Medicare & Medicaid Services). 2008. *2008 basic stand alone Medicare claims public use files.* http://www.cms.gov/Research-Statistics-Data-and-Systems/Statistics-Trends-and-Reports/BSAPUFS/Downloads/2008_BSA_PUF_Disclaimer.pdf (accessed December 19, 2014).

CMS. 2011. *BSA inpatient claims PUF.* http://www.cms.gov/Research-Statistics-Data-and-Systems/Statistics-Trends-and-Reports/BSAPUFS/Inpatient_Claims.html (accessed December 19, 2014).

Cohen, J. 1960. A coefficient of agreement for nominal scales. *Educational and Psychological Measurement* 20(1):37-46.

CORE (Center for Outcomes Research and Evaluation). 2014. *The YODA Project.* http://medicine.yale.edu/core/projects/yodap (accessed December 19, 2014).

Cox, L. H., and J. J. Kim. 2006. Effects of rounding on the quality and confidentiality of statistical data. In *Privacy in statistical databases,* edited by J. Domingo-Ferrer and L. Franconi. New York: Springer Berlin Heidelberg. Pp. 48-56.

Dankar, F., K. E. Emam, A. Neisa, and T. Roffey. 2012. Estimating the re-identification risk of clinical data sets. *BMC Medical Informatics and Decision Making* 12(1):66.

de Waal, A., and L. Willenborg. 1996. A view on statistical disclosure control for microdata. *Survey Methodology* 22(1):95-103.

Dryad. undated. *Dryad digital repository.* http://datadryad.org (accessed September 19, 2013).

El Emam, K. 2010. Risk-based deidentification of health data. *IEEE Security and Privacy* 8(3):64-67.

El Emam, K. 2013. *Guide to the deidentification of personal health information.* Boca Raton, FL: CRC Press (Auerbach Publications).

El Emam, K., and L. Arbuckle. 2013. *Anonymizing health data: Case studies and methods to get you started.* Sebastopol, CA: O'Reilly Media.

El Emam, K., F. Dankar, R. Vaillancourt, T. Roffey, and M. Lysyk. 2009. Evaluating patient re-identification risk from hospital prescription records. *Canadian Journal of Hospital Pharmacy* 62(4):307-319.

El Emam, K., A. Brown, P. AbdelMalik, A. Neisa, M. Walker, J. Bottomley, and T. Roffey. 2010. A method for managing re-identification risk from small geographic areas in Canada. *BMC Medical Informatics and Decision Making* 10(1):18.

El Emam, K., E. Jonker, L. Arbuckle, and B. Malin, 2011a. A systematic review of re-identification attacks on health data. *PLoS ONE* 6(12):e28071.

El Emam, K., D. Paton, F. Dankar, and G. Koru. 2011b. Deidentifying a public use microdata file from the Canadian national discharge abstract database. *BMC Medical Informatics and Decision Making* 11:53.

El Emam, K., L. Arbuckle, G. Koru, B. Eze, L. Gaudette, E. Neri, S. Rose, J. Howard, and J. Gluck. 2012. Deidentification methods for open health data: The case of the Heritage Health Prize claims dataset. *Journal of Medical Internet Research* 14(1):e33.

El Emam, K., G. Middleton, and L. Arbuckle. 2014. *An implementation guide for data anonymization.* Bloomington, IN: Trafford Publishing.

EMA (European Medicines Agency). 2014a. *European Medicines Agency policy on publication of clinical data for medicinal products for human use.* http://www.ema.europa.eu/docs/en_GB/document_library/Other/2014/10/WC500174796.pdf (accessed December 19, 2014).

EMA. 2014b. *Release of data from clinical trials.* http://www.ema.europa.eu/ema/index.jsp?curl=pages/special_topics/general/general_content_000555.jsp&mid=WC0b01ac0580607bfa (accessed December 19, 2014).

Erdem, E., and S. I. Prada. 2011. *Creation of public use files: Lessons learned from the comparative effectiveness research public use files data pilot project.* http://mpra.ub.uni-muenchen.de/35478 (accessed November 9, 2012).

Fung, B. C. M., K. Wang, R. Chen, and P. S. Yu. 2010. Privacy-preserving data publishing: A survey of recent developments. *ACM Computing Surveys* 42(4):1-53.

Gøtzsche, P. C. 2011. Why we need easy access to all data from all clinical trials and how to accomplish it. *Trials* 12(1):249.

Haggie, E. 2013. *PLoS Genetics partners with Dryad.* http://blogs.plos.org/biologue/2013/09/18/plos-genetics-partners-with-dryad (accessed September 19, 2013).

Harrison, C. 2012. GlaxoSmithKline opens the door on clinical data sharing. *Nature Reviews Drug Discovery* 11(12):891-892.

He, D., N. A. Furlotte, F. Hormozdiari, J. W. J. Joo, A. Wadia, R. Ostrovsky, A. Sahai, and E. Eskin. 2014. Identifying genetic relatives without compromising privacy. *Genome Research* 24(4):664-672.

Health Quality Council. 2004a. *Privacy code.* Saskatoon, Canada: Health Quality Council.

Health Quality Council. 2004b. *Security and confidentiality policies and procedures.* Saskatoon, Canada: Health Quality Council.

Health Research Authority. 2013. *The HRA interest in good research conduct: Transparent research.* http://www.hra.nhs.uk/documents/2013/08/transparent-research-report.pdf (accessed December 19, 2014).

Heatherly, R. D., G. Loukides, J. C. Denny, J. L. Haines, D. M. Roden, and B. A. Malin. 2013. Enabling genomic-phenomic association discovery without sacrificing anonymity. *PLoS ONE* 8(2):e53875.

Hede, K. 2013. Project data sphere to make cancer clinical trial data publicly available. *Journal of the National Cancer Institute* 105(16):1159-1160.

HHS (U.S. Department of Health and Human Services). 2000. *Standards for privacy of individually identifiable health information*. Washington, DC: HHS. http://aspe.hhs.gov/admnsimp/final/PVCFR05.txt (accessed March 31, 2015).

HHS. 2004. *Guidance on research involving coded private information or biological specimens*. Washington, DC: HHS.

HHS. 2008a. *Instructions for completing the limited data set data use agreement (DUA) (CMS-R-0235L)*. http://innovation.cms.gov/Files/x/Bundled-Payments-for-Care-Improvement-Data-Use-Agreement.pdf (accessed December 19, 2014).

HHS. 2008b. *OHRP: Guidance on research involving coded private information or biological specimens*. Washington, DC: HHS.

HHS. 2012. *Guidance regarding methods for deidentification of protected health information in accordance with the Health Insurance Portability and Accountability Act (HIPAA) Privacy Rule*. Washington, DC: HHS.

HIMSS Analytics. 2010. *2010 HIMSS Analytics report: Security of patient data*. Chicago, IL: HIMSS Analytics.

HIMSS Analytics. 2012. *2012 HIMSS Analytics report: Security of patient data*. Chicago, IL: HIMSS Analytics.

Homer, N., S. Szelinger, M. Redman, D. Duggan, W. Tembe, J. Muehling, J. Pearson, D. Stephan, S. Nelson, and D. Craig. 2008. Resolving individuals contributing trace amounts of DNA to highly complex mixtures using high-density SNP genotyping microarrays. *PLoS Genetics* 4(8):e1000167.

Hrynaszkiewicz, I., M. L. Norton, A. J. Vickers, and D. G. Altman. 2010. Preparing raw clinical data for publication: Guidance for journal editors, authors, and peer reviewers. *Trials* 11(1):9.

Humbert, M., E. Ayday, J.-P. Hubaux, and A. Telenti. 2013. Addressing the concerns of the Lacks family: Quantification of kin genomic privacy. *Proceedings of the 2013 ACM SIGSAC Conference on Computer and Communications Security* 1141-1152.

ICO (Information Commissioner's Office). 2012. *Anonymisation: Managing data protection risk code of practice*. http://ico.org.uk/~/media/documents/library/Data_Protection/Practical_application/anonymisation-codev2.pdf (accessed December 19, 2014).

ImmPort (Immunology Database and Analysis Portal). undated. *ImmPort: Immunology database and analysis portal*. https://immport.niaid.nih.gov/immportWeb/home/home.do?loginType=full (accessed September 19, 2013). .

IOM (Institute of Medicine). 2013. *Sharing clinical research data: Workshop summary*. Washington, DC: The National Academies Press.

ISO (International Organization for Standardization). 2008. *Health informatics—Pseudonymization*. ISO/TS 25237:2008. Geneva, Switzerland: ISO.

Jabine, T. 1993a. Procedures for restricted data access. *Journal of Official Statistics* 9(2):537-589.

Jabine, T. 1993b. Statistical disclosure limitation practices of United States statistical agencies. *Journal of Official Statistics* 9(2):427-454.

Jacobs, K. B., M. Yeager, S. Wacholder, D. Craig, P. Kraft, D. J. Hunter, J. Paschal, T. A. Manolio, M. Tucker, R. N. Hoover, G. D. Thomas, S. J. Chanock, and N. Chatterjee. 2009. A new statistic and its power to infer membership in a genome-wide association study using genotype frequencies. *Nature Genetics* 41(11):1253-1257.

Kantarcioglu, M., W. Jiang, Y. Liu, and B. Malin. 2008. A cryptographic approach to securely share and query genomic sequences. *IEEE Transactions on Information Technology in Biomedicine* 12(5):606-617.

Kayser, M., and P. de Knijff. 2011. Improving human forensics through advances in genetics, genomics and molecular biology. *Nature Reviews Genetics* 12(3):179-192.

Kennickell, A., and J. Lane. 2006. Measuring the impact of data protection techniques on data utility: Evidence from the survey of consumer finances. In *Privacy in statistical databases*, edited by J. Domingo-Ferrer and L. Franconi. New York: Springer Berlin Heidelberg. Pp. 291-303.

Knoppers, B. M., and M. Saginur. 2005. The Babel of genetic data terminology. *Nature Biotechnology* 23(8):925-927.

Kohn, L. A. P. 1991. The role of genetics in craniofacial morphology and growth. *Annual Review of Anthropology* 20(1):261-278.

Krumholz, H. M., and J. S. Ross. 2011. A model for dissemination and independent analysis of industry data. *Journal of the American Medical Association* 306(14):1593-1594.

Lechner, S., and W. Pohlmeier. 2004. To blank or not to blank?: A comparison of the effects of disclosure limitation methods on nonlinear regression estimates. In *Privacy in statistical databases*, edited by J. Domingo-Ferrer and V. Torra. New York: Springer Berlin Heidelberg. Pp. 187-200.

Li, G., Y. Wang, and X. Su. 2012. Improvements on a privacy-protection algorithm for DNA sequences with generalization lattices. *Computer Methods and Programs in Biomedicine* 108(1):1-9.

Lin, Z., M. Hewett, and R. Altman. 2002. Using binning to maintain confidentiality of medical data. *Proceedings of the American Medical Informatics Association Annual Symposium* 454-458.

Lin, Z., A. Owen, and R. Altman. 2004. Genomic research and human subject privacy. *Science* 305:183.

Loukides, G., A. Gkoulalas-Divanis, and B. Malin. 2010a. Anonymization of electronic medical records for validating genome-wide association studies. *Proceedings of the National Academy of Sciences of the United States of America* 107(17):7898-7903.

Loukides, G., J. C. Denny, and B. Malin. 2010b. The disclosure of diagnosis codes can breach research participants' privacy. *Journal of the American Medical Informatics Association* 17(3):322-327.

Lowrance, W., and F. Collins. 2007. Identifiability in genomic research. *Science* 317:600-602.

Machanavajjhala, A., J. Gehrke, and D. Kifer. 2007. l-Diversity: Privacy beyond k-anonymity. *Transactions on Knowledge Discovery from Data* 1(1):1-47.

Malin, B. 2005. Protecting genomic sequence anonymity with generalization lattices. *Methods of Information in Medicine* 44:687-692.

Malin, B., and L. Sweeney. 2000. Determining the identifiability of DNA database entries. *Proceedings of the AMIA Symposium* 537-541.

Malin, B., and L. Sweeney. 2004. How (not) to protect genomic data privacy in a distributed network: Using trail re-identification to evaluate and design anonymity protection systems. *Journal of Biomedical Informatics* 37(3):179-192.

Malin, B., G. Loukides, K. Benitez, and E. W. Clayton. 2011. Identifiability in biobanks: Models, measures, and mitigation strategies. *Human Genetics* 130(3):383-392.

Manitoba Center for Health Policy. 2002. *Privacy code*. http://umanitoba.ca/faculties/medicine/units/mchp/media_room/media/MCHP_privacy_code.pdf (accessed December 19, 2014).

Mello, M. M. J. K. Francer, M. Wilenzick, P. Teden, B. E. Bierer, and M. Barnes. 2013. Preparing for responsible sharing of clinical trial data. *New England Journal of Medicine* 369(17):1651-1658.

MRC (Medical Research Council). 2011. *Data sharing*. http://www.mrc.ac.uk/research/research-policy- ethics/data-sharing (accessed December 19, 2014).

NIH (U.S. National Institutes of Health). 2003. *Final NIH statement on sharing research data*. http://grants.nih.gov/grants/guide/notice-files/NOT-OD-03-032.html (accessed December 19, 2014).

Nisen, P., and F. Rockhold, 2013. Access to patient-level data from GlaxoSmithKline clinical trials. *New England Journal of Medicine* 369(5):475-478.

NRC (National Research Council). 1993. *Private lives and public policies: Confidentiality and accessibility of government statistics*. Washington, DC: National Academy Press.

Office of the Information and Privacy Commissioner of British Columbia. 1998. *Order No. 261-1998*. https://www.oipc.bc.ca/orders/496 (accessed December 19, 2014).

Office of the Information and Privacy Commissioner of Ontario. 1994. *Order P-644*. http://www.ipc.on.ca/images/Findings/Attached_PDF/P-644.pdf (accessed December 19, 2014).

Office of the Privacy Commissioner of Quebec (CAI). 1997. *Chenard v. Ministère de l'agriculture, des pêcheries et de l'alimentation (141)*.

Ohm, P. 2010. Broken promises of privacy: Responding to the surprising failure of anonymization. *UCLA Law Review* 57:1701.

OMB (Office of Management and Budget). 1994. *Report on statistical disclosure limitation methodology*. Working paper 22. Washington, DC: OMB.

Ontario Ministry of Health and Long-Term Care. 1984. *Corporate policy 3-1-21*. Toronto, ON: Ontario Ministry of Health and Long-Term Care.

Ou, X., J. Gao, H. Wang, H. Wang, H. Lu, and H. Sun. 2012. Predicting human age with bloodstains by sjTREC quantification. *PLoS ONE* 7(8):e42412.

Perun, H., M. Orr, and F. Dimitriadis. 2005. *Guide to the Ontario Personal Health Information Protection Act*. Toronto, ON: Irwin Law.

Purdam, K., and M. Elliot. 2007. A case study of the impact of statistical disclosure control on data quality in the individual UK samples of anonymised records. *Environment and Planning A* 39(5):1101-1118.

Rothstein, M. 2005. Research privacy under HIPAA and the Common Rule. *Journal of Law, Medicine & Ethics* 33:154-159.

Rothstein, M. 2010. Is deidentification sufficient to protect health privacy in research. *American Journal of Bioethics* 10(9):3-11.

Samarati, P. 2001. Protecting respondents' identities in microdata release. *IEEE Transactions on Knowledge and Data Engineering* 13(6):1010-1027.

Sandercock, P. A., M. Niewada, A. Członkowska, and the International Stroke Trial Collaborative Group. 2011. The International Stroke Trial database. *Trials* 12(1):101.

Sankararaman, S., G. Obozinski, M. I. Jordan, and E. Halperin. 2009. Genomic privacy and limits of individual detection in a pool. *Nature Genetics* 41(9):965-967.

Silventoinen, K., S. Sammalisto, M. Perola, D. I. Boomsma, B. K. Cornes, C. Davis, L. Dunkel, M. De Lange, J. R. Harris, J. V. B. Hjelmborg, M. Luciano, N. G. Martin, J. Mortensen, L. Nisticò, N. L. Pedersen, A. Skytthe, T. D. Spector, M. A. Stazi, G. Willemsen, and J. Kaprio. 2003. Heritability of adult body height: A comparative study of twin cohorts in eight countries. *Twin Research* 6(5):399-408.

Skinner, C. J. 1992. On identification disclosure and prediction disclosure for microdata. *Statistica Neerlandica* 46(1):21-32.

Skinner, C., and N. Shlomo. 2008. Assessing identification risk in survey microdata using log-linear models. *Journal of the American Statistical Association* 103(483):989-1001.

Statistics Canada. 2007. *Therapeutic abortion survey*. http://www23.statcan.gc.ca/imdb/p2SV.pl?Function=getSurvey&SurvId=1062&InstaId=31176&SDDS=3209 (accessed December 19, 2014).

Sweeney, L. 2002. *k*-anonymity: A model for protecting privacy. *International Journal on Uncertainty, Fuzziness and Knowledge-based Systems* 10(5):557-570.

Sweeney, L., A. Abu, and J. Winn. 2013. *Identifying participants in the personal genome project by name*. http://dataprivacylab.org/projects/pgp/1021-1.pdf (accessed December 19, 2014).

U.S. Department of Education. 2003. *NCES statistical standards*. http://nces.ed.gov/pubs2003/2003601.pdf (accessed December 19, 2014).

Vallance, P., and I. Chalmers. 2013. Secure use of individual patient data from clinical trials. *Lancet* 382(9898):1073-1074.

Wang, R., Y. F. Li, X. Wang, H. Tang, and X. Zhou. 2009. *Learning your identity and disease from research papers: Information leaks in genome wide association study.* http://www.informatics.indiana.edu/xw7/papers/gwas_paper.pdf (accessed December 19, 2014).

The Wellcome Trust. 2011. *Sharing research data to improve public health: Full joint statement by funders of health research.* http://www.wellcome.ac.uk/About-us/Policy/Spotlight-issues/Data-sharing/Public-health-and-epidemiology/WTDV030690.htm (accessed December 19, 2014).

Willenborg, L., and T. de Waal. 1996. *Statistical disclosure control in practice.* New York: Springer-Verlag.

Willenborg, L., and T. de Waal. 2001. *Elements of statistical disclosure control.* New York: Springer-Verlag.

Wjst, M. 2010. Caught you: Threats to confidentiality due to the public release of large-scale genetic data sets. *BMC Medical Ethics* 11:21.

Zubakov, D., F. Liu, M. C. van Zelm, J. Vermeulen, B. A. Oostra, C. M. van Duijn, G. J. Driessen, J. J. M. van Dongen, M. Kayser, and A. W. Langerak. 2010. Estimating human age from T-cell DNA rearrangements. *Current Biology* 20(22):R970-R971.

Appendix C

Legal Discussion of Risks
to Industry Sponsors

The committee examined, and in this appendix presents, the landscape of potentially relevant intellectual property protection laws encompassing trade secrets and confidential commercial information, data protection and exclusivity laws, and patents, as well as liability and antitrust. Because the legal and regulatory environment for medical devices may undergo significant change in the near future, the discussion focuses on small molecules and biologics.

INTELLECTUAL PROPERTY PROTECTION LAWS

Trade Secrets and Commercially Confidential Information

Outside the regulatory context, the issue of what constitutes a trade secret is addressed as an initial matter by state common law. The Uniform Trade Secrets Act (UTSA), which has been adopted in 47 states and the District of Columbia, defines a trade secret as

> Information, including a formula, pattern, compilation, program device, method, technique, or process, that: (i) derives independent economic value, actual or potential, from not being generally known to, and not being readily ascertainable by proper means by, other persons who can obtain economic value from its disclosure or use, and (ii) is the subject of efforts that are reasonable under the circumstances to maintain its secrecy.[1]

---

[1] Uniform Trade Secret Act, published 1979, amended 1985.

Under this definition, the categories of trade secrets and confidential commercial information overlap.

Trade secrets/confidential commercial information is typically protected from "misappropriation." The ultimate determination of competing claims as to whether particular information meets the UTSA definition is highly fact-specific and must be made by a court. However, as the UTSA reference to "efforts that are reasonable . . . to maintain . . . secrecy" would counsel, entities that regard information they possess as being a trade secret reveal it (if at all) only pursuant to agreements wherein the recipient agrees to keep the information confidential.

Public access to nonsummary clinical trial data generated by industry sponsors and submitted to government agencies is governed by federal statutory law. The two relevant statutes are the Freedom of Information Act (FOIA),[2] which addresses disclosure in response to citizen requests, and the Trade Secrets Act,[3] which addresses the limits of affirmative disclosure by the government.

Determining how the test for confidential commercial information applies to clinical trial data is often quite fact-intensive. An example is a 1999 case, *Public Citizen Health Research Group v. FDA,*[4] involving a FOIA request by Public Citizen for clinical study documents associated with trials that were discontinued because of serious safety concerns. The DC Circuit Court probed at some length the factual foundation for arguments made by the U.S. Food and Drug Administration (FDA) and Schering (the pharmaceutical firm in question) that document release would cause competitive harm. For four of the five investigational new drug applications (INDs) for which documents were sought, the court agreed with the FDA and Schering. For these INDs, the court focused on Schering's argument that it was testing successor drugs, the design of which was specifically based on information learned from the failed INDs. The court determined that in that context, releasing the IND information would "eliminate much of the time and effort that would otherwise be required to bring to market a product competitive with the product for which Schering filed its most recent IND." In contrast, in the fifth case, the court found Schering's argument regarding substantial competitive harm to be "conclusory and generalized," and rejected the applicability of Exemption 4. The arguments found to be conclusory and generalized included statements that the disclosure would reveal "disease models" as well as toxicology data and clinical protocols applicable beyond the failed drug in question.

---

[2] 5 U.S.C. § 552.

[3] 18 U.S.C. § 1905 (1982).

[4] *Public Citizen Health Research Group v. FDA,* 185 F.3d 898 (D.C. Cir 1999).

Similarly, in a 2010 case, a DC district court rejected arguments by the U.S. Department of Health and Human Services (HHS) and the FDA that release of certain clinical study data and contractor names with respect to the drug ciprofloxacin would result in substantial injury.[5] The court determined that blanket statements to the effect that the material could be used by a competitor to "support its own new drug application" were conclusory and generalized.

For the most part, discussion of the release of clinical trial data has focused on data associated with approved drugs. In the case of these data—as contrasted with the failed drug data at issue in the 1999 *Public Citizen* case[6]—the concern about data release leading competitors directly to successful alternative drugs may be diminished.

Under FOIA, which applies to clinical trial data submitted to the FDA for approval, a trade secret means "a secret, commercially valuable plan, formula, process, or device that is used for the making, preparing, compounding, or processing of trade commodities and that can be said to be the end product of either innovation or substantial effort."[7] Generally speaking, nonsummary clinical trial data should not include this type of formulation and manufacturing information or related information about analytical techniques used to characterize the intervention. If such information were included, it would be appropriate to redact it.

On the other hand, nonsummary clinical trial data may fall within the broader confidential commercial information provision of FOIA. Under the governing legal test, information is confidential if its release is likely "to cause substantial harm to the competitive position of the person from whom the information was obtained."

In its submission to the committee for this study, the biopharmaceutical firm AbbVie argues that data release on approved drugs could reveal "subjective" information about "study results, clinical development decisions, rationales for study designs, and processes for running clinical trials" that presumably could be useful to competitors attempting to develop alternatives.[8] According to AbbVie, however, this "subjective" commercially sensitive information can be segregated from other more "objective" information, including individual participant data. According to AbbVie, moreover, this "deliberative process and sponsor strategic decision-making information" are not necessary for purposes of conducting "useful re-analyses." Similarly, although the European Medicines

---

[5] *Government Accountability Project v. HHS*, 691 F. Supp. 2d 170 (D.D.C. 2010).

[6] *Public Citizen Health Research Group v. FDA*, 185 F.3d 898 (D.C. Cir 1999).

[7] 5 U.S.C. § 552.

[8] Personal Communication, M. D. Rivas, AbbVie Inc., to the Institute of Medicine Committee on Strategies for Responsible Sharing of Clinical Trial Data, regarding Written Testimony of AbbVie Inc., October 17, 2013.

Agency (EMA) recently indicated that information about company strategy with respect to future clinical studies and "exploratory endpoints," as well as company strategy with respect to regulators, could be confidential commercial information, the EMA's "redaction principles" rest on the supposition that this information can be segregated (EMA, 2014).

Data Protection and Exclusivity Laws

Submissions to the committee from the trade organization Pharmaceutical Research and Manufacturers of America (PhRMA) and AbbVie further focus on the concern that competitors with access to full data sets on approved drugs could seek to register identical drugs in countries without strong regulatory data protection (RDP) regimes.[9,10,11] Assume that, after a particular product had been approved by the FDA or the EMA, clinical data associated with that product were released. Pharmaceutical firms argue that in jurisdictions with limited RDP regimes, such as Australia, Brazil, and China, a competitor could take the data package and use it to submit a marketing application. According to PhRMA, "similar regimes are known to exist in several other South American countries including Chile, Mexico, and Peru, and in countries in the Middle East and Asia such as Egypt and Malaysia."[12]

---

[9] Ibid.

[10] Personal Communication, J. K. Francer, PhRMA, to the Institute of Medicine Committee on Strategies for Responsible Sharing of Clinical Trial Data, regarding Testimony of PhRMA, October 23, 2013.

[11] An evaluation of arguments about competitive harm and RDP requires a brief background discussion of international intellectual property, specifically Article 39.3 of the Trade-Related Aspects of Intellectual Property Rights ("TRIPS") agreement, to which all World Trade Organization (WTO) members must adhere. Article 39.3 of TRIPS mandates that member countries that require test data as a condition of marketing approval for pharmaceutical products "protect such data against disclosure, except where necessary to protect the public, or unless steps are taken to ensure that the data are protected from unfair commercial use." WTO members have interpreted the Article 39.3 obligation in different ways. In jurisdictions such as the United States, it has been interpreted as allowing the originator that submits data a period of exclusive marketing approval based on these data regardless of whether the data become publicly available. During that period, competitors with the same molecule (i.e., "generic" competitors) cannot enter the market with reliance on the data, even if no relevant patents exist. In the United States, exclusivity lasts 5 years for small molecules and 12 years for biologics. In the European Union, the period is 10 years for both small molecules and biologics. Other countries may afford originator data some protection from public disclosure by the government but do not afford the originator an exclusive marketing period, particularly if the data are otherwise publicly available.

[12] Personal Communication, W. W. Chin and J. K. Francer, PhRMA, to the Institute of Medicine Committee on Strategies for Responsible Sharing of Clinical Trial Data, regarding Discussion Framework for Clinical Trial Data Sharing, April 14, 2014.

These arguments have merit (see Box C-1); however, their merit depends to some extent on whether regulatory authorities in "limited RDP" regimes currently require data submission. As a practical matter, a detailed data package can benefit competitors only to the extent that regulatory authorities in the "limited RDP" jurisdictions actually require detailed submissions in the first instance. If competitors can rely for their marketing applications on approval of the molecule by the FDA or the EMA, data release may confer little marginal advantage to the competitor.

Patents

Release of clinical trial data also raises the issue of whether such release may compromise future patents. As might be expected, the patent law bars protection for inventions that are in the public domain or are "obvious" given what is in the public domain. To the extent that firms expect to secure additional patents based on data associated with approved drugs, release may compromise these additional patents.

The sample agreement for data sharing being utilized by GlaxoSmithKline and other pharmaceutical firms reflects concerns about future patents. Not only does the agreement maintain tight control over the data so as to prevent any argument about public domain status, but it also specifically addresses in detail (Section 3) ownership and assignment of future intellectual property.

The detailed provisions of this sample agreement notwithstanding, it is not clear how many economically significant future patents are likely to emerge from clinical trial data on approved drugs. For most drugs, the most important composition of matter patents and method of use patents is generally filed at the time clinical testing begins. Additional patents—for example, on the use of the drug for certain subpopulations—may be relatively weak and easy to circumvent (Rai, 2012). Even so, as the EMA's redaction principles for information regarding future uses make clear, measures to safeguard patentability are likely to be prudent.

To the extent that data release extends to abandoned applications, ensuring the possibility of future patent protection may be even more important. At least in the United States, use patents are more difficult to circumvent when the drug has not been approved for a prior use (Rai and Rice, 2014).

LIABILITY

Another concern raised by pharmaceutical firms is that broad availability of clinical data on approved drugs may yield analyses that increase liability risks. In recent years, mass tort claims, usually based on a theory

---

BOX C-1
Competitive Harm and Regulatory Data Protection

In the case of India, draft guidance issued in 2011 suggests that if a drug has been approved in jurisdictions such as Australia, Canada, the European Union, Japan, the United Kingdom, and the United States, approval in India is in fact based largely on approval in these other countries (CDSCO, 2011). Similarly, according to Raghu Cidambi, a former advisor to Dr. Reddy's Laboratories in Hyderabad, India, India's significant reliance on approval by other jurisdictions means that generic companies *currently* seek and obtain approval for molecules in India before (or without) originator entry (Kapczynski, 2014). "Generic-first" entry occurred, for example, with rasagiline mesylate, lenalidomide, and atomoxetine (Kapczynski, 2014). Similarly, according to a 2014 submission by Pharmaceutical Research Manufacturers of America (PhRMA) to the U.S. Trade Representative, "India conditions the approval of pharmaceutical products on prior approval by a regulatory authority in another country rather than requiring submission of the entire dossier for review by its regulatory authority. An applicant in India need only prove that the drug has been approved and marketed in another country and submit confirmatory test and other data from clinical studies on a very few (in some cases as few as 16) Indian patients" (PhRMA, 2014, p. 28).

China appears to provide another example of this dynamic. Although China nominally has 6 years of data exclusivity, the scope of this exclusivity appears to be restricted to originators that file first in China. Additionally, as PhRMA recently argued in its 2014 submission to the U.S. Trade Representative, China currently permits

> non-originator, or follow-on, applicants to rely on a foreign regulatory agency's approval of the originator product in another market during the RDP term in China. This practice gives an unfair commercial advantage to the follow-on manufacturer by permitting it to rely on the full clinical data submitted by an innovator to a foreign regulatory agency … while having to submit only a small amount of China-specific supplemental data to CFDA. (PhRMA, 2014, pp. 41-42)

---

of failure to warn of risks, have resulted in significant judgments against pharmaceutical companies. In a number of prominent cases, perhaps most notably the litigation over Fen-phen diet pills and Vioxx, companies have paid out $1 billion or more (Garber, 2013).

How much additional liability may be at issue is unclear, however. Many suits based on failure to warn rest upon risks that, even according to the plaintiffs' own theories, were identified only after the drug had been approved. In that situation, data generated during clinical trials are not relevant.

Although liability concerns are particularly salient for pharmaceutical companies, they may also arise for other actors in the clinical trial system,

Of course, in the case of both China and India, the competitor does have to conduct some small, country-specific trials. However, as the PhRMA submission to the U.S. Trade Representative suggests, the cost of these trials is not likely to be large.

In sum, as matters currently stand, data release and wholesale copying of the data by competitors are likely to cause additional competitive harm to originators primarily in those jurisdictions that require detailed data submissions but give only limited, or no, protection to originator data. In countries that do not require data submissions in the first instance, competitors gain no additional benefit. However, it is worth noting that biologics may differ from small molecules to the extent that countries with limited regulatory data protection regimes may be less likely to permit approval for biologics than for small molecules without some submission of clinical trial data. For example, although Brazil—which has no data exclusivity for either small molecule chemicals or biologics—may allow marketing approval for small molecules based on approval of the drug in a respected regulatory jurisdiction, it appears to require at least some clinical data for biologics.* Thus, in the case of biologics, having data copied from originators would actually help with marketing approval, and the additional competitive risk associated with data release would presumably be higher.

In sum, despite certain limitations on the additional competitive harm data release may cause, policies that guard against wholesale copying of originator data packages for purposes of seeking regulatory approval and maintain the confidentiality of the data, as with data use agreements, may be prudent. Such policies are also consistent with the Trade-Related Aspects of Intellectual Property Rights (TRIPS) obligation to protect data from "unfair commercial use."

---

*Personal communication, E. Lietzan, to the Institute of Medicine Committee on Strategies for Responsible Sharing of Clinical Trial Data, regarding report entitled "The Interaction Between Open Trial Data and Drug Regulation in Selected Developing Countries," May 23, 2014.

such as Data and Safety Monitoring Boards responsible for ensuring patient safety and study validity for subjects enrolled in research studies (DeMets et al., 2004; Tereskerz, 2010). That said, the liability issue appears to be primarily a U.S. phenomenon.[13] Judicial process rules adopted in other jurisdictions, especially the rule that losers pay the litigation costs of winners, tend to deter tort suits.

In general, positions on how to address liability risk turn significantly

---

[13] Virtual WebEx Open Session, L. Brown and G. Fleming, to the Institute of Medicine Committee on Strategies for Responsible Sharing of Clinical Trial Data, regarding clinical trial data sharing and product liability, April 9, 2014.

on the extent to which such risk is seen as a useful deterrent to socially undesirable corporate behavior. Proponents of the liability system argue that the FDA's regulatory process is insufficient to deter such behavior. Opponents argue that because the judicial process does not efficiently weed out spurious cases, pharmaceutical companies often are forced to expend large sums on these cases, with the result being increased drug prices and decreased innovation.

Even with respect to liability under the current system, in which clinical trial data are not widely available, the RAND Institute for Civil Justice recently concluded that "there is scant empirical evidence to support the claims asserted on either side of the debate" (Garber, 2013, p. xiv). The social impact of potentially greater liability under a system of greater data availability is even more difficult to discern.

ANTITRUST

Academic researchers' pooling of clinical trial data from multiple companies poses no obvious antitrust concerns. Some clinical trial data sharing activities may, however, involve direct collaborations between competitors. For example, public–private partnerships such as the Biomarkers Consortium (coordinated by the Foundation for the National Institutes of Health) involve companies in pooling placebo arm clinical trial data to develop models of disease progression. Whenever competitors collaborate, potential antitrust limits on such collaboration need to be addressed.

The U.S. Department of Justice and the Federal Trade Commission view most research and development collaborations between competitors as procompetitive and therefore evaluate them under the "rule of reason."[14] Rule of reason analysis focuses on whether the agreement in question "harms competition by increasing the ability or incentive profitably to raise price above or reduce output, quality, service, or innovation below what likely would prevail in the absence of the relevant agreement."

The Biomarkers Consortium has a publicly available document on antitrust policy and guidelines that may provide generally useful guidance for competitors seeking to share clinical trial data. This policy makes clear that the competitors in question are collaborating for the "precompetitive" purpose of "identification, validation, qualification, and commercial development of biological disease markers and related healthcare products." The policy also states clearly that the private-sector participants are free to engage in research and development on biomarkers outside the

---

[14] Antitrust Guidelines for Collaborations Among Competitors, Section 3.31(a).

Consortium, and that the Consortium will not attempt to exclude from the marketplace products or technology from non-Consortium members.

REFERENCES

CDSCO (Central Drugs Standard Control Organization). 2011. *Draft guidance on approval of clinical trials & new drugs*. http://www.cdsco.nic.in/writereaddata/Guidance_for_New_Drug_Approval-23.07.2011.pdf (accessed October 15, 2014).

DeMets, D. L., T. R. Fleming, F. Rockhold, B. Massie, T. Merchant, A. Meisel, B. Mishkin, J. Wittes, D. Stump, and R. Califf. 2004. Liability issues for data monitoring committee members. *Clinical Trials* 1(6):525-531.

EMA (European Medicines Agency). 2014. *Redaction principles.* http://www.google.com/url?sa=t&rct=j&q=&esrc=s&frm=1&source=web&cd=2&ved=0CCgQFjAB&url=http%3A%2F%2Fwww.ombudsman.europa.eu%2FshowResource%3FresourceId%3D1402406006491_INC2014-003908_2_Redaction%2520principles%2520DRAFT.pdf%26type%3Dpdf%26download%3Dtrue%26lang%3Den&ei=Qj9OVKPOO8uxyATzl4K YBw&usg=AFQjCNHYKYQJ1X47URHVduc2cr7gutNEEQ&bvm=bv.77880786,d.aWw (accessed October 27, 2014).

Garber, S. 2013. *Economic effects of product liability and other litigation involving the safety and effectiveness of pharmaceuticals*. Santa Monica, CA: RAND Corporation.

Kapczynski, A. 2014. The interaction between open trial data and drug regulation in selected developing countries. Paper commissioned by the Committee on Strategies for Responsible Sharing of Clinical Trial Data. www.iom.edu/datasharing (accessed December 19, 2014).

PhRMA (Pharmaceutical Research and Manufacturers of America). 2014. *Special 301 submission 2014*. http://www.phrma.org/sites/default/files/pdf/2014-special-301-submission.pdf (December 19, 2014).

Rai, A. 2012. Use patents, carve-outs, and incentives—a new battle in the drug-patent wars. *New England Journal of Medicine* 367(6):491-493.

Rai, A. K., and G. Rice. 2014. Use patents can be useful: The case of rescued drugs. *Science Translational Medicine* 6(248):248fs230.

Tereskerz, P. M. 2010. Data Safety Monitoring Boards: Legal and ethical considerations for research accountability. *Accountability in Research* 17(1):30-50.

Appendix D

Clinical Trial Data Sharing Policies: Top 1-12 Pharmaceutical Companies Ranked by 2013 Market Capitalization

The following tables were reproduced from [*Circulation: Cardiovascular Quality and Outcomes*, Harlan M. Krumholz, Cary P. Gross, Katrina L. Blount, Jessica D. Ritchie, Beth Hodshon, Richard Lehman, and Joseph S. Ross, 7, 499-504, 2014] with permission from BMJ Publishing Group Ltd.

TABLE D-1 Top 1 to 6 Pharmaceutical Companies, Ranked by 2013 Market Capitalization

Data-Sharing Parameters	PhRMA EFPIA Guidelines	Janssen Pharmaceuticals	Pfizer
Clinical trial data available for sharing	• CSR synopses should be available • Requests for full CSRs, IPD, and study-level data should be considered	• Data from interventional trials for products and indications approved in both the EU and United States (older studies may be difficult to access)	• Global trials that ended after September 2007 • Trials for which results are posted on ClinicalTrials.gov
Data not available for sharing	• Trials with possibility of re-identification (rare diseases, etc) • ICF restrictions • Legal restrictions to sharing, such as partnering agreements	• PhRMA EFPIA guidelines • Undue resources required to share (ie, older studies)	• PhRMA EFPIA guidelines • Trials for which results are not posted on ClinicalTrials.gov
Types of data provided	• Clinical trial materials for medicines and indications approved in United States and EU: —Anonymized IPD —Study-level clinical trial data —Protocols	• Deidentified IPD • Redacted full CSRs • CSR summaries (publicly available)** • Protocols and supporting documents	• Anonymized IPD • CSR summaries (publicly available)

Novartis	Roche	Sanofi	Merck
• January 2014 to present • Phase II–III trials for new medicines or indications approved by the EU and US regulatory agencies	• January 1999 to present • Trials from terminated programs • Phase II–III trials, and some phase IV trials, for new medicines that have been approved by the EU and US regulatory agencies	• January 2014 to present • Trials approved by EU and US regulatory agencies and accepted for publication	• September 2007 to present • Trials approved by EU and US regulatory agencies and accepted for publication • Trials for which results are posted on ClinicalTrials.gov
• PhRMA EFPIA guidelines • Studies supporting device registration • Phase I studies • Some phase IV studies	• PhRMA EFPIA guidelines • Substantial practical constraints (eg, large databases) • Undue resources required to share (eg, older studies)	• PhRMA EFPIA guidelines	• PhRMA EFPIA guidelines • Trials for which results are not posted on ClinicalTrials.gov • Phase I—Healthy participant trials • Consumer healthcare studies • Substantial practical constraints (eg, large databases)
• Anonymized IPD • Redacted full CSRs • CSR summaries (publicly available) • Protocols and supporting documents	• Anonymized IPD • Redacted full CSRs • CSR summaries (publicly available) • Protocols and supporting documents	• Anonymized IPD • Redacted full CSRs • Protocols and supporting documents	• Anonymized IPD • Redacted full CSRs

continued

TABLE D-1 Continued

Data-Sharing Parameters	PhRMA EFPIA Guidelines	Janssen Pharmaceuticals	Pfizer
Availability of CRFs	NA	• Blank CRF templates available	• Not stated
Data access fee	NA	• None	• None stated
Data application requirements of note	• Research proposal including hypothesis, data requested, and research rationale • Plans for analysis, publication and posting • Research team qualifications, experience, and any potential COIs • Potential for competitive use of the data • Funding sources • Researcher must not transfer shared data to individuals not listed on the proposal • Data must not be used for purposes not described in the proposal • No attempt should be made to reidentify participants	• PhRMA EFPIA guidelines • Scientific purpose is clearly described • Data requested will be used to create or materially enhance generalizable scientific and/or medical knowledge to inform science and public health • Proposed research can be reasonably addressed using the requested data • Proposals submitted for non-scientific purposes, such as in pursuit of litigation or for commercial interests, will not be approved	• PhRMA EFPIA guidelines • Rigorous statistical analysis plan • IRB documentation • CVs of all researchers

Novartis	Roche	Sanofi	Merck
• Blank CRF templates available	• Blank CRF templates available	• Blank CRF templates available	• Not stated
• None stated	• None stated	• None stated	• None stated
• PhRMA EFPIA guidelines	• PhRMA EFPIA guidelines • Biostatistician on research team • Detailed statistical analysis plan • Requestor seeks publication of their research results • Research Proposal is related to the medicine or disease researched in the selected studies • The names of 3 independent experts whom the independent review panel could consult regarding scientific merit, if requested	• PhRMA EFPIA guidelines • Any use of the data by a third party must address a scientific question in the same disease as the original trial unless the informed consent expressly allows broader use	• PhRMA EFPIA guidelines • CVs of all researchers • Biostatistician on research team

continued

TABLE D-1 Continued

Data-Sharing Parameters	PhRMA EFPIA Guidelines	Janssen Pharmaceuticals	Pfizer
Data request review process	• Review process should include external scientists and healthcare professionals, with identity and existing relationships publicly posted	• All data requests go directly to the YODA Project[†], which reviews for scientific merit and makes final decision • Janssen performs a due diligence assessment to determine its ability to make the data available to be shared externally • Reviewers are publicly named	• Internal Pfizer review committee reviews requests for data first • Independent Review Panel reviews requests that Pfizer declines and makes final decision • Reviewers are publicly named • Three of the 4 panel members are on the Pfizer external Bioethics Advisory Panel

Novartis	Roche	Sanofi	Merck
• Research proposals are checked by Novartis to make sure the information is complete and that they meet the requirements of this initiative and the sponsor's requirements for informed consent • They are then sent to an Independent Review Panel* that performs a high-level scientific review including qualifications of researchers and biostatistician and the scientific rationale and relevance of the proposed research to medical science or patient care • Researcher may be asked for names of 3 independent experts to perform an additional review • There is no appeal process • Reviewers are publicly named	• Roche reviews requests for data first to determine status of the requested data • Independent Review Panel* reviews for scientific merit and value, among other considerations	• Independent Review Panel* reviews for scientific merit, feasibility, and advancement of medical knowledge and public health • Reviewers are publicly named	• An internal Merck review committee reviews for feasibility, scientific validity of the request and the qualifications of the requesters • If there are questions regarding scientific validity, the request is forwarded to a non-Merck External Scientific Review Board (ESRB) for further review • A recommendation from the ESRB is then communicated to a Merck Steering Committee, which is composed of the research heads of clinical, regulatory, and biostatistics • Final decision is made by Merck Steering Committee • ESRB members are publicly named

continued

TABLE D-1 Continued

NOTE: COI indicates conflict of interest; CRF, case report form; CSR, clinical study report; CV, curriculum vitae; EFPIA, European Federation of Pharmaceutical Industries and Associations; EU, European Union; ICF, informed consent form; IPD, individual patient-level data; IRB, institutional review board; PhRMA, Pharmaceutical Research and Manufacturers of America; and YODA, Yale University Open Data Access.

TABLE D-2 Top 7 to 12 Pharmaceutical Companies, Ranked by 2013 Market Capitalization

Data-Sharing Parameters	PhRMA EFPIA Guidelines	GlaxoSmithKline	Bayer
Clinical trial data available for sharing	• CSR synopses should be available • Requests for full CSRs, IPD, and study-level data should be considered	• December 2000 to present • All global interventional clinical studies	• January 2014 to present • Data on new medicines and indications that have been approved by EU and/or US regulatory agencies without plans for further regulatory review or submissions • CSR summaries are publicly available back to 2005
Data not available for sharing	• Trials with possibility of re-identification (rare diseases, etc) • ICF restrictions • Legal restrictions to sharing, such as partnering agreements	• PhRMA EFPIA guidelines • Substantial practical constraints (e.g., large databases) • Undue resources required to share (e.g., older studies) • Studies of consumer healthcare products	• PhRMA EFPIA guidelines • Substantial practical constraints (e.g., large databases)

* Independent Review Panel is shared by ClinicalStudyDataRequest.com companies.
** Process for making CSR summaries publicly available is being developed.
† The YODA Project data request website is being developed. Those wishing to submit a request for Janssen data can visit http://www.clinicaltrialstudytransparency.com in the interim.

Bristol-Myers Squibb	AbbVie	Eli Lilly	AstraZeneca
• January 2008 to present • Phase I–IV interventional trials for medicines and indications approved in the United States and the EU	• All data for medicines and indications approved in the United States and the EU	• Interventional clinical studies for approved indications of medicines on the market in the United States and EU	• Not stated
• PhRMA EFPIA guidelines • Studies completed before 2008	• None stated	• PhRMA EFPIA guidelines	• Not stated

continued

TABLE D-2 Continued

Data-Sharing Parameters	PhRMA EFPIA Guidelines	GlaxoSmithKline	Bayer
Types of data provided	• Clinical trial materials for medicines and indications approved in United States and EU: —Anonymized IPD —Study-level clinical trial data —Protocols	• Anonymized IPD • Redacted full CSRs • Protocols and supporting documents	• Anonymized IPD • Redacted full CSRs • Protocols and supporting documents
Availability of CRFs	NA	• Blank CRF templates available	• Blank CRF templates available
Data access fee	NA	• None stated	• None stated
Data application requirements of note	• Research proposal including hypothesis, data requested, and research rationale • Plans for analysis, publication, and posting • Research team qualifications, experience, and any potential COIs • Potential for competitive use of the data • Funding sources • Researcher must not transfer shared data to individuals not listed on the proposal • Data must not be used for purposes not described in the proposal • No attempt should be made to re-identify participants	• PhRMA EFPIA guidelines • Biostatistician on research team • Researchers asked to certify IRB review in the DUA	• PhRMA EFPIA guidelines • Biostatistician on research team • Researchers asked to certify IRB review in the DUA

Bristol-Myers Squibb	AbbVie	Eli Lilly	AstraZeneca
• IPD • Study-level data • Redacted full CSRs • Protocols	• Anonymized IPD • Study-level data • Protocols	• Anonymized IPD	• IPD • Protocols
• Not stated	• Not stated	• Not stated	• Not stated
• None stated	• None stated	• None stated	• None stated
• PhRMA EFPIA guidelines • CVs of all research team members	• PhRMA EFPIA guidelines • Detailed statistical analysis plan • Biostatistician on research team • CV of lead researcher • Researchers asked to certify IRB review in the DUA	• PhRMA EFPIA guidelines • Biostatistician on research team	• Not stated

continued

TABLE D-2 Continued

Data-Sharing Parameters	PhRMA EFPIA Guidelines	GlaxoSmithKline	Bayer
Data request review process	• Review process should include external scientists and healthcare professionals, with identity and existing relationships publicly posted	• Research proposals are checked by GSK to make sure the information is complete and that they meet the requirements of this initiative and the sponsor's requirements for informed consent • They are then sent to an Independent Review Panel* that performs a high-level scientific review, including qualifications of researchers and biostatisticians and the scientific rationale and relevance of the proposed research to medical science or patient care • Researcher may be asked for names of 3 independent experts to perform an additional review • There is no appeal process • Reviewers are publicly named	• Research proposals are checked by Bayer to determine technical feasibility, make sure the information is complete, and that they meet the requirements of this initiative and the sponsor's requirements for informed consent • They are then sent to an Independent Review Panel* that performs a high-level scientific review, including qualifications of researchers and biostatisticians and the scientific rationale and relevance of the proposed research to medical science or patient care • Researcher may be asked for names of 3 independent experts to perform an additional review • There is no appeal process • Reviewers are publicly named

Bristol-Myers Squibb	AbbVie	Eli Lilly	AstraZeneca
• All requests reviewed internally by a qualified panel of Bristol-Myers Squibb experts and then passed to an Independent Review Committee (IRC) of external experts for review and final decision • Data requests evaluated based on the scientific rationale and methodology of the proposed research	• All requests managed by AbbVie, who may either grant or deny a request after reviewing the requestor's proposal • AbbVie will ensure that the proposal has clearly defined research questions, scientific merit, and that the researcher-directed analyses follow the research proposal • Access to Clinical Research Information Board (ATCRIB) reviews requests that AbbVie declines and makes a final decision • ATCRIB will be independent and publicly named	• Researcher first completes a request for availability of clinical study data form • Lilly reviews the request and determines whether the data are available for deidentification and sharing • If the data are available, a research proposal form is sent to the researcher and reviewed by Lilly once submitted • Data requests evaluated based on a scientific rationale that is relevant to medical science or patient care and a high-level review of the proposed research plan to meet the scientific objectives	• AstraZeneca considers requests for patient level data from other parties on a case-by-case basis, following consistent criteria to establish if and how the information provided will be used for valid scientific purposes and to benefit patients

continued

TABLE D-2 Continued

NOTE: COI indicates conflict of interest; CRF, case report form; CSR, clinical study report; CV, curriculum vitae; DUA, data use agreement; EFPIA, European Federation of Pharmaceutical Industries and Associations; EU, European Union; GSK, GlaxoSmithKline; ICF, informed consent form; IPD, individual patient-level data; IRB, institutional review board; and PhRMA, Pharmaceutical Research and Manufacturers of America.

* Independent Review Panel is shared by ClinicalStudyDataRequest.com companies.

Appendix E

Biosketches of Committee Members

Bernard Lo, M.D. (*Chair*), is currently president of the Greenwall Foundation. Previously, Dr. Lo was professor of medicine and director of the Program in Medical Ethics at the University of California, San Francisco (UCSF). Currently he is co-chair of the Standards Working Group of the California Institute of Regenerative Medicine, which recommends regulations for stem cell research funded by the state of California. Dr. Lo serves on the Board of Directors of the Association for the Accreditation of Human Research Protection Programs (AAHRPP) and on the Medical Advisory Panel of Blue Cross/Blue Shield. Formerly he was a member of the National Bioethics Advisory Commission under President Clinton, the U.S. National Institutes of Health (NIH) Recombinant DNA Advisory Committee and the Ethics Subcommittee, and the Advisory Committee to the Director of the Centers for Disease Control and Prevention. He served on a number of Data and Safety Monitoring Committees at NIH for HIV prevention and treatment, diabetes prevention, and oxygen treatment in chronic obstructive pulmonary disease. A member of the Institute of Medicine (IOM), Dr. Lo served on the IOM Council and chaired the Board on Health Sciences Policy. He chaired IOM committees on conflicts of interest in medicine and on confidentiality in health services research and has been a member of several other IOM committees. He currently is a member of the Board of Life Sciences of the National Academy of Sciences (NAS).

Dr. Lo and his colleagues have published approximately 200 peer-reviewed articles on ethical issues concerning decision making near the end of life, stem cell research, research with human participants and its oversight, the doctor–patient relationship, conflicts of interest, HIV infection, and public health. With colleagues on the UCSF stem cell research oversight committee, he has written articles on ethical issues in the procurement of embryos for research, oversight of stem cell lines derived in other institutions, informed consent for future research, and prohibiting the use of induced pluripotent stem cells for reproductive cloning. Dr. Lo is the author of *Resolving Ethical Dilemmas: A Guide for Clinicians* (5th ed., 2013) and of *Ethical Issues in Clinical Research* (2010). At UCSF he directed medical student teaching in ethics, chaired the hospital ethics committee, and served as an attending physician on the medicine inpatient service. He was co-director of the Policy and Ethics Core of the Center for AIDS Prevention Studies. He continues to serve as the primary care physician for a panel of general internal medicine patients.

Timothy Coetzee, Ph.D., is chief advocacy, services and research officer of the National Multiple Sclerosis Society. In this capacity he leads mission delivery in the areas of state and federal advocacy and service and care management programs for people with multiple sclerosis, as well as the Society's research program, which funds more than 375 academic and commercial research projects around the world. Most recently, he served as president of Fast Forward, a venture philanthropy of the National Multiple Sclerosis Society, where he was responsible for the Society's strategic funding of biotechnology and pharmaceutical companies, as well as partnerships with the financial and business communities. Prior to serving with Fast Forward, Dr. Coetzee led the Society's translational research initiatives on nervous system repair and protection in multiple sclerosis. He is a member of the IOM's Forum on Neuroscience and Nervous System Disorders and serves on the Board of Directors of the American Society of Experimental Neurotherapeutics. He also chairs the Integration Panel for the Multiple Sclerosis Research Program of the Department of Defense Congressionally Directed Medical Research Program. Dr. Coetzee received his Ph.D. in molecular biology from Albany Medical College in 1993 and has since been involved in the field of multiple sclerosis research. He has been with the National Multiple Sclerosis Society since fall 2000.

David L. DeMets, Ph.D., is currently Max Halperin professor of biostatistics and founder/former chair of the Department of Biostatistics and Medical Informatics at the University of Wisconsin–Madison. Since receiving his Ph.D. in 1970 from the University of Minnesota, he has been very active in the design, conduct, and analysis of clinical trials in several disease areas. Following a postdoctoral appointment at NIH (1970-1972), he spent 10 years (1972-1982) at the NIH National Heart, Lung, and Blood

Institute (NHLBI), where he became chief of the Biostatistics Research Branch. He has co-authored four texts on the topic of clinical trial design, interim monitoring, and analyses. Dr. DeMets is a recognized international leader in statistical research and methods for the analysis of clinical trials. He has collaborated in the development of statistical methods for the sequential analysis of outcome data and the design of clinical trials. He has extensive national and international clinical trial experience and has served on and chaired numerous NIH and industry-sponsored data safety and monitoring committees for clinical trials in diverse disciplines. He served on the Board of Scientific Counselors of the National Cancer Institute and Board of Directors of the American Statistical Association, and was president of the Society for Clinical Trials and of the Eastern North American Region (ENAR) of the Biometric Society. He is a fellow of the American Statistical Association, the International Statistics Institute, the Society of Clinical Trials, the American Medical Informatics Association, and the American Association for the Advancement of Science. Dr. DeMets has served on the Human Subjects Committee (1982-1987) and on several University of Wisconsin committees since 1990. He also has served on several of the university's search committees and graduate school committees.

Jeffrey Drazen, M.D., joined the *New England Journal of Medicine* (NEJM) as editor-in-chief in July 2000. At NEJM, Dr. Drazen's responsibilities include oversight of all editorial content and policies. His editorial background includes service as an associate editor or editorial board member for the *Journal of Clinical Investigation*, the *American Journal of Respiratory Cell and Molecular Biology*, and the *American Journal of Medicine*. A specialist in pulmonology, Dr. Drazen maintains an active research program. He has published more than 300 articles on such topics as lung physiology and the mechanisms involved in asthma. In 1999, he delivered the Amberson Lecture, the major research address at the annual meeting of the American Thoracic Society. In 2000, he received the Chadwick Medal from the Massachusetts Thoracic Society for his contributions to the study of lung disease. Dr. Drazen is distinguished Parker B. Francis professor of medicine at Harvard Medical School, professor of physiology at the Harvard School of Public Health, and a senior physician at Brigham and Women's Hospital. In 2003, he was elected to the IOM. He has served on numerous NIH committees and on the Veterans' Administration National Research Advisory Committee. He currently serves on the Global Initiative for Asthma Science Committee and the World Health Organization's Scientific Advisory Group on Clinical Trials Registration and co-chairs the IOM's Forum on Drug Discovery, Development, and Translation. Dr. Drazen earned his bachelor's degree and graduated summa cum laude from Tufts University. He received his medical degree from Harvard Medical School and completed his internship and residency at Peter Bent Brigham Hospital in Boston. He has received honorary degrees from the University of Ferrara, Italy, and the National and Kapodistrian University of Athens, Greece.

Steven N. Goodman, M.D., M.H.S., Ph.D., is associate dean for clinical and translational research and professor of medicine and health research and policy at Stanford University School of Medicine. He is the editor of *Clinical Trials: Journal of the Society for Clinical Trials* and is senior statistical editor of the *Annals of Internal Medicine*, where he has served since 1987. He has served previously on six IOM committees. Dr. Goodman is vice-chair of the Methodology Committee of the Patient-Centered Outcomes Research Institute and scientific advisor to the Medical Advisory Panel of the National Blue Cross/Blue Shield Technology Evaluation Center. He directs Stanford's Clinical and Translational Science Award (CTSA) research training programs and co-directs a new center focused on improving the validity and reproducibility of published medical research. Before joining Stanford in 2011, Dr. Goodman was professor of oncology in the Division of Biostatistics and Bioinformatics of the Johns Hopkins Kimmel Cancer Center, with appointments in the departments of Pediatrics, Biostatistics, and Epidemiology in the Johns Hopkins Schools of Medicine and Public Health. He was on the core faculties of the Johns Hopkins Center for Clinical Trials, the Berman Bioethics Institute, and the Graduate Training Program in Clinical Investigation and co-directed the epidemiology doctoral program. Dr. Goodman received an A.B. from Harvard and an M.D. from New York University, trained in pediatrics at Washington University, and received an M.H.S. in biostatistics and a Ph.D. in epidemiology from Johns Hopkins University. He writes and teaches on evidence evaluation and inferential, methodologic, and ethical issues in epidemiology and clinical research.

Patricia A. King, J.D., has expertise in the study of law, medicine, ethics, and public policy. She is also an adjunct professor in the Department of Health Policy and Management, School of Hygiene and Public Health, at Johns Hopkins University. She is the co-author of *Cases and Materials on Law, Science and Medicine*. She teaches family law courses and offers a seminar in bioethics and the law. She is a member of the American Law Institute and the IOM and a fellow of the Hastings Center. She is currently a member of the IOM's Board on Health Sciences Policy. Ms. King's work in the field of bioethics has included service on the Department of Health, Education, and Welfare (HEW) Recombinant DNA Advisory Committee; the President's Commission for the Study of Ethical Problems in Medicine and Biomedical and Behavioral Research; the National Commission for the Protection of Human Subjects of Biomedical and Behavioral Research; and the Ethics, Legal and Social Issues Working Group of the Human Genome Project. She is a former member of the Harvard Corporation and trustee emeritus of Wheaton College. Her professional experience before joining the Law Center faculty in 1973 was primarily in the civil rights field; she was deputy director of the Office of Civil Rights and special assistant to the chairman of the U.S. Equal Employment Opportunity Commission (EEOC). She also served as a deputy assistant attorney general in the Civil Division of the Department of Justice.

Trudie Lang, Ph.D., is a clinical trials research methodologist with specific expertise in capacity development and trial operations in low-resource settings. She currently leads the Global Health Network (GHN), a forum that seeks to help clinical researchers with trial design and methods, interpretation of regulations, and general operations. GHN conducts methodology research to identify the real barriers and issues involved in noncommercial trials, with the aim of developing best practice guidelines. Dr. Lang has worked in the field of clinical trials for 20 years and has experienced the benefits of working in the pharmaceutical industry, the World Health Organization, and academia. Ten years of managing trials in industry gave her strong capabilities in leading teams, dealing with regulations, managing complex projects, and conducting effective strategic planning and taught her the rigors of designing and operating clinical trials in varied settings. At Oxford she has further developed her expertise in the design, operation, and methodology of running trials in developing countries. Dr. Lang set up a clinical trial facility in Kenya with a strong focus on developing local research skills and engagement. More recently, she devised and set up Global Health Trials (www.globalhealth-trials.org), an online, research-led facility designed to support and guide research teams and used by more than 200,000 researchers. It evolved into The Global Health Network (www.theglobalhealthnetwork.org), a virtual science park that hosts 25 international collaborations across varied disease areas, all aiming to support research by sharing knowledge, research tools, and methods.

Deven McGraw, J.D., M.P.H., L.L.M., is a partner in the health care practice of Manatt, Phelps & Phillips, LLP. She provides legal, regulatory, and strategic policy and business counsel to health care providers, payers, and other health care organizations with respect to the adoption and implementation of health information technology (IT) and electronic health information exchange. Her areas of focus include Health Insurance Portability and Accountability Act (HIPAA)/privacy advice and compliance, data security, data governance, research and health data analytics, health information technology (IT) policy, and patient engagement. Previously, Ms. McGraw was director of the Health Privacy Project at the Center for Democracy & Technology (CDT). In this role, she led efforts to develop and promote workable privacy and security protections for electronic personal health information. Ms. McGraw's background includes service on a number of committees established by the U.S. Department of Health and Human Services (HHS) and other work groups to provide guidance on a wide array of health IT, privacy and security policy, and business issues. She was one of three people appointed by former HHS Secretary Kathleen Sebelius to serve on the Health Information Technology Policy Committee, a federal advisory committee established under the American Recovery and Reinvestment Act of 2009. Ms. McGraw also served on two key work groups of the American Health Information Community, the federal advisory body established by HHS in the Bush administration to develop recommendations on how to facilitate use of health IT to improve health. She also served on the Policy Steering Committee of the eHealth Initiative and currently serves on its Leadership Committee. She serves as well on the Steering Committee of the Electronic Data Methods Forum and leads the privacy policy work for the Patient-Centered Outcomes Research Network. Prior to her service with CDT, Ms. McGraw was chief operating officer at the National Partnership for Women & Families. Earlier in her career, she was an associate in the public policy and health care groups of two international law firms. She also served as deputy legal counsel to the governor of Massachusetts and taught in the Federal Legislation Clinic at the Georgetown University Law Center.

Elizabeth Nabel, M.D., has served as president of Harvard-affiliated Brigham and Women's Hospital (BWH) since 2010. A cardiologist and distinguished biomedical researcher, Dr. Nabel is professor of medicine at Harvard Medical School. She brings a unique perspective to health care based on her experience as a physician, research scientist, academic medicine leader, and wellness advocate. At BWH, she led the development of a comprehensive strategic plan that defines a new model of medicine characterized by cross-disciplinary collaboration, patient-inclusive care, and innovation. Initiatives include a new translational medical facility; patient-centered intensive care unit (ICU) care; and a $1 billion campaign to advance innovation, patient care, and community health. Dr. Nabel has a long record of advocacy for health and for broadening access to care. As director of NHLBI from 2005 to 2009, she leveraged a $3 billion research portfolio to establish pioneering scientific programs in genomics, stem cells, and translational research. One of her signature advocacy efforts was the Red Dress Heart Truth campaign, which raises heart awareness in women through innovative partnerships. Throughout her career, Dr.

Nabel has been a champion for global health. At NHLBI, she established centers of excellence in developing countries to combat cardiovascular and lung diseases. At BWH she helped create a national teaching hospital in Haiti and is advancing training for clinicians in underresourced countries. An accomplished physician-scientist, Dr. Nabel has conducted work on the molecular genetics of cardiovascular diseases that has produced 17 patents and more than 250 scientific publications. Her colleagues elected her to the American Academy of Arts and Sciences and the IOM, and she is a fellow of the American Association for the Advancement of Science. Her honors include the Willem Einthoven Award from Leiden University in the Netherlands, two Distinguished Achievement Awards from the American Heart Association, and six honorary doctorates. Dr. Nabel attended Weill Cornell Medical College and completed her cardiology training at BWH.

Arti Rai, J.D., is an internationally recognized expert in intellectual property (IP) law, administrative law, and health policy. She has also taught at the Harvard, Yale, and University of Pennsylvania law schools. Her research on IP law and policy in biotechnology, pharmaceuticals, and software has been funded by NIH, the Kauffman Foundation, and the Woodrow Wilson Center. She has published more than 50 articles, essays, and book chapters on IP law, administrative law, and health policy. Her publications have appeared in both peer-reviewed journals and law reviews. She is the editor of *Intellectual Property Law and Biotechnology: Critical Concepts* (Edward Elgar, 2011), co-author of a 2012 Kauffman Foundation monograph on cost-effective health care innovation, and co-author of a casebook on law and the mental health system. From 2009 to 2010, Ms. Rai served as administrator of the Office of External Affairs at the U.S. Patent and Trademark Office (USPTO). Prior to that, she served on President-Elect Obama's transition team reviewing the USPTO. Before entering academia, Ms. Rai clerked for the Honorable Marilyn Hall Patel of the U.S. District Court for the Northern District of California, was a litigation associate at Jenner & Block, and was a litigator in the U.S. Department of Justice's Civil Division. Ms. Rai regularly testifies before Congress and relevant administrative bodies on IP law and policy issues and advises federal agencies on IP policy issues raised by the research they fund. She is a member of the National Advisory Council for Human Genome Research and of an Expert Advisory Council to the Defense Advanced Projects Research Agency. She is a public member of the Administrative Conference of the United States, a member of the American Law Institute, and co-chair of the IP Committee of the Administrative Law Section of the American Bar Association. In 2011, Ms. Rai won the World Technology Network Award for Law. She graduated from Harvard College, magna cum laude, with a B.A. in biochemistry and history; attended Harvard Medical School for the 1987-1988 academic year; and received her J.D., cum laude, from Harvard Law School in 1991.

Ida Sim, M.D., Ph.D., is professor of medicine; co-director of biomedical informatics at UCSF's Clinical and Translational Science Institute; and co-founder of Open mHealth, a nonprofit organization that is breaking down barriers to mobile health app and data integration through an open software architecture. Her primary research work is on knowledge-based technologies for evidence-based practice, especially in the ontological representation of clinical trials for data sharing and scientific computation. In 2005, Dr. Sim was founding project coordinator of the World Health Organization's International Clinical Trials Registry Platform. She led the establishment of the first global policy on clinical trial registration, including the development of the Trial Registration Data Set, the common 20-item data set adhered to by all registries worldwide. She has also published on clinical trial reporting bias, new models of scientific epublication of clinical research, and other policies and practices of trial reporting and registration. Dr. Sim was a member of the National Research Council committee that produced a report on computational technology for effective health care. She is a recipient of the United States Presidential Early Career Award for Scientists and Engineers, a fellow of the American College of Medical Informatics, and a member of the American Society for Clinical Investigation. She is also a practicing primary care physician.

Sharon Terry, M.A., is president and CEO of Genetic Alliance, a network of more than 10,000 organizations, 1,200 of which are disease advocacy organizations. Genetic Alliance engages individuals, families, and communities to transform health. Ms. Terry also is founding CEO of PXE International, a research advocacy organization for the genetic condition pseudoxanthoma elasticum (PXE). As co-discoverer of the gene associated with PXE, she holds the patent for ABCC6 to act as its steward and has assigned her rights to the foundation. She developed a diagnostic test for the condition and conducts clinical trials. She is the author of 140 peer-reviewed papers, 30 of which are PXE clinical studies. Ms. Terry also is a co-founder of the Genetic Alliance Registry and Biobank. In the forefront of consumer participation in genetics research, services, and policy, she serves in a leadership role for many of the major international and national organizations in this area. She serves as well on the editorial boards of several journals and is an editor of *Genome*. She led the coalition that was instrumental in the passage of the Genetic Information Nondiscrimination Act. Ms. Terry received an honorary doctorate from Iona College for her work in community engagement in 2006, the first Patient Service Award from the University of North Carolina at Chapel Hill Institute for Pharmacogenomics and Individualized Therapy in 2007, the Research!America Distinguished Organization Advocacy Award in 2009, and the Clinical Research Forum and Foundation's Annual Award for Leadership in Public Advocacy in 2011. In 2012, she became an honorary professor of Hebei United University in Tangshan, China, and also received the Facing Our Risk of Cancer Empowered (FORCE) Spirit of Empowerment Advocacy Award. She was named one of the U.S. Food and Drug Administration's "30 Heroes for the Thirtieth Anniversary of the Orphan Drug Act" in 2013. In 2012 and 2013, Ms. Terry won first prizes in three large competitions for the Platform for Engaging Everyone Responsibly (PEER), which was awarded a $1 million contract from the Patient-Centered Research Outcomes Institute in 2014. She also is an Ashoka fellow.

Joanne Waldstreicher, M.D., is chief medical officer, Johnson & Johnson. In this role, she has oversight for epidemiology and safety of all Johnson & Johnson products worldwide across all sectors, including pharmaceuticals, devices, and consumer products. In addition, she plays a leadership role for internal and external partnerships and collaborations, including the development of corporate science and technology policies. Dr. Waldstreicher also chairs the Pharmaceuticals R&D Development Committee, which reviews all late-stage development programs in the pharmaceutical pipeline. Previously, she was chief medical officer of the pharmaceutical sector and head of Asia Pacific medical sciences. Prior to that, she was head of global drug development for the Johnson & Johnson Pharmaceutical Research & Development, LLC (J&JPRD) Central Nervous System/Internal Medicine business unit. Prior to joining J&JPRD in 2002, Dr. Waldstreicher was head of the endocrinology and metabolism clinical research group at Merck Research Laboratories. During that time, she received numerous distinctions, including the Merck Research Laboratory Key Innovator Award. Dr. Waldstreicher received the Jonas Salk and Belle Zeller scholarships from the City University of New York and graduated summa cum laude from Brooklyn College and cum laude from Harvard Medical School. She completed her fellowship in endocrinology and metabolism at Massachusetts General Hospital, has won numerous awards and scholarships, and has authored numerous papers and abstracts.

IOM ANNIVERSARY FELLOW

Scott D. Halpern, M.D., Ph.D., is assistant professor of medicine, epidemiology, and medical ethics and health policy at the Perelman School of Medicine, University of Pennsylvania. He is founding director of the

Fostering Improvement in End-of-Life Decision Science (FIELDS) program, deputy director of the Center for Health Incentives and Behavioral Economics, and a practicing critical care medicine doctor. The FIELDS program, which Dr. Halpern founded in 2012, includes scholars from multiple health-related disciplines who are united by the belief that untoward influences on how patients, family members, and providers make choices contribute to the high intensity of care that many patients receive near the end of their life. Dr. Halpern's research is supported by NIH, the Robert Wood Johnson Foundation, the Gordon and Betty Moore Foundation, and the American Heart Association. Most of his funding supports randomized trials of behavioral and health system interventions. He has received the United States' most prestigious awards for young academics in two different disciplines: the Greenwall Foundation Faculty Scholar Award (2008) in bioethics and AcademyHealth's Alice S. Hersh New Investigator Award (2011) in health services research. In 2012, Dr. Halpern was recognized with a Young Leader Award from the Robert Wood Johnson Foundation as 1 of 10 people aged 40 or under "who offer great promise for leading the way to improved health and health care for all Americans." He is an anniversary fellow at the IOM and a member of the editorial board of the *Annals of Internal Medicine*. Dr. Halpern is the author of more than 100 scientific articles and has consulted on ethical and scientific matters for NIH, the Centers for Disease Control and Prevention, the United Network for Organ Sharing, The World Bank, and two advisory committees to the U.S. Secretary of Health and Human Services.